Adult Leukemias 1

# Cancer Treatment and Research  5

WILLIAM L. MCGUIRE, *series editor*

1. R. B. Livingston, ed., Lung Cancer 1. 1981. ISBN 90-247-2394-9.
2. G. Bennett Humphrey, Louis P. Dehner, Gerald B. Grindey and Ronald T. Acton, eds., Pediatric Oncology 1. 1981. ISBN 90-247-2408-2.
3. Jerome J. DeCosse and Paul Sherlock, eds., Gastrointestinal Cancer 1. 1981. ISBN 90-247-2461-9.
4. John M. Bennett, ed., Lymphomas 1, including Hodgkin's Disease. 1981. ISBN 90-247-2479-1.

*series ISBN 90-247-2426-0.*

# Adult Leukemias   1

*edited by*

CLARA D. BLOOMFIELD

*University of Minnesota, Minneapolis*

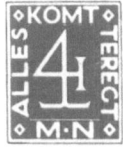

1982

MARTINUS NIJHOFF PUBLISHERS

THE HAGUE / BOSTON / LONDON

*Distributors:*

*for the United States and Canada*

Kluwer Boston, Inc.
190 Old Derby Street
Hingham, MA 02043
USA

*for all other countries*

Kluwer Academic Publishers Group
Distribution Center
P.O. Box 322
3300 AH Dordrecht
The Netherlands

---

**Library of Congress Cataloging in Publication Data**　　　　　　　　　　　　　　ᴄɪᴘ

Adult leukemias.

  (Cancer treatment and research ; v. 5-   )
  Includes index.
  1. Leukemia.  I. Bloomfield, Clara D.  II. Series:
Cancer treatment and research ; v. 5, etc.  [DNLM:
1. Leukemia--Period.  W1 CA693 v. 5 etc.]
RC643.A33     616.99'419     81-18950
ISBN 90-247-2478-3 (v. 1)    AACR2

ISBN-13: 978-94-009-7435-7        e-ISBN-13: 978-94-009-7433-3
DOI: 10.1007/978-94-009-7433-3

# Contents

# Cancer Treatment and Research

## Foreword

Where do you begin to look for a recent, authoritative article on the diagnosis or management of a particular malignancy? The few general oncology textbooks are generally out of date. Single papers in specialized journals are informative but seldom comprehensive; these are more often preliminary reports on a very limited number of patients. Certain general journals frequently publish good indepth reviews of cancer topics, and published symposium lectures are often the best overviews available. Unfortunately, these reviews and supplements appear sporadically, and the reader can never be sure when a topic of special interest will be covered.

Cancer Treatment and Research is a series of authoritative volumes which aim to meet this need. It is an attempt to establish a critical mass of oncology literature covering virtually all oncology topics, revised frequently to keep the coverage up to date, easily available on a single library shelf or by a single personal subscription.

We have approached the problem in the following fashion. First, by dividing the oncology literature into specific subdivisions such as lung cancer, genitourinary cancer, pediatric oncology, etc. Second, by asking eminent authorities in each of these areas to edit a volume on the specific topic on an annual or biannual basis. Each topic and tumor type is covered in a volume appearing frequently and predictably, discussing current diagnosis, staging, markers, all forms of treatment modalities, basic biology, and more.

In Cancer Treatment and Research, we have an outstanding group of editors, each having made a major commitment to bring to this new series the very best literature in his or her field. Martinus Nijhoff Publishers has made an equally major commitment to the rapid publication of high quality books, and world-wide distribution.

Where can you go to find quickly a recent authoritative article on any major oncology problem? We hope that Cancer Treatment and Research provides an answer.

WILLIAM L. MCGUIRE
Series Editor

# Preface

Rapid advances have been made recently in our understanding of adult leukemia. These advances have resulted in our progressing in less than 15 years from an era where fewer than 25% of adults with acute myelogenous leukemia achieved remission and almost all were dead within a year to a time where we now expect 70 to 90% of patients to achieve remission and 15 to 20% to be cured.

With these rapid advances even the specialist has difficulty remaining current. Oncology textbooks are generally out of date by the time they are published. Timely in-depth reviews periodically appear but they can not be found in a single volume and the date and times of their publication are unpredictable. The purpose of the present series is to provide a regularly published single volume where recent advances in adult leukemia are authoritatively and comprehensively summarized and interpreted. These volumes will review current basic and clinical research in leukemia with an emphasis on application to the control of leukemia in adults. They will hopefully help bridge the gap between basic and clinical science and treatment of the patient.

Although the series will cover adult leukemia in general, this first volume considers only acute leukemia. Twelve different topics ranging from the viral induction of leukemia to its cure by intensive combination chemotherapy are lucidly discussed by internationally recognized experts in their respective fields. Most of the chapters consist of comprehensive state-of-the-art reviews which are accompanied by extensive up-to-date bibliographies and often useful detailed tabulations of previously published data. Several articles also include large amounts of previously unpublished data. Brief outlines at the front of each chapter should provide the reader with a rapid review of each chapter's contents and assist in locating specific information.

The scope of this volume is indicated by scanning the table of contents.

The first three chapters consider various aspects of leukemogenesis. Gallo and his colleagues lucidly summarize for the nonvirologist some of the exciting new data supporting a role for viruses in the etiology of human leukemia. Smith expands on a provocative area, briefly introduced by Gallo,—the potential role of the newly recognized growth factors (in particular T-cell growth factor) in leukemogenesis. Coltman provides a detailed survey and tabulation of the literature on chemotherapy- and radiotherapy-induced leukemia.

Chapters four through eight focus on various aspects of adult acute myeloid leukemia (AML). Bennett and Golomb review, respectively, morphologic and cytogenetic characteristics of the malignant cell from the viewpoint of clinical significance. Preisler, in a most provocative chapter, discusses new approaches to the treatment of AML based primarily on *in vitro* growth characteristics and drug sensitivities of the leukemic cell. Peterson presents the first in-depth consideration of leukemia in the elderly since the routine use of intensive chemotherapy. The data suggesting cure in a substantial fraction of adults with AML are analyzed by Keating with an emphasis on risk factors which predict for responsiveness to treatment.

Chapters nine and ten focus on adult acute lymphoblastic leukemia (ALL). Bloomfield provides the first comprehensive synthesis of studies of biologic characteristics of the malignant cell in adult, as distinct from childhood, ALL with an emphasis on the clinical utility of immunologic phenotype. Esterhay and Wiernik summarize the results of therapy for adult ALL.

The last two chapters consider aspects of therapy that apply to both adult AML and ALL. Strauss and Connett survey and critically analyze recent data regarding the role of granulocyte transfusions during induction chemotherapy. Kay discusses the current status and future potential of bone marrow transplantation as therapy for adults with acute leukemia.

Overall, these 12 chapters, although written by 16 authors from 11 different institutions, provide a comprehensive and remarkably consistent picture of what we now know about, and what we need to learn to better understand and treat, adult leukemia. It is hoped that this volume will be a valuable reference for all who study and treat acute leukemia and provocative and exciting reading for the generalist in medicine and science.

# List of Contributors

BENNETT, John M., University of Rochester, School of Medicine and Dentistry, Department of Medicine and Cancer Center, 601 Elmwood Avenue, Box 704, Rochester, NY 14642, U.S.A.

BLOOMFIELD, Clara D., Section of Medical Oncology, Department of Medicine, University of Minnesota School of Medicine, Mayo Memorial Building, Box 277, Minneapolis, MN 55455, U.S.A.

COLTMAN, Charles A., Jr., Division of Oncology, University of Texas Health Science Center at San Antonio, 7703 Floyd Curl Drive, San Antonio, TX 78284, U.S.A.

CONNETT, John E., Division of Biometry, School of Public Health, University of Minnesota, Minneapolis, MN 55414, U.S.A.

ESTERHAY, Robert H., Jr., Baltimore Cancer Research Center, University of Maryland Hospital, 22 South Greene Street, Ninth Floor, Baltimore, MD 21201, U.S.A.

GALLO, Robert C., Laboratory of Tumor Cell Biology, National Cancer Institute, Building 37, Room 6B04, Bethesda, MD 20205, U.S.A.

GOLOMB, Harvey M., Department of Medicine, Section of Hematology/Oncology, The University of Chicago. The Division of the Biological Sciences and The Pritzker School of Medicine, 950 East 59th Street, Box 420, Chicago, IL 60637, U.S.A.

KAY, H. E. M., The Royal Marsden Hospital, Fulham Road, London SW3 6JJ, England

KEATING, Michael J., Department of Developmental Therapeutics, M.D. Anderson Hospital and Tumor Institute, 6723 Bertner, Houston, TX 77030, U.S.A.

PETERSON, Bruce A., Section of Medical Oncology, Department of Medicine, University of Minnesota Health Sciences Center, Mayo Memorial Building, Box 348, Minneapolis, MN 55455, U.S.A.

PREISLER, Harvey D., Department of Medical Oncology, Roswell Park Memorial Institute, 666 Elm Street, Buffalo, NY 14263, U.S.A.

RUSCETTI, Francis, Laboratory of Tumor Cell Biology, National Cancer Institute, Building 37, Room 6B04, Bethesda, MD 20205, U.S.A.

SMITH, Kendall A., The Immunology Program, Norris Cotton Cancer Center, Dartmouth Medical School, Hanover, NH 03755, U.S.A.

STRAUSS, Ronald G., Division of Hematology/Oncology, Department of Pediatrics, University of Iowa Hospitals and Clinics, Iowa City, IA 52242, U.S.A.

WIERNIK, Peter H., Baltimore Cancer Research Center, University of Maryland Hospital, 22 South Greene Street, Ninth Floor, Baltimore, MD 21201, U.S.A.

WONG-STAAL, Flossie, Laboratory of Tumor Cell Biology, National Cancer Institute, Building 37, Room 6B04, Bethesda, MD 20205, U.S.A.

# 1. Viruses and Adult Leukemia — Lymphoma of Man and Relevant Animal Models

ROBERT C. GALLO, FLOSSIE WONG-STAAL and FRANCIS RUSCETTI

CONTENTS

## 1. INTRODUCTION

RNA tumor viruses (or 'retroviruses') are the causative agents of leuke-mogenesis in several animal species. There is strong evidence that this group of viruses produces leukemias, lymphomas, and other hematopoietic neo-plasias in chickens, wild mice, cows, cats, and gibbon apes. In these well-studied animal model systems, infectious retroviruses can usually, but not always, be isolated from tumor material. Isolates of infectious retroviral particles clearly of human origin have not been reproducibly obtained from human tumors. The questions then are, do viruses in the conventional sense or viral genetic information in the more recently understood sense (see later section) have a role in human leukemogenesis, and if so, how do they par-take in these events, and why has it been so difficult to elucidate? In attempting to answer these questions, one should look at the accumulated data derived from studying human leukemia as well as the rapidly expand-ing information available on viral structure, 'transforming proteins' and cellular transformation from animal model systems.

Like most diseases the development of leukemia and lymphoma are mul-tifactorial and, as a result, epidemiologists have looked for different risk factors. Epidemiological studies related to human leukemia have not proven that leukemias are *commonly* caused by radiation, environmental chemical carcinogens, or inherited abnormalities although they clearly can increase risk. In contrast, they tend to emphasize the rather diffuse geographic dis-tribution of these diseases, their general failure to show cluster patterns, and a lack of clear genetic susceptibility. Similarly, such studies clearly show that the leukemias of man are not an *acute* infectious disease transmitted direct-ly from patients [1]. On the other hand, and as emphasized before [2], these studies do not rule out a transmissible agent in the cause of the disease. Epidemiological patterns can be obscured by several circumstances. For example, if a virus is transmitted vertically, e.g., by congenital infection of the developing embryo or even of the egg or sperm, no infectious pattern may be discernible, especially if there is a long latency period. Long latency may even obscure detection of classical horizontal infections. Also, such patterns may be difficult to discern if factors other than the transmissible agent are etiologically required. In fact, all these epidemiological complications do occur in one or another leukemia of animals. RNA tumor viruses are sometimes transmitted vertically. Sometimes they infect the germ cell (egg or sperm) or the developing embryo. In other instances they can be transmitted in the DNA of the germ line from generation to generation without visible evidence of virus in a manner identical to cellular genes (true endogenous retroviruses).

The latency of leukemia induction by retroviruses is variable and depends on the virus and the host. However, as in the case with most carcinogens, latency is usually relatively long. For instance, infection of a gibbon ape with gibbon ape leukemia virus may not induce leukemia until a few years later [3]. Clearly, there must be requirements other than virus for disease induction in many instances of animal leukemia. These factors may primarily be host factors, e.g., newborn animals are generally more susceptible to virus than adults and many animals may carry virus without getting disease. Risk to virus may be increased by specific genetic changes. Those genetic factors presently known to affect the incidence of animal leukemia tend to be those which relate to the control of virus replication. Host chromosomal changes can be associated with the risk of leukemia, e.g., the congenital syndromes like Fanconi's anemia and Down's syndrome are associated with an increase in the risk of developing leukemia. A striking example of the role of congenital and/or hereditory factors being involved in human leukemia is the high concordance of childhood leukemia in an identical twin of a child who already developed leukemia [4]. Whether or not any genetic factors cause an increased risk of leukemia by way of affecting the expression, replication, or susceptibility to virus in humans is unknown. Finally, it should be noted that a virus which is ubiquitous may still be pathogenic, but in that situation there can be problems in epidemiological inferences. EBV involvement in Burkitt's lymphoma is an excellent example. Is the reason for disease in some infected people and not in others due to strain variation in virus, genetics of the host, or environmental factors? In this case, it may be all three since various strains of EBV are now known to be variable in their transforming capacity, the geographic limits of the disease strongly imply other environmental factors are needed, and genetic susceptibility is suggested by the very high prevalence of specific chromosomal translocations which may be required for final stages of cell transformation [5].

Our objectives here will be to summarize some of the evidence that specific kinds of viruses are involved in the cause of naturally occurring animal leukemias, to discuss some of the basic features of these viruses and to consider the evidence that such viruses are also present in the human population, to consider whether the data imply etiological relevance and which (if any) results may be clinically useful. Although it has been suggested that infection of mothers by some common non-transforming viruses is associated with an increased risk of childhood leukemia, we will consider only classes of viruses which are known to be true tumor viruses, i.e., for which there is evidence for either *in vitro* cell transformation or *in vivo* experimental tumor production, and naturally occurring animal models.

## 2. EPSTEIN-BARR VIRUS

We will not consider EBV in detail here because it has been recently and extensively reviewed in a series of excellent articles by workers in the field [6]. However, it is important to emphasize that this complex member of the herpes DNA virus group induces a mitogenic effect on human B-lymphocytes *in vitro*, sometimes can produce malignant lymphomas after inoculation into some primates, causes infectious mononucleosis, and appears to be involved in at least the early phase of African Burkitt's lymphoma as well as some nasopharyngeal carcinomas. Recent reports also suggest that EBV causes some rare acute and fatal lymphoproliferative diseases in a genetically susceptible group of children who may have a defect in their immune response to EBV [7]. The molecular mechanisms by which EBV induces cell growth is poorly understood, but there is evidence that its effect in Burkitt's lymphoma may chiefly be as an initiating event in the mitogenic stimulation of B-cells, whereas other factors are required for frank malignant conversion. These other factors may be genetic susceptibility, malaria, or chromosomal changes developing for unknown reasons. On the other hand the fatal acute lymphoproliferative diseases in an immunologically compromised child may be directly and solely caused by EBV [7]. There have also been intermittent suggestions that EBV is involved in the cause of Hodgkin's disease. This speculation is based on the following considerations: 1) Some epidemiological considerations led to the suggestion that Hodgkin's disease is due to a common human virus causing an uncommon event. EBV, of course, fits that description. 2) The incidence of Hodgkin's disease is higher after infectious mononucleosis and sometimes it appears that infectious mononucleosis leads into Hodgkin's disease. 3) Sometimes high EBV antibody titers are found in the sera of patients with Hodgkin's disease. 4) Some epidemiological results suggest that Hodgkin's disease follows an epidemiological pattern similar to infectious mononucleosis (higher socioeconomic groups) [8]. However, all these arguments are equally consistent with alternative interpretations, as for example, that infectious mononucleosis and Hodgkin's disease are caused by different agents which follow similar modes of transmission, and infectious mononucleosis can lead to an increased risk for Hodgkin's disease by reducing host defenses [9]. In fact, direct examination of the neoplastic cells of Hodgkin's disease (Reed-Sternberg cells) has failed to reveal any evidence for EBV [10]. There is no evidence whatsoever for a role for EBV in the more common human leukemias and lymphomas, and there is much direct evidence against it. For these diseases we must consider causes other than viruses or in some cases the possibility of causes by viruses other than EBV. The most important group of viruses in this regard are the type-C retroviruses because they cause leukemia in many species, and there is some recent evidence for their association with certain forms of leukemia and lymphoma of man. Moreover, and as we will discuss in this report, they may be important tools for unravelling the pathogenesis of human leukemias and lymphomas even when they are not the cause.

## 3. RETROVIRUSES AND LEUKEMOGENESIS: BASIC CONSIDERATIONS

### 3.1. Modes of Transmission

Retroviruses are either endogenous or exogenous to a species with which they are naturally associated. Endogenous viruses are carried in the germ line of their hosts, usually as a multigene family, and are vertically transmitted from parent to progeny. They are usually xenotropic, i.e., they have lost the capacity to infect their hosts. Furthermore, endogenous retroviruses are rarely associated with pathogenicity. Many species, including higher primates, harbor endogenous virus genomes. It was calculated that a tenth percent of the mouse genome was comprised of endogenous viral genes. Their ubiquity had prompted speculations that these genes may play an essential role in normal cellular functions. However, the concept of endogenous viruses has been greatly modified in recent years. First, analysis of the genetic loci containing these genomes showed that these are multiple and variable from individual to individual, in contrast to loci of cellular genes which are invariant [11]. This observation is indicative of random integration of the virus genomes after relatively recent exogenous infection, i.e., after speciation. Their acquisition after speciation seems to be generally applicable to endogenous virus genomes [12, 13], including those of the baboon endogenous virus [14] in contrast to earlier speculation that they were introduced into primates at least thirty million years ago [15]. Second, a rare but completely normal and healthy chicken was found to be devoid of the endogenous virus RAV-O. This argues against any essential role for RAV-O, the only known endogenous virus of chickens in development and growth of the animal.

Besides germ line transmission, retroviruses can also be spread by infection *in utero,* or horizontally among individuals. All of the retroviruses that cause leukemias and sarcomas are exogenous, i.e., the population at large does not carry complete genetic information that codes for these viruses. Infection with the exogenous viruses sometimes, but not always, leads to virus production and/or disease. Genetic and immunological factors of the hosts may play a role in determining the course of these events.

## 3.2. Structures and Replication of the Genomes of Non-defective Viruses

All retroviruses share a similar genetic structure. The retrovirus genomes contain two identical subunits of 30–35 S RNA bound together at the 5′ end by a 'dimer-linkage structure' to form a 60–70 S RNA complex [16]. The genomic RNA resembles cellular messenger RNA in that it has a cap structure of $5′-M^7GpppG^m$ at its 5′ end [17] and a stretch of poly(A) of approximately 200 residues at its 3′ end [18]. Immediately before the poly(A), there is a short region that is repeated at the 5′ terminus. All non-defective viruses have coding capacity for at least three gene products: *gag* (for group specific antigens), a precursor protein which is cleaved into four core proteins of the virion; *pol,* the virion RNA directed DNA polymerase (reverse transcriptase); and *env,* the virion envelope glycoproteins. These gene products are necessary, and probably sufficient for virus replication. A fourth region, *C* (for 'common'), is present near the 3′ end, and it is probably not codogenic. The order of these genes has been determined to be 5′-*gag-pol-env-C*-3′.

The mechanism of retrovirus replication has been the subject of many recent reviews [19, 20] and will only be briefly dealt with here (see above reviews for references). Shortly after infection, a DNA copy (called the provirus) of the retrovirus RNA genome is synthesized. For this synthesis to occur the catalytic role of the virion DNA polymerase, reverse transcriptase, is needed. Like all DNA polymerases, reverse transcriptase can not initiate without a 'primer' molecule. Primers are nucleic acids (RNA or DNA) which are hydrogen bonded to the template nucleic acid at regions of base complementarity. The polymerase extends the primer by adding deoxyribonucleotides to its 3′ end (see Figure 1 for schematic illustration). The natural 'primer' for the reverse transcriptase reaction is a tRNA molecule, which binds at a defined distance from the 5′ end. The first DNA product then is a piece of DNA extending from the 3′-OH end of the tRNA to the 5′ terminus of the viral RNA. The length of this DNA (often called strong-stop DNA) is specific for a given family of viruses [21], e.g., 100–105 nucleotides for avian viruses and 135–145 nucleotides for murine viruses. The strong stop DNA terminates in a sequence that is repeated at the 3′ end of the genome. To synthesize the rest of the virus genome, the enzyme reverse transcriptase

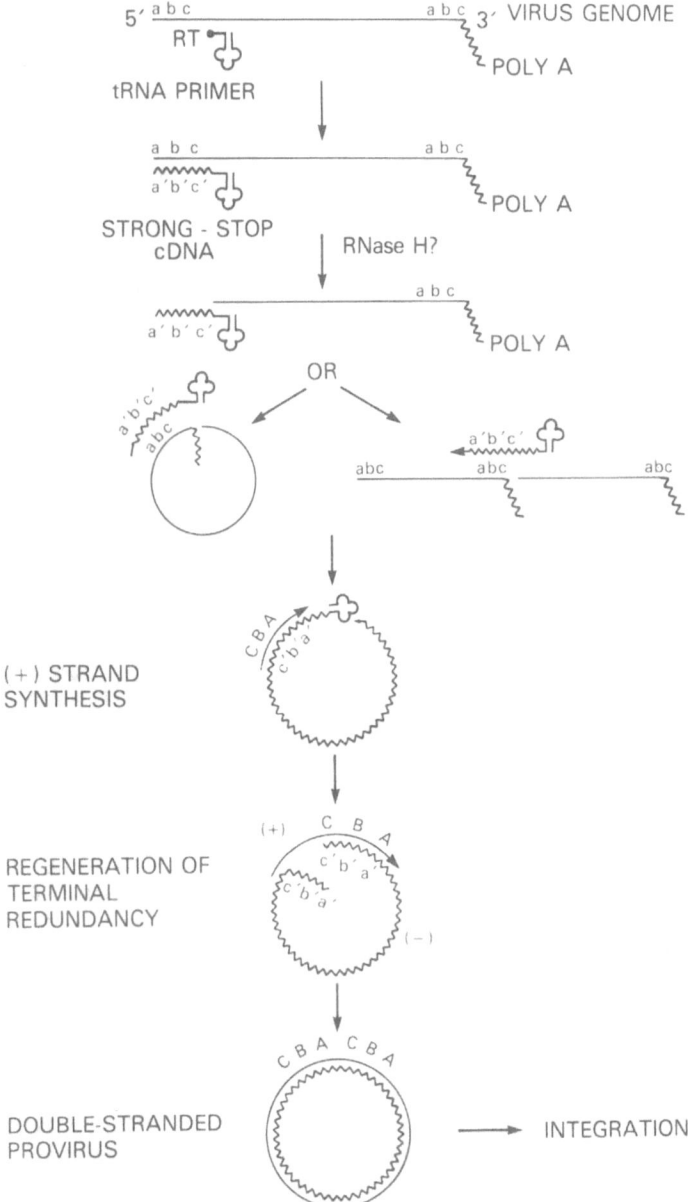

*Figure 1.* Synthesis of double-stranded provirus. Possible sequence of events for synthesis of double-stranded viral DNA intermediates. See text for description. A tRNA primer molecule binds to the viral RNA genome at a site 100–150 nucleotides from the 5'-end. The enzyme reverse transcriptase then extends 3'-OH of this molecule and copies up to the 5'-terminus of the template RNA. The resultant DNA (strong stop DNA) terminates in a sequence that is repeated at the 3'-end of the genome. The redundancy may provide means for circularization or dimer formation so that the rest of the RNA fenome may be copied. Plus strand synthesis commences before completion of the negative strand.

must be able to jump from the 5' end of one 35 S viral RNA subunit to the 3' end of the other 35 S subunit (see Figure 1) or to the 3' end of the same subunit by circularization of the subunit (see Figure 1). The short terminally redundant sequences potentially provide means for such mechanisms of circularization or dimer formation. The integrated provirus as well as some of the proviral DNA intermediate forms have the C region as well as sequences 5' of the primer binding site (strong stop DNA sequences) duplicated at both ends (or adjacent to each other in circular molecules). Each repeat unit containing the 3' and 5' derived sequences is termed an LTR unit (long terminal repeat). The LTR unit contains recognition sites for initiation of transcription (i.e., promotor sites) and signaling sequences for polyadenylation [22]. There are many striking parallels between LTRs and bacterial insertion elements: the presence of both direct and inverted repeat sequences at the ends, the content of regulatory elements such as RNA polymerase binding sites, the ability to 'flip-flop' and cause inversions and deletions of adjacent cellular DNA sequences and their location in bracketing other gene(s) as in transposons [23]. The implication of the duplicated LTR units on both ends of the integrated provirus for possible mechanisms of leukemogenesis will be discussed later.

Several forms of viral DNA intermediates are found in the early infected cells: linear viral DNA and circular DNA with one or two LTR units. It is not known which is the integrating form. The integrated provirus is colinear with viral RNA except for the duplicated LTR units at the virus-cell junction. Integration sites are multiple with respect to cellular DNA, with no apparent sequence specificity. As a result of the integration, several nucleotides of cell DNA sequences are duplicated at the junctions [22]. This phenomenon again parallels integration of bacterial insertion elements.

## 3.3. Genetic Structures of Defective, Acutely Transforming Viruses

Some retroviruses are defective for replication and need a non-defective 'helper' virus. An important group of defective viruses is the acutely transforming retroviruses which had acquired specific genes for transformation (onc genes) at the expense of one or more viral structural genes. These viruses have been isolated in association with nondefective helper viruses from animals with sarcomas, leukemias, and carcinomas. When their genomes were analyzed by oligonucleotide mapping and compared to those of their helper viral RNA [24, 25] or by direct heteroduplex analysis of RNA of the defective transforming component and cDNA (complementary DNA) of the helper component [26, 27], certain salient features emerged: 1) The defective viruses have a smaller genome of approximately 6–7 kilobases (Kb) compared to 8–10 Kb for non-defective viruses. 2) The 5' and 3' termini of the defective viruses are homologous to the helper viruses. These terminal sequences constitute a unit that is repeated at both ends of the unintegrated or integrated viral DNA, and may be important for viral functions like integration or expression. 3) Varying portions of the structural genes of the helper virus may be retained. 4) With the exception of the Friend virus, all defective transforming viruses contain an internal portion of 1–3 Kb that is specific for transformation. Members of the defective transforming viruses include all of the sarcoma viruses except Rous sarcoma virus, which is replication competent and contains all three replicative genes in addition to the transforming gene, the avian erythroblastosis virus (AEV), viruses that cause myelocytomatosis (e.g., MC29, MH2, CM11) or myeloblastosis in chickens (AMV), and the murine Friend and Abelson leukemia viruses. Figure 2 illustrates the genetic structure of some of these viruses.

Analyses of the gene products of the transforming viruses revealed two general structures. Viruses that have retained part of the *gag* gene of the helper virus immediately preceding the *onc* (transformation-specific) gene synthesize a fused *gag*-X polyprotein, X being derived from the *onc*-specific information. Examples of these are the feline sarcoma viruses [28], Abelson murine leukemia virus [29], and the avian viruses AEV [30], MC29 [24], and FSV [31]. Viruses that have alternative location for the *onc* gene synthesize a transforming protein containing no recognizable viral structural peptides. Such is the case with the transforming proteins of Rous sarcoma virus (pp60 src), Harvey murine sarcoma virus (p21), and probably those of the avian myeloblastosis virus, Moloney sarcoma virus, and simian sarcoma virus, although the *onc* gene product has not been unambiguously identified for these viruses.

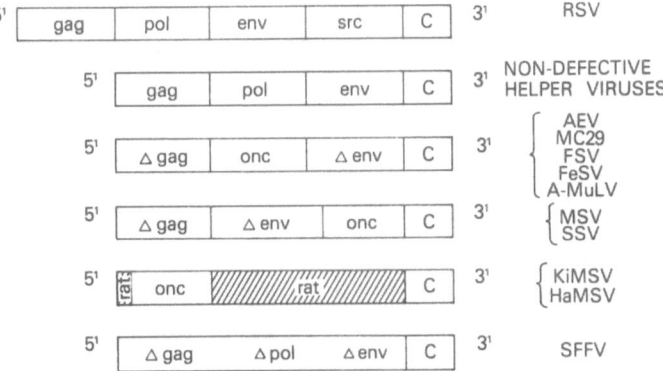

*Figure 2.* Genetic structures of some acutely transforming retroviruses. Abbreviations are: RSV, Rous sarcoma virus; AEV, avian erythroblastosis virus; MC29, avian myelocytomatosis virus; FSV, avian sarcoma virus, Fujinami strain; FeSV, feline sarcoma virus; A-MuLV, Abelson murine leukemia virus; MSV, Moloney murine sarcoma virus; SSV, simian sarcoma virus; KiMSV, Kirsten murine sarcoma virus; HaMSV, Harvey murine sarcoma virus; SFFV, spleen focus-forming virus. Δ indicates a deletion in the genome in the region indicated.

It is of interest to note that several of the transforming proteins are found to have an associated protein kinase activity that phosphorylates specifically tyrosine residues [29, 32, 33]. However, not all transforming proteins are protein kinases.

### 3.4. Cellular Origin of the Transforming Genes

The earliest characterization of a transforming gene (generically designated as *onc* gene) was that of the Rous sarcoma virus *src* gene. This virus is helper independent and contains all the replicative genes in addition to the *src* gene. Spontaneous, transformation-defective mutants of RSV (td-RSV) later became available. By comparison to the wild-type, these mutants were found to be identical to RSV except for deletion of the *src* gene. Transformation specific sequences were obtained by recycling RSV cDNA against tdRSV RNA to remove the sequences of the viral structural genes. Hybridization of these sequences to chicken DNA showed that these sequences are homologous, though not necessarily identical, to a set of host cell DNA sequences [34]. A similar approach was taken to generate *onc* specific sequences of defective, transforming viruses by recycling against helper viral RNA. In all cases, the *onc*-specific sequences have homologues in normal host cell DNA [35–37]. Therefore, the acutely transforming viruses are genetic recombinants containing portions of retrovirus genomes and cellular genes. The cellular *onc* sequences probably code for similar protein product(s) as the viral *onc* genes. Wang *et al.* [38] were able to recover transformation competent avian sarcoma virus (ASV) from chicken microinjected with transformation-defective mutants of ASV. The td-ASV mutants have deletions of a portion of the *src* gene. Apparently, the recovered ASVs have regained these sequences from the host. There is also direct proof that the ASV-related cellular *onc* gene is expressed in normal cells. Antiserum specific for the ASV protein (pp60$^{src}$) immunoprecipitated a 60 000 dalton polypeptide from normal cells [39].

There are now a number of transforming genes identified, and these have been derived from chicken, mouse, rat, cat, and primate species. Table 1 summarizes the different viral *onc* genes and their species of origin. The most recently characteried *onc* gene is that of the simian sarcoma virus, SSV. Although the helper virus SSAV has a rodent origin, SSV has acquired its *onc* gene from primates, specifically from woolly monkey [40]. Another interesting feature of the cellular *onc* genes is that they are highly conserved among vertebrates. By Southern blot hybridization [41], unique genetic loci containing cellular sequences homologous to the various *onc* genes could be located in all vertebrate DNA [40, 42, 43]. In most cases, the cellular *onc* loci contain coding sequences interrupted by several introns [42, 44, 45]. The *onc* genes of diverse species probably have similar functions. The same

*Table 1.* Comparison of the acutely transforming viruses.

| Virus prototype | Genetic origin of *onc* gene | *onc* gene product | Protein kinase activity | Target cells of *in vitro* transformation | Diseases found *in vivo* |
|---|---|---|---|---|---|
| AEV | Chicken | 75K fusion protein | ? | Erythroblasts Fibroblasts | Erythroblastosis Sarcomas |
| MC29 | Chicken | 110K fusion protein | ? | Macrophages Fibroblasts | Myelocytomatosis Carcinomas Sarcomas |
| AMV | Chicken | ? | ? | Myeloblasts | Myeloid leukemia |
| RSV | Chicken | 60K protein | + | Fibroblasts | Sarcomas |
| FSV | Chicken | 140K fusion protein | + | Fibroblasts | Sarcomas |
| A-MuLV | Mouse | 120K fusion protein | + | B-lymphocytes Fibroblasts | Lymphomas Plasmacytomas |
| M-MSV | Mouse | ? | ? | Fibroblasts | Sarcomas |
| Ha-MSV Ki-MSV | Rat | 21K protein | − | Fibroblasts | Sarcomas |
| FeSV (ST & GA) | Cat | 85–95K fusion protein | + | Fibroblast | Fibrosarcomas Melanomas |
| FeSV(SM) | Cat | 130K fusion protein | − | Fibroblast | Fibrosarcomas |
| SSV | Primate | ? | ? | Fibroblast | Fibrosarcomas |

related *onc* gene in two species, chicken and cat, was incorporated into the genomes of the Fujinami avian sarcoma virus and two strains of feline sarcoma virus (Snyder-Theilen and Garnder-Arnstein strains) [46]. The *onc* gene products for all three viruses exhibit tyrosine kinase activity [31, 33, 47].

### 3.5. Possible Mechanisms of Leukemogenesis

*3.5.1. Acute Leukemia Viruses.* Acute leukemia viruses cause leukemias rapidly *in vivo* and transform hematopoietic cells *in vitro*. Members of this group include the avian erythroblastosis virus (AEV), viruses that cause myelocytomatosis (e.g., MC29, MH2, CM11) or myeloblastosis in chickens (AMV), and the murine Friend and Abelson leukemia viruses. With the exception of the Friend virus, these viruses contain transformation specific (*onc*) genes and are structurally similar to defective sarcoma viruses. As a matter of fact, some of the viruses in this group, namely AEV, the MC29 group, and Abelson-MuLV, not only interact with and affect the growth of hematopoietic cells but are also capable of transforming fibroblasts *in vitro* and inducing sarcomas and carcinomas *in vivo*. Cells transformed by these viruses express a noval type of protein consisting of part of the *gag* gene product and a portion coded by the RNA sequences unique to the acute leukemia viruses [24, 25], i.e., the *onc* sequences. Mutants defective in transformation synthesize an altered *gag*-X polyprotein with diminished protein kinase activity [48, 49]. These results suggest that the *onc* genes are essential for transformation.

The acute leukemia viruses show considerable target cell specificity *in vivo* and *in vitro*. As an example, three classes of avian viruses show different target specifications. Avian myeloblastosis virus (AMV) induces myeloid leukemia, avian erythroblastosis virus (AEV) induces acute erythroleukemia, and myelocytomatosis virus (e.g., strain MC29) induces myelocytomatosis (marked increase in the proliferation of myeloid cells of the macrophage monocyte lineage) and tumors of predominantly epitheloid origin [48]. *In vitro* cell transformation is indicated by the proliferation capacity of the cells and their inability to adhere to the substrate. Cells transformed by these viruses *in vitro* exhibit different morphology and express markers for different states of hematopoietic differentiation. AMV-transformed cells are myeloblastic, i.e., they express high ATPase activity and myeloblast antigen and low levels of phagocytic activity, Fc receptors, and macrophage antigen. MC29-transformed cells resemble macrophages in that they strongly express phagocytic activity, Fc receptors, and macrophage cell surface antigen. Finally, AEV-transformed cells resemble erythroblasts since they are negative for all myeloid parameters but rather display erythroid markers such as histone H5 and erythroblast antigen, and to a lesser extent, hemoglobin, carbonic anhydrase, and erythrocyte antigens. Therefore, the types of cells transformed *in vitro* are the same as the types of cells transformed *in vivo*.

The same virus or different strains of the same virus can alter the expression of the differentiation program in the same cell lineage so that the final differentiated phenotype of the cell can vary. Abelson leukemia virus, whose target cell is a pre-B lymphoid cell, can transform cells expressing no immunoglobulin chain, heavy chain, or both heavy and light chains, three distinct stages of differentiation [49]. One strain of SFFV, whose target cell is an erythroid progenitor, transforms erythroid bursts, which contain no hemoglobin thereby leading to anemia in the animal, while another strain transforms erythroid bursts containing hemoglobin which leads to a polycythemia in the animal [50]. These results raise intriguing questions. What is the origin of target-cell specificity? Is a single genetic entity responsible for multiple forms of disease? Do all tumors arise from a final common pathway?

The cellular *onc* genes of the acute leukemia viruses may be expressed at low levels in normal cells. Using antibodies raised against the *gag*-related protein pl20 of Abelson murine leukemia virus, and absorbing the antibodies with the helper virus proteins, Witte *et al.* [51] found that antibodies specific for the non-*gag* region of pl20 precipitated a protein from extracts of normal mouse thymus, bone marrow, and spleen cells but not that of liver cells. This normal cell protein has a molecular weight of 150 000. It is not clear how expression of an apparently normal cell protein directed by a leukemia virus genome could cause malignant transformation. One may envision several possible mechanisms (Figure 3); first, by transduction of a normal cell gene, the virus now places that gene under different regulatory elements and may cause it to be expressed inopportunely or at unacceptably high levels. Alternatively, the viral coded protein may be altered from the normal cell protein by recombination or mutation. If the normal cell protein is necessary in some pathways of differentiation, the viral analogue could compete with it and block cell differentiation. The latter model has been proposed by Graf *et al.* [48] to explain the specific *in vitro* transformation of various hematopoietic target cells by the different avian acute leukemia viruses, but this fails to explain how the same virus can sometimes cause remarkably unrelated neoplasias, e.g., AEV not only causes avian erythroblastosis but may also cause sarcoma and MC29 not only causes a myeloid leukemia, it may also produce carcinomas. We think the first model is more

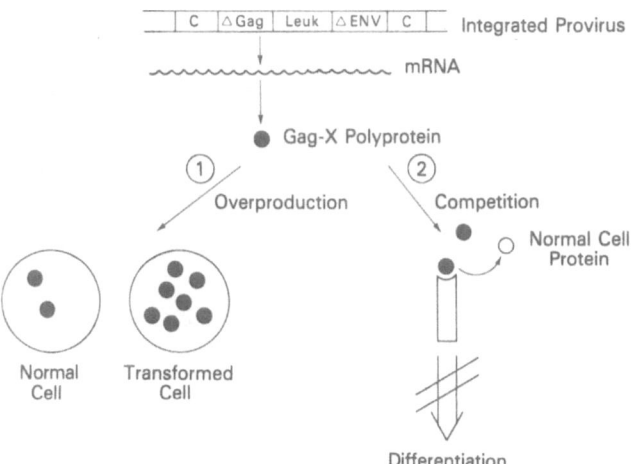

*Figure 3.* Leukemogenesis with acute leukemia viruses. Diagram illustrating the possible mechanisms of leukemogenesis by acute leukemia viruses: 1) overproduction of a normal cell protein, 2) synthesis of an analogue protein that competes with a normal cell protein.

likely, especially in view of what we understand about how the chronic leukemia viruses may induce leukemias.

3.5.2. *Chronic Leukemia Viruses.* Chronic leukemia viruses induce a wide spectrum of diseases in animals after long latent periods. They are non-defective viruses which do not appear to carry '*onc*' genes distinguishable from the three viral genes *gag, pol,* and *env.* However, recent data suggest that they may induce disease by promoting expression of cellular *onc* genes. Most of the relevant data are derived from studies of the exogenous avian leukosis virus. The endogenous and exogenous avian leukosis viruses have closely related genomes, but the endogenous viruses are entirely nonpathogenic, while the exogenous leukosis viruses can cause a wide spectrum of diseases after some latent periods. The C region of exogenous viruses ($C^X$) confers a growth advantage on the viruses since recombinant viruses containing endogenous *gag, pol, env,* and $C^X$ grow better than the endogenous viruses and as well as the exogenous viruses [52]. Comparing the oncogenic potential of viruses which had $C^X$ but endogenous or exogenous *env* genes, Robinson *et al.* [53] found that viruses of both types show the same incidence of diseases. This result suggests that C regions, not envelope antigens, play a role in the non-acute diseases. As mentioned earlier, it is unlikely that the C regions code for a transforming protein. By nucleotide sequencing of the LTR of Rous sarcoma virus, they found sequences that resemble promotor sites for RNA polymerases II and III. Yamomoto *et al.* [54] have identified a functional promotor in the C region.

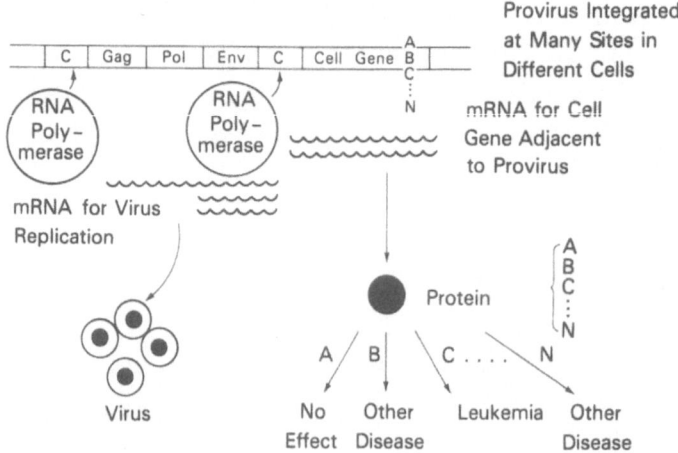

*Figure 4.* Leukemogenesis with chronic leukemia viruses. Diagram illustrating that the C region of an integrated provirus could act as promotor of adjacent cellular genes. One of of the consequences may be leukemogenesis.

One can speculate how a promotor in the C region can have disease potential (Figure 4). Since the C region is duplicated at the 5′ end of the integrated provirus [55], the promotor for viral RNA transcription should be at the 5′ end. At the same time, the 3′ C region could serve as promotor for cell genes downstream on the chromosome. Therefore, a strong promotor ($C^X$) may *cause inopportune expression of normal cell genes* more efficiently than a weak promotor ($C^N$), and have more disease-causing potential. Indeed, chicken fibroblast cells have been shown to transcribe 1000 new transcription units including the globin gene when infected with different avian viruses [56]. In studying B-cell lymphoma-induced avian leukosis virus, information relating to the MC29 *onc* gene was found fused with 5′ leader sequences of ALV [57]. DNA from these lymphomas was able to transform fibroblasts [58]. These studies provide direct evidence that chronic and acute leukemia viruses may ultimately share the same pathway for leukemogenesis. The lower efficiency of the chronic leukemia viruses may be due to requirement for integration of the provirus adjacent to the proper cellular *onc* genes, while the acute viruses have already acquired the *onc* genes in the requisite proximity of viral promotors.

*3.5.3. Recombinant Viruses.* Study of the mechanism of leukemogenesis by murine retroviruses has focused on a class of viruses called MCF (mink-cell focus-forming) viruses. MCF viruses emerge in the thymus of the AKR mouse at about five months of age, shortly before the onset of the disease. Based on their dual host range (i.e., they grow in both mouse and foreign cells), serologic cross-reactivity and interference with both xenotropic and ecotropic mouse viruses, they were suspected to be recombinants of these two types of murine viruses [59]. Analysis of the viral envelope glycoproteins [60] confirmed that the MCF viruses constitute a diverse family of *env* gene recombinants.

Another leukemia virus, the Friend spleen focus-forming virus (SFFV), is defective but contains no cell-derived *onc* gene even though it induces erythroleukemia in mice with high efficiency. SFFV transformed non-producer cells express a subgenomic mRNA which is translated into a 55 K glycoprotein that resembles serologically the *env*-gene products of ecotropic and xenotropic viruses [61].

Thus, two separate virus recombinants in the *env* gene are leukemogenic. The exact mechanism of leukemogenesis by these viruses is still not clear. It is possible that the altered host range, due to the recombination event, allows the virus to infect cells at a critical and vulnerable stage. Another possibility is that the envelope glycoprotein can interact with host cells and alter the membrane properties of the cells, leading to transformation.

4.  RETROVIRUSES AND SPONTANEOUS LEUKEMOGENESIS: ANIMAL MODEL
    SYSTEMS (summarized in Table 2)

## 4.1. Avian Leukemia

Up to 20% of all chicken flocks develop spontaneous leukemia, predominantly manifested as a lymphoproliferative disease of B-cell origin located
in the visceral organs. Retroviruses isolated from these tumors when inoculated into chickens would cause a variety of neoplasms, predominantly lymphatic leukemia, and the virus was called avian leukosis virus. However,
osteopetrosis, nephroblastomas, myeloblastosis, erythroblastosis, sarcomas,
and endotheliomas could also be induced [62]. Subsequently, it was shown
that different retroviruses were involved. Most of these viruses are non-
defective viruses, which are endemic in all commercial chicken flocks.
Transmission of the so-called avian leukosis virus can be horizontal or congenital through the egg. In the absence of maternal antibody in the egg, the
embryo can become persistently infected. In such cases, the newly hatched
chicken will not develop antiviral immunity and subsequently will become
leukemic. It is believed that this congenital transmission is the major route
for disease spread, while horizontal transmission usually results in immun-

*Table 2.* Retrovirus-associated naturally occurring leukemias in animals.

| Species | Etiologic agent | Disease | Target cell | Major routes of transmission |
|---|---|---|---|---|
| Chicken | Avian leukosis virus | Leukemia | B-lymphocyte | Congenital (egg) |
| Wild mice (Lake Casitas) | Amphotropic MuLV | Lymphoma | Non-thymic B-cell | Congenital (milk) |
| Cat | FeLV | Leukemia, Lymphoma | T-lymphocyte B-lymphocyte myeloid cell, Erythroid | Horizontal (saliva) Congenital (unknown route) |
| Cattle | BLV | Leukemia, Lymphoma | B-lymphocyte (and/or mixed) | Horizontal (insect vectors; and unknown route) Congenital (milk and possibly transplacental) |
| Gibbon ape | GaLV | Leukemia, Lymphoma | Lymphoblast, Myeloblast | Horizontal (saliva; urine; feces) Congenital (transplacental?) |

ity [63]. Recent studies showed that the disease begins as a polyclonal disease but then develops as a monoclonal tumor [64].

## 4.2. Leukemia-Lymphoma in Wild Mice

Although most of our knowledge of viral leukemogenesis in mice pertains to laboratory animals, there have been recent studies of leukemia in natural populations of wild mice. While the incidence of spontaneous leukemia and expression of indigenous retroviruses vary widely among these populations, one population at Lake Casitas (LC), California was found to be high virus excretors with a high incidence (18 %) of associated lymphoma. The etiological agent was identified as an 'amphotropic' MuLV [65], i.e., the virus grows well in non-murine and murine cells. The LC wild mouse model is remarkably similar to avian lymphatic leukemia (leukosis) in nature. Congenital infection is the major route of virus transmission in both cases. In about 85 % of LC mice, MuLV is transmitted by maternal congenital infection especially via the milk. As a consequence, these mice are persistently infected and are immunologically tolerant to the virus. In most cases, the lymphoma apparently arises in the spleen, which is also the site for early virus replication and involves cells of nonthymic B-cell origin [66].

## 4.3. Feline Leukemia

The etiology and epidemiology of leukemia and lymphoma in domestic cats are probably the most extensively studied among all outbred animal species. After the discovery and subsequent isolation of feline leukemkia (FeLV) from cats with lymphosarcoma, the nature and mode of transmission of these viruses was thoroughly studied [67, 68]. FeLV is widely distributed among domestic cats. The primary mechanism of transmission is direct contact, since virus is excreted in high titers in the saliva of viremic cats [69], and cats frequently groom or lick each other. However, epigenetic transmission, i.e., in utero or via the milk probably also occurs. Due to the immune response, only a few of the animals remain persistently viremic. The immune response is directed toward both the virus and/or a cell surface antigen (FOCMA) [70]. The nature of FOCMA antigens present in leukemia cells remains to be determined. Development of antibody against FOCMA appears to be an effective immune surveillance mechanism against tumorigenesis. Viremic cats with no FOCMA antibody are at high risk of developing leukemia while viremic cats having circulatory FOCMA antibody are resistant. Among uninfected cats, the presence of FeLV neutralizing antibody protects them against FeLV replication but not leukemia and the presence of FOCMA antibody protects them against leukemia but not virus infection. Therefore, only cats with both types of antibodies are resistant to virus infection and disease. Unlike the avian and murine systems, FeLV induced lymphoma and leukemia occur commonly in several morphologic forms. The most common forms are acute lymphoblastic leukemia, thymic lymphoma, multicentric lymphoma, and alimentary lymphoma. In the thymic lymphomas, the multicentric lymphomas, as well as most cases of acute lymphoblastic leukemia, the target cell is a T-cell. In the alimentary form, the target cell is usually a B-cell. Occasionally, myeloid and erythroid leukemias also occur.

Although exogenous feline leukemia virus (FeLV) is recognized as the etiological agent in most of the spontaneous leukemias and lymphomas where virus or viral antigens are readily detectable, a significant percentage (30–40%) of leukemic cats have no detectable virus or viral components [71]. These virus-negative tumors are clinically indistinguishable from the virus-positive tumors. There is an epidemiological association between exposure to FeLV and the occurrence not only of virus positive but also of virus negative tumors. The incidence of virus negative leukemias in cats sharing households with virus positive excretor cats is significantly higher than in cats from carrier-free households and parallels that of virus-positive leukemias within such environments [71]. When DNA from multiple tissues of virus-negative leukemic cats was examined by liquid hybridization for FeLV-related sequences and compared to virus-positive and normal uninfected animals, it was found that tumor DNA of virus-negative leukemic cats hybridized the same amount of FeLV probes as DNA from other tissues of the same animal and DNA from normal, uninfected animals [72]. The results ruled out the presence of a complete exogenous FeLV in every tumor cell. When analyzed by restriction enzymes and Southern blot hybridization, there was also no evidence for exogenous infection or expression of FeLV or FeSV related sequences [73–75]. However, there are multiple copies of endogenous viral genes that are partially homologous to the exogenous FeLVs and these endogenous sequences may obscure detection of exogenous small subgenomic viral fragments or complete provirus in a subpopulation of cells.

If FeLV is indeed etiologically associated with virus-negative tumors, novel mechanisms have to be invoked to explain its role: 1) integration of a very small fragment of FeLV (e.g., the LTR) which can initiate some cellular gene(s) for transformation; 2) a 'hit and run' mechanism whereby FeLV transiently infects the cell, turns on some cellular genes and induces transformation, but maintenance of the provirus is not necessary for the transformed phenotype; 3) infection of nontarget cells which may consequently produce an abnormal or excessive amount of a cell protein (e.g., growth factor) that regulates growth and differentiation of other leukocytes. Thus, the tumor cells themselves may have no detectable viral information, and the infected cells may be too rare to detect. In fact, these very mechanisms have been previously invoked for a possible viral role in human leukemias [76] where type-C viral information is only rarely detected.

## 4.4. Bovine Leukemia

Seroepidemiologic and transmission studies on controlled herds have identified a retrovirus, bovine leukemia virus (BLV), as the causative agent of two related lymphoproliferative diseases in cattle: the enzootic form of lymphoid leukemia lymphosarcoma and persistent lymphocytosis. The latter is in itself a benign condition but frequently ends with a lymphosarcoma [77, 78]. Besides the adult form of lymphosarcoma, which is the most common manifestation, three other clinical forms also occur: the juvenile form, affecting the visceral organs as well as nearly all lymph nodes, and more rarely, the thymic form and the cutaneous or skin form. Although in nature BLV has only been identified as the adult form of lymphosarcoma-leukemia of cattle, sheep experimentally inoculated with BLV may develop any of the four forms of disease with high frequency [79].

BLV is a retrovirus exogenous to the bovine genus. Infected cattle contain integrated provirus only in lymphoid target cells. The target cell is apparently a B-cell [80]. Restriction enzyme analysis of the integrated BLV provirus suggests that lymphocytes from cattle with persistent lymphocytosis are polyclonal and contain a mixture of normal and infected cells while tumor cells from cattle with lymphosarcoma are monoclonal with respect to the virus integration sites [81]. Thus, as in avian lymphoid leukemia, it appears that bovine lymphoid leukemia may initiate as a polyclonal, relatively benign disorder but progress in some cases to a malignant monoclonal disease.

Like other non-defective retroviruses, the BLV genome codes for all the viral structural proteins. The major *gag* protein cleavage products are p24 (equivalent to p30 of murine viruses), p12 and p15. The major envelope glyprotein has a molecular weight of 50–60 thousand (gp51). However, BLV is unique in many respects. Its genome has no detectable homology with other retrovirus genomes as assayed by molecular hybridization [82]. While most exogenous viruses can be traced to their more recent species of origin (e.g., SSAV to mouse, FeLV to rat), BLV probes do not hybridize significantly to cell DNA of any species tested [83]. The uniqueness of BLV is further demonstrated by lack of serological reactivity of any of its proteins with proteins of other retroviruses, including the major core protein, p24 [84], even though p30 of other viruses contains antigenic determinants well conserved among mammalian retroviruses [85]. As shown in a subsequent section, a virus isolated from a human T-cell lymphoma cell line

(HTLV) also shows minimal relatedness to all previously known retrovirus isolates.

It appears that most cattle infected with BLV develop antibodies against BLV, predominantly to the major core protein p24 and the envelope glyco-protein gp51 [86]. *In vivo, neither infected lymphocytes nor saliva produces BLV.* This may be the reason that BLV infection in cattle is persistent despite the continuous presence of virus-neutralizing antibodies. However, there is evidence for horizontal transmission of BLV. Lymphosarcoma and persistent lymphocytosis can spread from enzootic to leukosis-free herds. More definitive information comes from a longitudinal study on a well-characterized multiple-case herd [87]. Eighteen percent of the calves were infected at birth, suggesting congenital infection (e.g., transplacental) as one of the possible routes of transmission. However, by three years of age, almost all of the cattle in this herd were infected with BLV. When BLV-free calves nursed on BLV-free dams were raised with infected cattle, more than 90% of the exposed animals became infected. Since viruses are rarely re-leased by cells *in vivo*, it is believed that infected lymphocytes transmitted through the milk are the source of secondary infection.

## 4.5. Gibbon Ape Leukemia

Spontaneous tumors are very rare among primates, with the exception of gibbons in captivity. Gibbon colonies at different locations had a high inci-dence of hematopoietic neoplasms, including lymphosarcoma [88, 89], acute lymphoblastic leukemia [90], and granulocytic leukemias very similar to human chronic myelogenous leukemia [91]. Several strains of gibbon ape leukemia viruses (GaLV) were isolated from some of these neoplasms. $GaLV_{SF}$ was isolated from lymphosarcomas of two gibbons in the San Fran-cisco Medical Center [92]. $GaLV_{SEATO}$ was isolated from tissues of five gib-bons with granulocytic leukemia [93, 94]. $GaLV_H$ was isolated from a gib-bon with acute lymphoblastic leukemia (null cell type) from a colony on Hall's Island, Bermuda [95]. Inoculation of gibbons with $GaLV_{SEATO}$ in-duced viremia and myelogenous leukemia in young gibbons [3, 96]. In addi-tion, similar viruses have been isolated from brain extracts [97, 98] of a few non-leukemic gibbons. All the isolates of GaLV are closely related, but they are distinguishable from each other [99]. This means that the GaLV isolates form a group. This group also includes a closely related virus, the woolly monkey virus, which consists of a replication competent virus and a defec-tive sarcoma component which transforms fibroblasts. The complex, often called simian sarcoma associated virus and simian sarcoma virus (SSAV/SSV), was isolated only once from a woolly monkey, a pet which developed myelofibrosis and fibrosarcoma [100]. Inoculation of SSAV/SSV into marmosets produces sarcomas [101]. All these viruses are exogenous to primates since genomes of these viruses have no detectable homology with normal primate cellular DNA. Therefore, they must enter primates by infection. In animals infected postnatally, provirus could be detected in target tissues and some non-target tissues. Muscles and brain seem to be most resistent to virus infection [95]. Those rare animals infected early *in utero* contain provirus in all tissues [102].

Both horizontal and congenital infections occur. Animals lacking virus neutralizing antibody are more susceptible to infection. Kawakami and associates [93] studied a group of more than 200 gibbons and found 9% of the animals were viremic, and another 16% had antibodies to GaLV. In contrast, 14 orangutans, 58 chimpanzees, 14 gorillas, 134 macaques, 6 woolly monkeys, and 26 marmosets had no GaLV or GaLV antibodies. Thus, gibbons seem more susceptible to infection by these viruses than other primates. However, it is not known whether gibbons in the wild are also infected with GaLV.

GaLV and the related viruses SSV/SSAV are of particular interest among retroviruses because: 1) they are the only primate retroviruses which are known to be associated with naturally occurring neoplasms; 2) some produce CML extremely similar to the disease in humans and which to our knowledge is the only animal CML model of its kind; 3) viral markers related to these viruses are occasionally detected in humans, suggesting that viruses related to them might be present at low levels in man (see later section); and 4) viruses of this group can markedly enhance growth of human peripheral blood lymphocytes [103; and see later section].

## 5. RETROVIRUSES AND HUMAN LEUKEMIAS-LYMPHOMAS

In the absence of infectious viral isolates from human cells, the main approach has been to probe for the presence of virus in human cells by using sensitive biochemical assays (e.g., reverse transcriptase, molecular hybridization with viral nucleic acids). Positive findings may be indications for the presence of a retrovirus in the diseases examined, where whole virus may not be detected or isolated because they are few or defective, or at least difficult to transmit. However, though the findings may stimulate further investigations to determine if retroviruses are involved in the etiology of these disorders, in themselves they do not constitute definitive proof of virus. The isolation of intact virus must be achieved to produce the appropriate viral nucleic acid probes and antigens for molecular and sero-epidemiological surveys. We shall examine the available evidence for 1) influence on growth and differentiation of human hematopoietic cells of primate viruses, 2) retrovirus markers in man, and 3) actual virus isolations from cultured human cells. Special attention will be given to several related virus isolates from cultured human T-cell lymphomas which appear novel and unrelated to previous known virus isolates.

## 5.1. Biological Effects of Primate Type-C Viruses on Human Hematopoietic Cells

Fresh leukocytes from the peripheral blood and bone marrow of normal donors and leukemic patients usually survived 2 to 4 weeks in culture. However, exposure of these cultures to SSAV/SSV or GaLV resulted in immortalization of the cells with much higher frequency (50–60% with virus versus 5% for spontaneous immortalization). Other viruses tested, including BaEV and FeLV, had no growth effect, although some cultures showed evidence of productive infection. The established cell cultures were shown to be B-lymphoblasts by several biological, immunological, and biochemical assays [103]. Although all the cell lines are EBV-positive, the cells transformed by SSAV-GaLV are different from EBV-transformed B-lymphoblasts in one important respect: newly established lymphoblast cell lines from non-lymphoma sources obtained either spontaneously or following exposure to EBV were reported to be non-tumorigenic after subcutaneous inoculation into nude mice and to grow poorly in semisolid media; lymphoma cell lines after extensive culture or when obtained from Burkitt's lymphoma are tumorigenic, but the tumorigenicity is always accompanied by chromosomal abnormalities [104]. In contrast, approximately 80% of the B-lymphoblast cell lines newly established by exposure to SSAV/GaLV induced tumors in athymic nude mice and formed colonies in semisolid medium while retaining a normal human diploid karyotype [103]. When the cells were analyzed for genetic information (proteins, RNA, DNA) related to SSAV/GaLV, it became apparent that only a subpopulation of the cells have complete provirus and express viral RNA and protein [105]. Analysis of the cells by restriction enzyme and Southern [41] hybridization failed to reveal subgenomic viral fragments in a major fraction of the cells [105]. Therefore, SSAV/GaLV apparently can influence the growth characteristics of human lymphoblastoid cells without being permanently associated with all cells.

## 5.2. Viral Markers in Human Leukemic Cells

The earliest evidence for virus-like components in human cells was derived from studies of reverse transcriptase activities. Retroviruses contain a unique DNA polymerase (reverse transciptase or RT) which utilized an RNA template. Search for similar enzyme actvities in human tumor tissues has led to repeated detection of an RT-like activity in some leukemic cells or tissues. Gallo and associates [106, 107] were able to partially purify an

RT-like enzyme activity from approximately 30% of leukemic patients. In some cases of acute myelogenous leukemia, the RT was shown to be antigenically related to the RT of SSAV and GaLV [108, 109]. Using another approach, Jacquemin *et al.* [110] detected IgG eluted from the surfaces of human leukocytes (normal and leukemic) that specifically inhibited purified RT of mammalian retroviruses. IgG from some leukemic and normal blood cells inhibited SSAV and GaLV RTs more than other viral RTs and cellular polymerases not at all. In a high percentage of blast phase CMLs, the eluted IgG mainly inhibited RT from FeLV. Similar enzymes were purified by Chandra and associated from the spleen of a patient with myelofibrosis which later turned into AML [111], and from an orbital chloroma of a patient with acute myelomonocytic leukemia [112]. The latter result is particularly interesting since orbital chloromas in cases of acute myelomonocytic leukemia occur in clusters near Ankara, Turkey. The simplest and most significant interpretation of these results is that the enzyme is indicative of a virus like these primate retroviruses in these diseases. However, it is also possible that the enzyme is a normal cell gene product that is preferentially expressed in some leukemias, and the immunologic relatedness to the viral enzymes of the primate viruses is fortuitous.

There is evidence that the RT activity in leukemic cells is physically associated with intracytoplasmic particles with biophysical and biochemical properties of tumor viruses. The particles have a buoyant density in sucrose of 1.15–1.18 g/ml and a sedimentation constant of ~600 S [112, 113]. Radiolabeled cDNA synthesized using an endogenous reaction hybridized most frequently to RNA from the infectious primate retrovirus group [113] and to some murine viruses [114].

Studies have also been undertaken to examine human tumor cells for the presence of viral genetic information, expression of other viral antigens and to assay human sera for antibodies against defined viral antigens. A survey of many tumors and normal human tissues for the presence of type-C viral genetic information indicates that positive results are rare [76]. Infrequent DNA samples from leukemic patients show significantly higher hybridization to probes of BaEV [115], MuLV [116], and SSAV [117]. The results suggest that occasional humans can be infected by these viruses, but the low frequency at which the viral sequences can be detected can not be construed as evidence for or against an etiological role of these viruses in human leukemia. Similarly, antigens related to proteins of the primate and murine viruses were detected in some human tumor samples as assayed by an immunofluorescence reaction with purified viral proteins, or by competitive radioimmunoassay [99]. However, the results are somewhat controversial and in none of these studies has the putative viral antigen been purified and characterized.

## 5.3. Human Virus Isolates Related to Other Primate Retroviruses

Isolation of complete infectious virus from cultured human cells remains a rare event despite intense efforts from many laboratories. So far, six of seven human virus isolates are found to be closely related to the primate retroviruses SSAV-GaLV and BaEV (see Table 3). In some cases, many experimental data argue against laboratory contamination as a source of the virus, e.g., repeated isolation of the virus from different samples of the same patient and detection of viral components in fresh uncultured cells of the same patient [76]. Also, although human cells are permissive for growth for a wide range of mammalian retroviruses, the human virus isolates are almost always related to the primate viruses (especially SSAV-GaLV). This fact would suggest that these viruses are in the human population. However, the close relatedness of the human virus isolates to laboratory virus strains makes it difficult to absolutely rule out contamination. Therefore, isolation

*Table 3.* Recent reports of retroviruses isolated from human cells.

| Reference | Source | Type | Characteristics * |
|---|---|---|---|
| 1. Gallagher and Gallo [137] | Adult myeloid leukemia cells (one case × 3) | C | SSAV & BaEV |
| 2. Panem *et al.* [138] | Embryo (one case, many times) | C | SSAV |
| 3. Nooter *et al.* [139] | Childhood lymphatic leukemia cells (two cases) | C | SSAV |
| 4. Gabelman *et al.* [140] | Adult lymphatic leukemia cells (B lymphocytes) (one case) | C | SSAV |
| 5. Kaplan *et al.* [141] | Histocytic lymphoma cells (two cases) | C | SSAV |
| 6. Bronson *et al.* [142] | Testicular embryonal carcinoma (one case) [†] | C? | ? [‡] (possibly BaEV) |
| 7. Poiesz *et al.* [127] | Cutaneous T-cell lymphoma and Leukemia (two cases × 3) | C | Novel [§] |

* Describes relatedness to known animal RNA tumor viruses. Isolates 1 to 4 are *very* closely related to SSAV. Kaplan's isolate is related to viruses of SSAV-GaLV group but appears distinct. SSAV is woolly monkey (simian) sarcoma associated virus, GaLV is gibbon ape leukemia virus. BaEV is baboon endogenous virus.

[†] Presently 8 cases have been detected by these authors (Bronson DL and Fraley E, personal communication), but only one isolation.

[‡] This isolate is so far very poorly characterized because of low production. Early results show relatedness to BaEV.

[§] Not detectably related to any known animal virus.

of a novel virus from human T-cell lymphomas (see Table 3, last entry) is a significant advance in the demonstration of retrovirus in man. These studies will be presented in detail in the next section.

### 5.4. Recent Isolation of Novel Type-C Retroviruses from Cutaneous Human T-Cell Leukemia-Lymphomas

5.4.1. The Continuous Growth of Normal Functional Mature Human T-Cells. The ability to continuously grow normal human mature T-cells in liquid suspension culture was achieved for the first time about 5 years ago [118–121] and is now almost routinely employed in laboratories interested in T-cell biology. The system has extremely interesting and important features. *First* of all, despite long-term culture the cells remain normal in karyotype, have maintained functional (e.g., cytotoxic) activity, and remain strictly dependent on a factor termed T-cell growth factor (TCGF) for their growth (see below). *Second,* cells specifically activated for one function can be cloned and used as immunobiological reagents. *Third,* there is rationale for their clinical use. For example, by the combination of cloning techniques and the use of TCGF, autologous cytotoxic T-cells for a tumor may be obtained in large numbers and used in immunotherapy. *Fourth,* the availability of purified TCGF [122] and its specific interaction with activated T-cells makes it possible to study the interaction of a pure growth factor with a cloned population of cells newly cultured from clinical specimens. *Fifth,* as discussed later, this system recently led to the establishement of several new kinds of neoplastic T-cell lines, and the available information suggests that T-cell-TCGF changes in the normal production and/or response to TCGF may be involved in the abnormal proliferation characteristic of T-cell leukemias and lymphomas. Some of the new cell lines also led to the isolation of new kinds of type-C retroviruses (see below).

5.4.2. Components of the System. Normal leukocytes are obtained from blood, bone marrow, or spleen and the mononuclear fraction separated from other leukocytes by nylon column chromatography [123, 124]. The cells are stimulated with lectin/antigen (generally PHA). This leads to blastogenesis (activation) of a subset of T-cells involving synthesis of DNA, some cell division, and if left as such, termination of the culture. After the exposure to the lectin/antigen TCGF is released into the media, probably by a subset of T-cells different from those which respond to TCGF. Eventually, TCGF release ceases and the cultured cells terminate their growth unless there is intervention. Apparently, macrophages mediate the T-cell release of TCGF. After their interaction with lectin/antigen, the macrophages release a factor termed lymphocyte activating factor which induces the T-cells to release TCGF. Thus, some adherent cells are required. If exogenous TCGF is added every 3 to 4 days to the cultured cells, the T-cells proliferate indefinitely [125]. It is now abundantly clear that with normal cells TCGF can only induce growth after the T-cells are activated [122]. It is therefore the second signal in the immune response of T-cells which is solely responsible for the clonal expression of the activated cells.

Human TCGF was recently purified from lymphocyte conditioned media prepared mitogen-stimulated peripheral blood cells incubated for 72 hours in germ-free media. The details of the purification scheme have been published [122]. TCGF is a protein of 13–14 K daltons with a pI of 6.8. An interesting feature of human TCGF is that it has little species specificity. It will stimulate T-cell growth in primates, cows, cats, horses, and rodents but it has an apparent cell specificity, interacting only with activated T-lymphocytes.

*5.4.3. Direct Growth of Neoplastic T-Cell with TCGF.* Recently, it was found that T-cells from patients with leukemias and lymphomas of mature T-cells *directly* respond to purified TCGF [126]. This suggests that these cells differ from normal T-cells by maintaining TCGF receptors while normal cells must first be activated *in vitro* (unless, of course, there has been a recent substantial antigenic *in vivo* stimulation to the normal cells). This might mean that these neoplastic T-cells are chronically exposed to some antigens or that in the process of neoplastic transformation a membrane change occurs which makes available a previously 'cryptic' TCGF receptor.

When crude TCGF was used, growth of the neoplastic T-cells was generally maintained for only 2–4 weeks. There are inhibitors of TCGF activity in the crude and even partially purified fractions. These include interferon, PHA (which inhibits the long-term growth effect of TCGF), and other unidentified substances. When the more purified TCGF was used, growth was maintained and in some cases cell lines independent of TCGF were established [126]. These cell lines were established from patients with cutaneous T-cell leukemias and lymphomas (Sézary syndrome and mycosis fungoides, respectively), and they have several interesting features. They have characteristics of mature T-cells (E-rosette positive) but also are positive for nonspecific esterase, a macrophage marker. The cultured cells include 1–15% giant multinucleated cells often surrounded by smaller mono- or binucleated cells in rosette-like fashion. Some cells have convoluted nuclei as Sézary lymphocytes. The chief characteristics are summarized in Table 4.

*5.4.4. Isolation of New Type-C Viruses.* Type-C viruses were recently isolated from four of these cell lines. Three viruses were from different clinical

*Table 4.* Characteristics of T-cells cultured from patients with mature T-cell leukemias and lymphomas indicative of neoplastic origin.

| | |
|---|---|
| 1. Morphology | Some giant multinucleated cells. |
| 2. Karyotype | Same in each case as primary tumor (3 possessing karyotypic anomalies). |
| 3. Response to TCGF | Direct (no lectin or antigen *in vitro* activation required). |
| * 4. Histochemistry | In case of cutaneous T-cell leukemias and lymphomas—non-specific esterase positive. |
| 5. Virus | Three lines release a type-C retrovirus (HTLV) not found in any normal T-cell line. |
| 6. TCGF Independent Growth | Two lines became TCGF independent and produce their own TCGF. |

* Normal T-cells and those from patients with ALL fresh or grown in culture are non-specific esterase negative.

specimens obtained from one patient with cutaneous T-cell lymphomas (mycosis fungoides) [127, 128]. One was isolated from a cell line established from a patient with Sézary leukemia [128]. These viruses are closely related and possibly identical to each other and collectively we call them HTLV (human T-lymphomas-leukemia virus). Detailed analysis of the reverse transcriptase of HTLV has shown that immunologically it is not detectably related to reverse transcriptase of any previously isolated animal retrovirus [129]. This strongly suggests that HTLV is a novel retrovirus rather than a laboratory contaminant. This indication has in our opinion been recently and conclusively established by analysis of other proteins of HTLV [130], by analysis of HTLV nucleic acid sequences [131], and by demonstrating that nucleic acids of or closely related to HTLV can be found in the DNA of *fresh uncultured* tumor specimens from some people with T-cell leukemia-lymphoma, including one out of one tested adult with T-cell ALL. Only a few specimens have been examined. It could be that HTLV is commonly involved in mature T-cell leukemias and lymphomas. Since the viral (provirus) nucleic acid sequences were not found in normal human DNA, we can conclude that HTLV is not an endogenous human virus, i.e., not genetically transmitted. Rather, it must be acquired by some kind of an as yet unknown infection event.

Like most other viruses derived from outbred animals, HTLV does not appear to be transforming *in vitro*. Attempts to establish productive infection in secondary cultures have been unsuccessful. Normal T-cells (3 out of 15 cases) dependent on TCGF for growth have been productively infected whereas their normal B-cell counterparts have not (Figure 5). However, the virus produced by these T-cells is still poorly infectious.

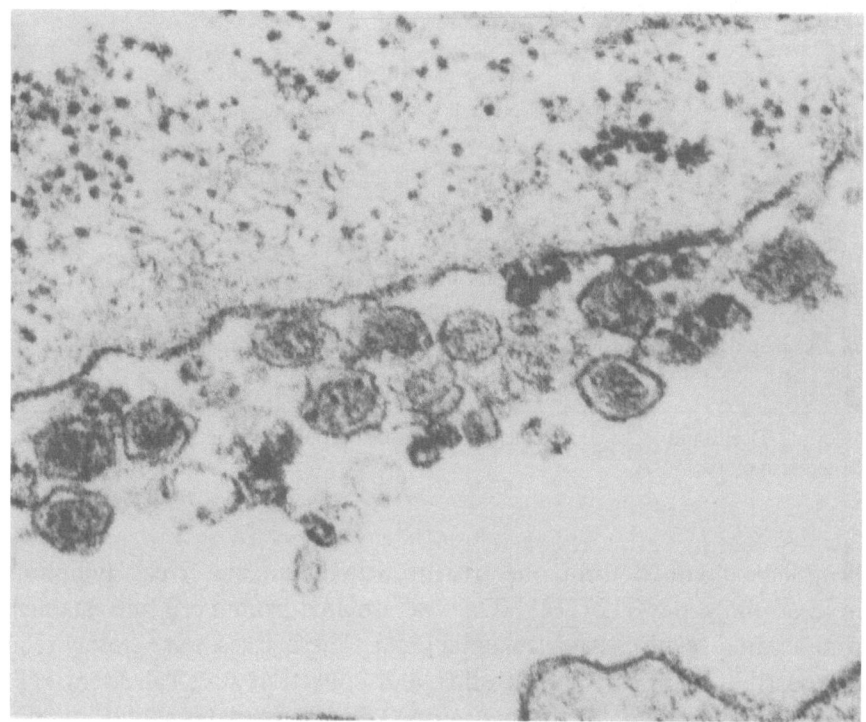

*Figure 5.* Electron micrograph of the type-C retrovirus, HTLV from normal T-cells growing in vitro productively infected with HTLV. Note the mature virions released from the cells. The virus size is variable but approximates 1000 Å.

These phenomena with HTLV are reminiscent of bovine leukemia-lymphoma and bovine leukemia virus (BLV). As noted in an earlier section, BLV was not detected until the last decade when the tumor cells were first successfully grown in culture [132]. Moreover, the bovine disease sometimes manifests cutaneous lesions, and when BLV is inoculated into sheep, one of the diseases which develops is a cutaneous lymphoma [79].

In summary, HTLV are tumor viruses recently isolated from some human T-cell lymphomas and a T-cell (Sézary) leukemia. Both of these diseases exhibited cutaneous manifestations. HTLV are novel oncornaviruses which are not endogenous to humans and must enter by some kind of infection. It is reasonable to assume that HTLV may be involved in the etiology of these diseases. Other studies are in progress to further delineate their role in human T-cell leukemias and lymphomas.

*5.4.5. The Possible Role of TCGF and HTLV in the Pathogenesis of Lymphomas and Leukemias of Mature T-Cells.* The two cutaneous T-cell lymphoma cell lines which chronically produce HTLV were originally dependent on TCGF for proliferation. After 6-8 subdivisions in culture, they became independent of the need for exogenous TCGF. They both are now producing and responding to their own growth factors [133]. Material constitutively released by these cell lines and material eluted from their cell membranes will support the growth of activated but not unactivated T-cells. Both cell lines will absorb TCGF in a time, temperature, and cell concentration-dependent manner and will also increase its proliferative response in the presence of TCGF. These results have been confirmed by demonstrating that single cell clones of one of the cell lines produce HTLV and TCGF and

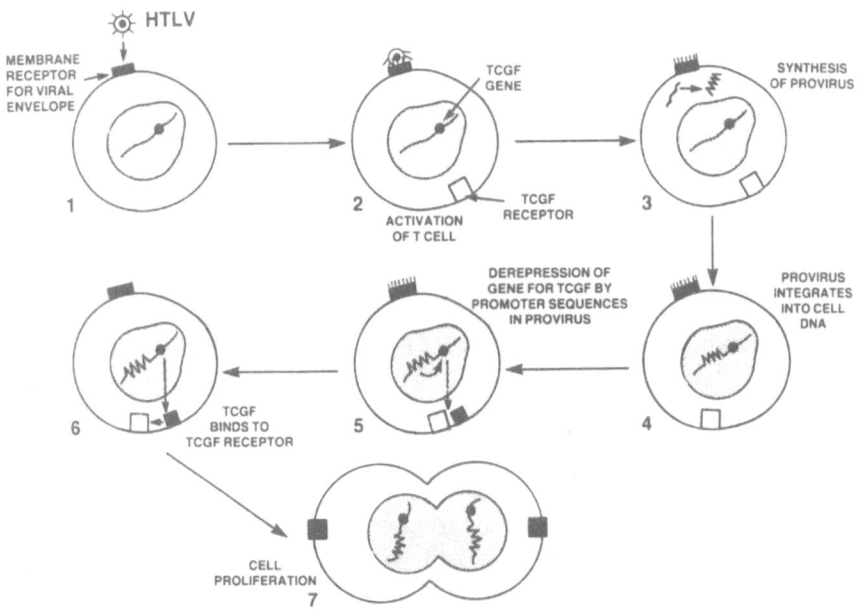

*Figure 6.* A schematic and simple model for the first stage of T-cell leukemic transformation. We propose that the target cell is a mature T-cell with an antigen receptor site, which in the case of a proposed viral induced disease, recognizes an envelope protein of HTLV. This leads to the recently known antigen effect of inducing the availability of receptors for TCGF. Concomitantly, nucleic acid sequences contained in the HTLV genome which are integrated into the host cell DNA include sequences which can act as promotors for expression of certain cell genes. (Much evidence suggests that this may be the case in animal models with animal retroviruses.) We suggest that this leads to an abnormal expression of the gene for TCGF. We think the available data indicate that separate subsets of T-cells usually make and respond to TCGF under normal circumstances. The above model of a cell both making and responding to TCGF may lead to uncontrolled proliferation. In turn, this may subsequently lead to an increase in the likelihood of mutational events which 'fix' the transformed state. Later in the progression of leukemogenesis, cells which express virus may be selected against by immune mechanisms, making finding them rare and difficult by the time of frank disease.

also respond to TCGF (Maeda and Gallo, unpublished). This is different from the normal situation where a subset of T-cells needs lectin/antigen stimulation plus an accessory cell to produce TCGF [134, 135]. These results suggested a model for the interaction between HTLV, TCGF and mature T-cells (Figure 6).

In this model an HTLV protein (presumably the envelope) interacts with a very specific group of T-cells (those which have receptors for the envelope). This mimics an antigen stimulation of blastogenesis. The T-cell is one normally designed to develop TCGF receptors and does so. However, promotor-like sequences contained in the integrated HTLV provirus triggers derepression of the TCGF gene, leading to TCGF release and auto-stimulation. This may be an early step in the transformation. Subsequently, the increase in proliferation leads to an increased incidence of mutation with fixation of the transformed state. Virus expressing cells are selected against by immune mechanisms so that one may only rarely identify virus by the time overt leukemia occurs. Other initiators (non-viral) may be involved in the early stages of other forms of T-cell lymphomas and leukemias, but even in these cases, abnormalities in TCGF production or response may be central to the pathogenesis of these diseases.

Recently, specific antibodies to HTLV were found in the sera of a few patients with cutaneous T-cell lymphoma [136]. One positive result was with serum from C.R., the first patient from whom HTLV was isolated. These antibodies were detected by both ELISA (enzyme linked immunoassay) and RIP (radioimmunoprecipitation) assays and in both cases, competition assays showed remarkable specificity (see summary of specificity data in Table 5). The presence of antibodies is perhaps more suggestive of an exogenous entry of HTLV, i.e., by some kind of a poorly understood infection. However, antibodies can occur to endogenous viruses so the question of its origin must remain open. It will be important to look globally for clusters of patients with these types of leukemias and lymphomas. A careful study of disease clusters and of family studies combined with information generated from molecular biological studies with HTLV reagents may lead to a better understanding of the origin of these diseases.

## 5.5. Human onc Genes: Implications and Future Directions

As described in section 3.4, most acutely transforming retroviruses contain onc genes that are derived from a set of well-conserved vertebrate genes. Although the function of these genes is still not well defined, accumulating data point to a significant role for them in regulation of cellular growth and differentiation. In fact, these genes may be effectors of a 'universal' pathway of leukemogenesis, not only by the acute and nonacute

*Table 5.* Specificity of natural antibodies from serum of patients with cutaneous T-cell lymphoma against HTLV: competition in RIP and ELISA assays. *

| Patient source of serum antibody | Test of competing antigen | | | | | | | | | |
|---|---|---|---|---|---|---|---|---|---|---|
| | Proteins from viruses | | | | | Proteins from human cell lysates | | | | |
| | FCS | BSA | HTLV_CR | HTLV_MB | Numerous animal retorviruses | HUT-102 † | CTCL-2 † | Normal T-cells | B-cell lines | Normal transformed T-cell lines not producing HTLV |
| CTCL-CR ‡ | – | – | + | + | – | + | + | – | – | – |
| CTCL-4 ‡ | – | – | + | + | – | + | + | – | – | – |

* CTCL = cutaneous T-cell lymphoma, HTLV = human T-cell lymphoma-leukemia virus, RIP = radioimmunoprecipitation, ELISA = enzyme linked immunoassay, FCS = fetal calf serum, BSA = bovine serum albumin.

† Cell lines produce HTLV.

‡ CTCL-CR is the patient from whom cell line HUT-102 was established. The virus HTLV_CR was first isolated from T-cells. CTCL-4 is another patient with a similar stage of disease as patient CTCL-CR.

viruses as discussed in section 3.5, but also by nonviral agents such as chemical carcinogens. The fact that humans have homologues of these *onc* genes spurs us to examine more closely their nature and function in different human tumor and non-tumor cells. There are now several human *onc* genes molecularly cloned and characterized (our unpublished data); simultaneous efforts are directed at studying expression of these genes in different cell types and characterization of the cellular *onc* gene products in several laboratories, including our own. The next decade of research may provide some basic answers to the mechanisms of leukemogenesis in man.

## 6. SUMMARY AND CONCLUSIONS

It seems increasingly important for people in leukemia research to have some interest and understanding of a major group of viruses, called retroviruses or RNA tumor viruses. It is now clear that in the interaction of these viruses with host cells they sometimes lose portions of their genome and in so doing, can acquire cellular nucleotide sequences. Sometimes these sequences impart the transforming activity of the retrovirus, converting a poorly oncogenic or non-oncogenic virus into one with high potential for neoplastic conversion. Genetic information acquired from cells by retroviruses (*onc* genes) may be genes important to cell growth, and by studying these genes, basic aspects of cell growth and of leukemic transformation may be approached at the molecular level. Thus, one way retroviruses appear to cause neoplastic conversion is by bringing into the cell a cell gene (or cell-related gene since some diversity is generated in the evolution of the virus) which directly affects cell growth, perhaps by having it integrated into host DNA sequences at the wrong location or in numerous copies so that its expression is not properly controlled. Other leukemia viruses (those with long latency periods) apparently do not contain such cellular sequences, and how they cause leukemia is not completely understood. There is increasing realization that sequences near the ends of the viral genome (the LTR units) are similar to sequences of insertion elements and transposons. These sequences may move about in the host DNA, and since they may carry promotor sequences, they may act by altering the normal expression of certain host sequences, specifically the *onc* genes. The long period for leukemia development characteristic of these viruses may be the time needed for a random integration of the kind which would lend to proper alignment of the viral LTR to the target cellular genes.

Even if these viruses were not the direct causes of leukemia, they have provided us with purified cellular genes, the studies of which will be useful and applicable to leukemogenesis whatever the primary cause, particularly, if there is some final common pathway. However, retroviruses are indeed involved in the cause of naturally occurring leukemia. In fact, to our knowledge they are the chief known cause of naturally occurring leukemias of animals. This includes leukemias of chickens, mice, cats, cows, and apes. Moreover, the forms of leukemia encompass erythroleukemias, B-lymphoblastic leukemia and lymphoma, myeloid leukemias (both AML and CML), and T-lymphoblastic leukemia and lymphoma. The latter are among the most common virus induced leukemia of animals.

Retroviruses have recently been identified in humans. Two types appear at this time to merit special interest: those related to the woolly monkey virus, especially those reported by Kaplan and his co-workers in diffuse histiocytic lymphoma and called DHL viruses, and the novel class of retroviruses isolated recently from T-cells of Sézary leukemia and mycosis fungoides, known as HTL virus or HTLV. We can not predict that studies with retroviruses will lead to improved diagnostic methods, better prognostic forecasts, or better therapy. Nevertheless, we can predict that this knowledge will lead to a better understanding of these diseases and hope that this will have practical ramifications.

REFERENCES

1. Miller RW: Epidemiology of leukemia. In: Modern trends in human leukemia III. Neth R, Gallo RC, Hofschneider PH, Mannweiler K (eds). New York: Springer-Verlag, 1978, pp 37–52.
2. Gallo RC: Viruses and the pathogenesis of human leukemia. Schweiz Med Wochenschr 107:1436–1440, 1977.
3. Kawakami TG, Kollias G, Holmberg C: Oncogenicity of gibbon type-C myelogenous leukemia virus. Int J Cancer 25:641–646, 1980.
4. MacMahon B, Levy M: Prenatal origin of childhood leukemia: evidence from twins. N Engl J Med 270:1082–1085, 1964.
5. Rowley JD: Chromosome abnormalities in leukemia. In: Modern trends in human leukemia III. Neth R, Gallo RC, Hofschneider PH, Mannweiler K (eds). New York: Springer-Verlag, 1978, pp 43–52.
6. Klein G: Viral oncology. New York: Raven Press, 1980.
7. Purtilo DT, Paquin L, DeFlorio D, Virzi F, Sakhuja R: Immunodiagnosis and immunopathogenesis of the X-linked recessive lymphoproliferative syndrome. Semin Hematol 4(16):309–343, 1979.
8. Gutensohn N, Cole P: Childhood social environment and Hodgkin's disease. N Eng J Med 204:135–140, 1980.
9. Gallo RC, Gelmann EP: In search of a Hodgkin's disease virus. N Eng J Med 304:169–170, 1981.
10. Schaadt M, Diehl V, Stein H, Fonatsch C, Kirchner HH: Two neoplastic cell lines with unique features derived from Hodgkin's disease. Int J Cancer 26:723–731, 1980.
11. Hughes SH, Payvar F, Spector D, Schimke RT, Robinson HL, Payne GS, Bishop JM,

Varmus HE: Heterogeneity of genetic loci of chickens: analysis of endogenous viral and nonviral genes by cleavage of DNA with restriction endonucleases. Cell 18:347–359, 1979.

12. Astrin SM: Endogenous viral genes of the white leghorn chicken: common site of residence and sites associated with specific phenotypes of viral gene expression. Proc Nat Acad Sci USA 75:5941–5945, 1978.

13. Cohen JC, Varmus HE: Endogenous mammary tumor virus DNA varies among wild mice and segregates during inbreeding. Nature 278: 418–423, 1979.

14. Wong-Staal F, Josephs SF: Baboon endogenous virus genomes in four species of baboons and five other genera of Old World monkeys: evidence for infection post speciation. Virology 112:289–295, 1981.

15. Benveniste RE, Todaro GJ: Evolution of type-C viral genes. I. Nucleic acid from baboon type-C virus as a measure of divergence among primate species. Proc Nat Acad Sci USA 71:4513–4518, 1974.

16. Bender W, Davidson N: Mapping of poly (A) sequences on the electron microscope reveals unusual structure of type-C oncornovirus RNA molecules. Cell 7:595–599, 1976.

17. Furuichi Y, Shatkin AJ, Stravenzer E, Bishop JM: Blocked methylated 5′-terminal sequences in avian sarcoma virus RNA. Nature 257:618–621, 1975.

18. Gillespie DH, Marshall S, Gallo RC: RNA of RNA tumor viruses contains poly A. Nature New Biol 236:227–229, 1972.

19. Bishop JM: Retroviruses. Ann Rev Biochem 47:35–88, 1978.

20. Coffin J: Structure, replication, and recombination of retrovirus genomes: some unifying hypotheses. J Gen Virol 42:1–26, 1979.

21. Haseltine WA, Klied DG: A method for classification of 5′-termini of retroviruses. Nature 273:358–364, 1978.

22. Dhar R, McClements NL, Enquist LW, Vande Woude GF: Nucleotide sequences of integrated Moloney sarcoma provirus long terminal repeats and their host and viral junctions. Proc Nat Acad Sci USA 77:3937–3941, 1980.

23. Calos MP, Miller JH: Transposable elements. Cell 20:579–595, 1980.

24. Mellon P, Pawson A, Bister K, Martin GS, Duesberg PH: Specific RNA sequences and gene products of MC29 avian leukemia virus. Proc Nat Acad Sci USA 75:5874–5879, 1978.

25. Baltimore D, Shields A, Otto G, Goff S, Besmer P, Witte O, Rosenberg N: Structure and expression of the Abelson murine leukemia virus genome and its relation to a normal cell gene. In: Viral oncogenes. Cold Spring Harbor Symposium Quant Biol, Vol XLIV, 1979, pp 849-854.

26. Hu S, Lai MMC, Vogt PK: Genome of avian myelocytomatosis virus MC29: analysis by heterduplex mapping. Proc Nat Acad Sci USA 76:1265–1270, 1979.

27. Shields A, Goff S, Paskind M, Otto G, Baltimore D: Structure of the Abelson murine leukemia virus genome. Cell 18:955–962, 1979.

28. Ruscetti SF, Turek LP, Sherr CJ: Three independent isolates of feline sarcoma virus code for three distinct gag-X polyproteins. J Virol 35:259–264, 1980.

29. Witte ON, Dasgupta A, Baltimore D: Abelson murine leukemia virus protein is phosphorylated in vitro to form phosphotyrosine. Nature 283:826–831, 1980.

30. Hayman MJ, Royer-Pokora B, Graf T: Defectiveness of avian erythroblastosis virus: synthesis of a *gag* related protein. Virology 92:31-39, 1979.

31. Feldman RA, Hanafusa T, Hanafusa H: Characterization of protein kinase activity associated with the transforming gene product of Fujinami sarcoma virus. Cell 22:757–765, 1980.

32. Erikson RL, Brugge JS, Erikson E, Collett MS: Studies on the structure and function of the avian sarcoma virus transforming gene product. In: Modern trends in human leukemia III,

Neth R, Gallo RC, Hofschneider PH, Mannweiler L (eds). New York: Springer-Verlag, 1978, pp 261–270.

33. Barbacid M, Bolognesi D, Aaronson SA: Humans have antibodies capable of recognizing oncoviral glycoproteins demonstriction that these antibodies are formed in response to cellular modification of flycoproteins rather as consequence of exposure to virus. Proc Nat Acad Sci USA 77:1617–1621, 1980.

34. Stehelin D, Varmus HE, Bishop JM: DNA related to the transforming gene(s) of avian sarcoma virus is present in normal avian DNA. Nature 260:170–172, 1976.

35. Frankel AE, Fischinger PJ: Nucleotide sequences in mouse DNA and RNA specific for Moloney sarcoma virus. Proc Nat Acad Sci USA 73:3705–3709, 1976.

36. Frankel AG, Gilbert JH, Porzig KJ, Scolnick EM, Aaronson SA: Nature and distribution of feline sarcoma virus nucleotide sequences. J Virol 30:821–827, 1979.

37. Roussel M, Saule S, Lagrou C, Rommens C, Beug H, Graf T, Stehelin D: Defective avian leukemia viruses. Three new viral oncogenes of cellular origin specific for three types of hematopoietic cell transformation. Nature 281:452–455, 1979.

38. Wang LH, Galpern CC, Nadel M, Hanafusa H: Recombination between viral and cellular sequences generates transforming sarcoma virus. Proc Nat Acad Sci USA 75:5812, 1978.

39. Collett MS, Brugge JS, Erikson RL: Characterization of a normal avian cell protein related to the avian sarcoma virus transforming gene product. Cell 15:1363–1369, 1978.

40. Wong-Staal F, Gelmann E, Dalla-Favera R, Manzari, V, Szala S, Josephs S, Gallo RC: The v-sis transforming gene of simian sarcoma virus is a new onc gene of primate origin. Nature 294:273–275, 1981.

41. Southern EM: Detection of specific sequences among DNA fragments separated by gel electrophoresis. J Mol Biol 98:503–517, 1975.

42. Goff SP, Gilboa E, Witte ON, Baltimore D: Structure of the Abelson murine leukemia virus genome and the homologous cellular gene: studies with cloned viral DNA. Cell 22:777–785, 1980.

43. Ellis RW, Defeo D, Maryak JM, Young HA, Shih TY, Chang EH, Lowy DR, Scolnick EM: Dual evolutionary origin for the rat genetic sequences of Harveymurine sarcoma virus. J Virol 36:408–420, 1980.

44. Franchini G, Even J, Sherr CJ, Wong-Staal F: Onc sequences (v-fes) of Snyder-Theilen feline sarcoma virus are derived from discontiguous regions of a cat cellular gene (c-fes). Nature 290:154–157, 1981.

45. Dalla-Favera R, Gallo RC, Gelmann E, Wong-Staal F: A human onc gene homologous to the transforming gene (v-sis) of simian sarcoma virus. Nature 292:31–35, 1981.

46. Shibuya M, Hanafusa T, Hanafusa H, Stephenson JR: Homology exists among the transforming sequences of avian and feline sarcoma viruses. Proc Nat Acad Sci USA 77:7536–6540, 1980.

47. Van de Ven WMJ, Reynolds FW, Stephenson JR: The nonstructural components of polyproteins encoded by replication – defective mammalian transforming retroviruses are phosphorylated and have associated protein kinase activity. Virology 101:185–197, 1980.

48. Graf T, Beug H, von Kirchbach A, Hayman MJ: Three new types of viral oncogenes in defective leukemia viruses II. Biological, genetical and immunochemical evidence. In: Cold Spring Harbor Symp Quant Biol, Vol XLIV, 1979, pp 1225–1234.

49. Rosenberg NE, Clark DR, Witte ON: Abelson murine leukemia virus mutants deficient in kinase activity and lymphoid cell transformation. J Virol 36: 766–774, 1980.

50. Hankins WD, Troxler D: Polycythemia and anemia-inducing erythroleukemia viruses exhibit differential erythroid transforming effects in vitro. Cell 22:693–699, 1980.

51. Witte ON, Rosenberg N, Baltimore D: A normal cell protein cross reactive to the major Abelson murine leukemia virus gene product. Nature 281:396–398, 1979.
52. Tsichlis PN, Coffin JM: Recombination between the defective component of an acute leukemia virus and RAV-O, an endogenous virus of chickens. Proc Nat Acad Sci USA 76:3001, 1979.
53. Robinson HL, Pearson MN, DeSimone DW, Tsichlis PN, Coffin JM: Subgroup E avian leukosis virus associated disease in chickens. In: Viral oncogenes, Cold Spring Harbor Symp Quant Biol, Vol XLIV, 1979, pp 1133–1142.
54. Yamamoto T, Jay G, Pastan I: Unusual features in the nucleotide sequence of a cDNA clone derived from the common region of avian sarcoma virus messenger RNA. Proc Nat Acad Sci USA 77:176–180, 1980.
55. Sabran JL, Hsu TW, Yeater C, Kaji A, Mason WS, Taylor JM: Analysis of integrated Avian RNA tumor virus DNA in transformed chicken, duck and quail fibroblasts. J Virol 29:170–176, 1979.
56. Groudine M, Weintraub H: Activation of cellular genes by avian RNA, tumor viruses. Proc Nat Acad Sci USA 77:5351–5354, 1980.
57. Hayward WS, Neel BG, Astrin SM: Induction of lymphoid leukosis by Avian leukosis virus: activation of a cellular 'onc' gene by promoter insertion. Nature 290:475–480, 1981.
58. Cooper GM, Neiman P: Transforming genes of neoplasms induced by Avian leucosis virus. Nature 287:656–657, 1980.
59. Hartley JW, Wolford NK, Old LJ, Rowe WP: A new class of murine leukemia virus associated with development of spontaneous lymphomas. Proc Nat Acad Sci USA 74:789, 1977.
60. Elder JH, Gautsch JW, Jensen FC, Lerner RA, Hartley JW, Rowe WP: Biochemical evidence that MCF murine leukemia viruses are envelope (env) gene recombinants. Proc Nat Acad Sci USA 74:4676–4680, 1977.
61. Dresler, S, Ruta M, Murray MJ, Kabat D: Glycoprotein encoded by the Friend spleen focus-forming virus. J Virol 30:564, 1979.
62. Burmester BR, Fredrickson TN: Transmission of virus from field cases of avian lymphomatosis I isolation of virus in line 15 I chickens. J Nat Cancer Inst 32:37–63, 1964.
63. Weyl KG, Dougherty RM: Contact transmission of avian leukosis virus. J Nat Cancer Inst 58:1019–1025, 1977.
64. Neiman PE, Payne LN, Jordan L, Weiss RA: Malignant lymphoma of the bursa of fabricius: analysis of early transformation. In: Viruses in naturally occurring cancer, 7th Cold Spring Harbor Symposium on Cell Proliferation, Essex M, Todaro GJ, zur Hausen H (eds.). New York Cold Spring Harbor Press, 1980, pp 519–528.
65. Gardner MB, Henderson BE, Estes JD, Ronjey RW, Casagrande J, Pike M, Huebner RJ: The epidemiology and virology of C-type virus-associated hematological cancers and related diseases in wild mice. Cancer Res 36:574–581, 1976.
66. Blankenhorn EP, Gardner MB, Estes JD: Immunogenetics of a thymus antigen in lymphoma-prone and lymphoma-resistant colonies of wild mice. J Nat Cancer Inst 54:665–672, 1975.
67. Jarrett WF, Jarrett O, Mackey L, Laird W, Hardy WD, Essex M: Horizontal transmission of leukemia virus and leukemia in the cat. J Natl Cancer Inst 51:833–841, 1973.
68. Hardy ND, Hess GW, MacEwen EG, McClelland AJ, Zuckerman EE, Essex M, Cotter SM, Jarrett O: Biology of feline leukemia virus in the natural environment. Cancer Res 36:582–588, 1976.
69. Francis DP, Essex M, Hardy WD: Excretion of feline leukemia virus by naturally infected pet cats. Nature 269:252–254, 1977.

70. Essex M, Sliski AH, Worley M, Grant CK, Snyder H, Hardy WD, Chen LB: Significance of the feline oncornavirus associated cell membrane antigen (FOCMA) in the natural history of feline leukemia. In: Viruses in naturally occurring cancers, 7th Cold Spring Harbor Symposium on Cell Proliferation. Essex M, Todaro GJ, zur Hausen H (eds). New York: Cold Spring Harbor Press, 1980, pp 589-602.

71. Hardy WD, Zuckerman AJ, McClelland HW, Synder HW, Essex M, Francis D: The immunology and epidemiology of FeLV non-producer feline lymphosarcoma. In: Viruses and naturally occurring cancer, 7th Cold Spring Harbor Symposium on Cell Proliferation, Essex M, Todaro GJ, zur Hausen H (eds). New York: Cold Spring Harbor Press, 1980, pp 677-698.

72. Koshy R, Wong-Staal F, Gallo RC, Hardy W, Essex M: Distribution of FeLV sequences in DNA of normal and leukemia domestic cats. Virology 99:135-144, 1979.

73. Wong-Staal F, Koshy R, Gallo RC: Feline leukemia virus genomes associated with the domestic cat: a survey of normal and leukemic animals. In: Viruses in naturally occurring cancers, 7th Cold Spring Harbor Symposium on Cell Proliferation, Essex M, Todaro GJ, zur Hausen H (eds). New York, Cold Spring Harbor Press, 1980, pp 623-634.

74. Wong-Staal F, Franchini G, Gallo RC: Some studies of the nature and expression of viral genetic information in cells from normal and leukemic cats. In: Feline leukemia virus, Hardy WD, Essex M, McClelland AJ (eds). New York: Elsevier North-Holland, 1980, pp 381-391.

75. Koshy R, Gallo RC, Wong-Staal F: Characterization of the endogenous feline leukemia virus related DNA sequences in cats and attempts to identify exogenous viral sequences in tissues of virus-negative leukemia animals. Virology 103:454-455, 1980.

76. Gallo RC, Saxinger WC, Gallagher RE, Gillespie DH, Ruscetti F, Reitz MS, Aulakh GS, Wong-Staal F: Some ideas on the origins of leukemia in man and recent evidence for the presence of type-C viral related information. In: Origins of human cancer, Cold Spring Harbor Conference, Watson JD, Winsten JA (eds). New York: Cold Spring Harbor Press, Vol 4, 1977, pp 1253-1286.

77. Burny A, Bex F, Chantrenne H, Cleuter Y, Dekegel D, Ghysdael G, Kettmann R, Leclercq M, Leunen J, Mammerickx M, Portetelle D: Bovine leukemia virus involvement in enzootic bovine leukosis. In: Advances in cancer research, Klein G, Weinhouse S (eds). New York: Academic Press, 1978, pp 251-259.

78. Ferrer JF, Abt DA, Bhatt DM, Marshak RR: Studies on the relationship between infection with bovine C-type virus, leukemia and persistent lymphocytosis in cattle. Cancer Res 34:893-898, 1974.

79. Olson C: Progress for control of bovine leukosis. Bovine Practitioner 14:115-120, 1979.

80. Paul PS, Pomeroy KA, Johnson DW, Muscoplat CC, Handwerger BS, Soper FS, Sorensen DK: Evidence for the replication of bovine leukemia virus in the B-lymphocytes. Am J Vet Res 38:873, 1977.

81. Kettmann R, Meunier-Rotival M, Marbaix G, Cortadas J, Mammerickx M, Burny A, Bernardi G: Genomic integration of bovine leukemia provirus. In: Viruses in naturally occurring cancers, 7th Cold Spring Harbor Symposium on Cell Proliferation, Essex M, Todaro GJ, zur Hausen H (eds). New York: Cold Spring Harbor Press, 1980, pp 927-942.

82. Kettmann R, Portetelle D, Mammerickx M, Cleuter Y, Dekegel D, Galorex M, Ghysdael J, Burny A, Chantrenne H: Bovine leukemia virus: an exogenous RNA oncogenic virus. Proc Nat Acad Sci USA 73: 1014-1418, 1976.

83. Callahan R, Lieber MM, Todaro GJ, Graves DC, Ferrer JF: Bovine leukemia virus genes in the DNA of leukemic cattle. Science 192: 1005-1007, 1976.

84. Devare SG: Bovine lekemia virus: an etiologic agent associated with lymphosarcoma of domestic cattle. In: Viruses in naturally occurring cancers, Cold Spring Harbor Conference

on Cell Proliferation, Essex M, Todaro G, zur Hausen H (eds). New York: Cold Spring Harbor Press, Vol 7, 1980, pp 943–952.

85. Gilden RV: Interrelationships among RNA tumor viruses and host cells. Adv Cancer Res 22:157–202, 1975.

86. Devare SL, Chander S, Samagh BS, Stephenson JR: Evaluation of radioimmunoprecipitation for the detection of bovine leukemia virus. J Immunol 119:277–282, 1977.

87. Piper CE, Abt DA, Ferrer JF, Markshah RR: Seroepidemiological evidence of the horizontal transmission of the bovine C-type virus. Cancer Res 35:2714–1716, 1975.

88. Johnson DO, Wooding WL, Tanticharoenyos P, Bourgeois Jr CH: Malignant lymphoma in the gibbon. J Am Vet Med Assoc 159:563–566, 1971.

89. Newberne JW, Robinson VB: Spontaneous tumors in primates: a report of two cases with notes on the apparent low incidence of neoplasms in subhuman primates. Am J Vet Res 21:150–155, 1960.

90. De Paoli A, Garner FM: Acute lymphocytic leukemia in a white cheeked gibbon (*Hylobates concolor*). Cancer Res 28:2559–2561, 1968.

91. De Paoli A, Johnsen DO, Noll WW: Granulocytic leukemia in white-handed gibbons. J Am Vet Med Assoc 163:624–628, 1973.

92. Kawakami T, Huff S, Buckley P, Dungworth D, Synder S, Gilden R: C-type virus associated with gibbon lymphosarcoma. Nature New Biol 235:170–172, 1972.

93. Kawakami TG, Buckley PM: Antigenic studies on gibbon type-C viruses. Transplant Proc 6:193–196, 1974.

94. Kawakami TG, Buckley PM, De Paoli A, Nall W, Bustad LK: Studies on the prevalence of type-C virus associated with gibbon hematopoietic neoplasms. In: Comparative leukemia research, 1973, Ito Y, Dutcher RM (eds). Basel: Karger, 1975, pp385–389.

95. Gallo RC, Gallagher RE, Wong-Staal F, Aoki T, Markham PD, Schetters H, Rescetti F, Valerio M, Walling M, O'Keefe RT, Saxinger WC, Smith RG, Gillespie DH, Reitz MS: Isolation and tissue distribution of type-C virus and viral components from a gibbon ape (*Hylobates lar*) with lymphocytic leukemia. Virology 84:359–373, 1978a.

96. Sun L, Kawakami TG, Matoba SI: Genomic stability of gibbon oncornavirus. Virology 28:767–771, 1978.

97. Todaro GJ, Lieber MM, Benveniste RE: Infectious primate type-C viruses: three isolates belonging to a new subgroup from the brains of normal gibbons. Virology 67:335–357, 1975.

98. Kawakami TG, Sun L, McDowell TS: Distribution and transmission of primate type-C virus. In: Advances in comparative leukemia research, Bentvelzen P, Hilgers J, Yohn DS (eds). Amsterdam: Elsevier North-Holland, 1977, pp 33–36.

99. Gallo RC, Wong-Staal F: Molecular biology of primate retroviruses. In: Viral oncology, Klein G (ed). New York: Raven Press, 1980, pp 399–431.

100. Theilen GH, Gould D, Fowler M, Dungworth DL: C-type virus in tumor tissue of a wolly monkey (*Lagothrix spp*) with fibrosarcoma. J Nat Cancer Inst 47:881–889, 1971.

101. Deinhardt F: Biology of primate retroviruses. In: Viral oncology, Klein G (ed). New York: Raven Press, 1980, pp 357–398.

102. Kawakami TG, Sun L, McDowell TS: Distribution and transmission of primate type-C virus. In: Advances in comparative leukemia research, Bentvelzen P, Hilgers J, Yohn DS (eds). Amsterdam: Elsevier North-Holland, 1978, pp 33–36.

103. Markham PD, Ruscetti F, Salahuddin SZ, Gallagher RE, Gallo RC: Enhanced induction of growth of B-lymphoblasts from fresh blood by primate type-C retroviruses (gibbon ape leukemia virus and simian sarcoma virus). Int J Cancer 23:148–156, 1979.

104. Nilsson K, Giovanella BC, Stehelin JS, Klein G: Tumorigenicity of human hematopoietic cell lines in athymic nude mice. Int J Cancer 19:337–344, 1977.

105. Gallo RC, Wong-Staal F, Markham PD, Ruscetti F, Kalyanaraman VS, Ceccherini Nelli L, Dalla Favera R, Josephs S, Miller NR, Reits Jr MS: Recent studies with infectious primate retroviruses: evidence for a human origin of the sarcoma genome of simian sarcoma virus and some biological effects on fresh human blood leukocytes by simian sarcoma virus and gibbon ape leukemia virus. In: Viruses in naturally occurring cancer, Essex M, Todaro G, zur Hausen H (eds). New York: Cold Spring Harbor Press, 1980, pp 753–774.

106. Gallo RC, Yang SS, Ting RC: RNA dependent DNA polymerase of human acute leukaemic cells. Nature 228:927–929, 1970.

107. Sarngadharan MG, Sarin PS, Reitz MS, Gallo RC: Reverse transcriptase activity of human acute leukemic cells: purification of the enzyme, response to AMV 70S RNA, and characterization of the DNA product. Nature New Biol 240:67–72, 1972.

108. Todaro GJ, Gallo RC: Immunological relationship of DNA polymerase from human acute leukemia cells and primate and mouse leukemia virus reverse transcriptase. Nature 244:206–209, 1973.

109. Gallo RC, Gallagher RE, Miller NR, Mondal H, Saxinger WC, Mayer RJ, Smith RG, Gillespie DH: Relationships between components in primate RNA tumor viruses and in the cytoplasm of human leukemic cells: implications to leukemogenesis. In: Cold Spring Harbor Symposium on Quantitative Biology: tumor viruses. New York: Cold Spring Harbor Press, Vol 39, 1975, pp 933–961.

110. Jacquemin P, Saxinger C, Gallo RC: Surface antibodies of human myelogenous leukaemia leukocytes reactive with specific type-C viral reverse transcriptase. Nature 276:230–236, 1978.

111. Chandra P, Steel LK, Laube H, Kornduber B: Expression of C-type viral information in tissues of patients with preleukemic disorders: myelofibrosis and granulocytic sarcoma associated with acute myelomonocytic leukeia (AMML) of children. In: Antiviral mechanisms for the control of neoplasia, Chandra P (ed). New York: Plenum Press, 1978, pp 177–198.

112. Chandra P, Steel LK, Caudar AO: Evidence for the presence of an oncronaviral reverse transcriptase in an orbital tumor associated to acute myelomonocytic leukemia in children: biochemical and immunological characterization of the enzyme. In: Moderns trends in human leukemia III, Neth R, Gallo RC, Hofschneider P, Mannweiler K (eds). New York: Springer-Verlag, 1979, pp 497–500.

113. Gallo RC, Miller NR, Saxinger WC, Gillespie D: Primate RNA tumor virus-like DNA synthesized endogenously by RNA-dependent DNA polymerase in virus-like particles from fresh human acute leukemic blood cells. Proc Nat Acad Sci USA 70:3219–7224, 1973.

114. Baxt WG, Spiegelman S: Nuclear DNA sequences present in human leukemic cells and absent in normal leukocytes. Proc Nat Acad Sci USA 69:3737–3741, 1972.

115. Wong-Staal F, Gillespie D, Gallo RC: Proviral sequences of baboon endogenous type-C RNA virus in DNA of leukemic tissues from seven patients with myelogenous leukemia. Nature 262:190–194, 1976.

116. Aulakh GS, Gallo RC: Rauscher leukemia virus related sequences in human DNA presence in some tissues of some patients with hematopoietic neoplasias and their absence in DNA from other tissues. Proc Nat Acad Sci USA 74:353–357, 1977.

117. Prochownik EV, Kirsten WH: Nucleic acid sequences of primate type-C viruses in normal and neoplastic human tissues. Nature 267:175–177, 1977.

118. Morgan DA, Ruscetti FW, Gallo RC: Selective in vitro growth of T-lymphocytes from normal bone marrows. Science 193: 1007–1008, 1976.

119. Ruscetti FW, Morgan D, Gallo RC: Functional and morphological characterization of human T-cells continuously grown in vitro. J Immun 119:131–138, 1977.

40

120. Smith KA: T-cell growth factor. Immunol Rev 51:337–357, 1980.
121. Ruscetti FW, Gallo RC: Human T-lymphocyte growth factor: regulation of growth and function of T-lymphocytes. Blood 57:379–393, 1981.
122. Mier JW, Gallo RC: Purification and some characteristics of human T-cell growth factor (TCGF) from PHA-stimulated lymphocyte conditioned media. Proc Nat Acad Sci USA 77:6134–6138, 1980.
123. Riddick DH, Gallo RC: The transfer RNA methylases of human lymphocytes: II. Delayed induction by PHA in lymphocytes. Blood 37:293–298, 1971.
124. Prival J, Paran M, Gallo RC, Wu AM: Colony-stimulating factors in cultures of human peripheral blood cells. J Nat Cancer Inst 53:1583–1588, 1974.
125. Ruscetti FW, Gallo RC: Human T-lymphocyte growth factor: the second signal in the immune response. (editorial review) Blood 1980b 57:379–393.
126. Poiesz BJ, Ruscetti FW, Mier JW, Woods AM, Gallo RC: T-cell lines established from human T-lymphocytic neoplasias by direct response to T-cell growth factor. Proc Nat Acad Sci USA 77:6815–6819, 1980a.
127. Poiesz BJ, Ruscetti FW, Gazdar AF, Bunn PA, Minna JD, Gallo RC: Isolation of type-C retrovirus particles from cultured and fresh lymphocytes of a patient with cutaneous T-cell lymphoma. Proc Nat Acad Sci USA 77:7415–7519, 1980b.
128. Poiesz BJ, Ruscetti FW, Gallo RC: Unpublished data, 1981.
129. Rho HM, Poiesz B, Ruscetti FW, Gallo RC: Characterization of the reverse transcriptase from a new retrovirus (HTLV) produced by a human cutaneous T-cell lines. Virology 112:355–358, 1981.
130. Kalyanaraman VS, Sarngadharan MG, Poiesz BJ, Ruscetti FW, Gallo RC: Immunological properties of a type-C retrovirus isolated from cultured human T- lymphoma cells and comparison to other mammalian retroviruses. J Virol 38:906–913, 1981.
131. Reitz MS, Poiesz BJ, Ruscetti FW, Gallo RC: Characterization and distribution of nucleic acid sequences of a novel type-C retrovirus isolated from neoplastic human T-lymphocytes. Proc Nat Acad Sci USA 78:1887–1891, 1981.
132. Ferrer JF, Avila L, Stock ND: Serological detection of type C viruses found in bovine cultures. Cancer Res 32:1864–1980, 1972.
133. Gootenberg JE, Ruscetti FW, Mier JW, Gazdar A, Gallo RC: Human cutaneous T-cell lymphoma cell lines produce and respond to T-cell growth factor activity. J Exp Med 154:1403–1408, 1981.
134. Schrier MH, Iscove NN, Tees R, Aaedon L, von Boehmer H: Clones of killer and helper T-cells: growth requirements, specificity and retention of function in long-term cultures. Immunol Rev 51:315–334, 1980.
135. Ruscetti FW, Gallo RC: Production of T-cell growth factor by cultured human T-lymphocytes. Behring Inst Mitt 67:240–244, 1980b.
136. Posner LE, Robert-Guroff M, Kalyanaraman VS, Poiesz BJ, Ruscetti FW, Bunn PA, Minna JD, Gallo RC: Natural antibodies to the retrovirus HTLV in patients with cutaneous T-cell lymphomas. J Exp Med 154:333–336, 1981.
137. Gallagher RE, Gallo RC: Type-C RNA tumor virus isolated from cultured human acute myelogenous leukemia cells. Science 187:350–353, 1975.
138. Panem S, Prochownik EV, Reale Fr, Kirsten WH: Isolation of C-type virions from a normal human fibroblast strain. Science 189:297–299, 1975.
139. Nooter K, Aarssen AM, Bentvelzen P, d'Groot FG: Isolation of an infectious C-type oncornavirus from human leukemic bone marrow cells. Nature 256:595–597, 1975.
140. Gabelman N, Waxman S, Smith W, Douglas SD: Appearance of C-type virus-like particles after co-cultivation of a human tumor cell line with rat (XC) cells. Int J Cancer 16:355–356, 1975.

141. Kaplan HS, Goodenow RS, Epstein AL, Gartner S, DeCleve A, Rosenthal PN: Isolation of type-C RNA virus from an established human histiocytic lymphoma cell line. Proc Nat Acad Sci USA 74:2564–2568, 1977.
142. Bronsan DL, Ritzi DM, Fraley EE, Dalton AJ: Morphologic evidence for retrovirus production by epithelial cells derived from a human testicular tumor metastasis—brief communication. J Nat Cancer Inst 60:1305–1308, 1978.

# 2. T-cell Growth Factor-Dependent Leukemic Cell Growth: Therapeutic Implications *

KENDALL A. SMITH

CONTENTS

## 1. INTRODUCTION: THE POSSIBLE ROLE OF GROWTH FACTORS IN LEUKEMIA

As an outgrowth of tissue culture studies with sarcoma and carcinoma cell lines, it has been proposed recently that malignant cells respond to growth-promoting factors they themselves elaborate [1, 2]. In leukemia and lymphoma it has long been appreciated that nutritional and/or growth promoting factors might be associated with the maintenance of viable malignant cells, especially as they appear to persist and expand *in vivo*, yet invariably die out when cultured in artificial media. Malignant cell lines that do grow *in vitro* may be viewed as highly selected variants of the malignant clone, in that they are able to survive and grow in culture media deficient in growth

* Supported in part by National Cancer Institute grants CA-17643, Ca-17323, CA-23108, CA-26273; American Cancer Society grant CH-167; and National Cancer Institute Contract N01-CB-74141.

factors. It has also been found that only a small fraction of the malignant cell population persists as a self-renewing compartment, whereas the majority of the progeny persist in $G_0$ [3]. Accordingly, it can be visualized that the self-replicating malignant 'stem cells' proliferate in response to physiological stimuli, possibly the very same ones responsible for replication of normal cells of the same lineage. If true, this concept could explain the difficulties encountered in initiating and maintaining leukemic cells *in vitro*: the majority of cells, unresponsive to growth-promoting factors, would have a limited life-span both *in vivo* and *in vitro*, whereas the growth factor-dependent stem cells would also die when placed *in vitro* as a consequence of the absence of adequate quantities of growth-promoting substances. It follows that the rare cells or variants that survive under *in vitro* conditions would be capable of both producing and responding to their own growth factors.

In seeking to explore further this line of reasoning, we initiated a series of experiments with T-cell growth factor (TCGF), a protein released from antigen/lectin-activated T-cells that is responsible for normal T-cell clonal expansion [for review see 4, 5]. In this chapter, I will summarize our present knowledge of the immunophysiology of TCGF, as well as recent experimental work that points towards TCGF as being involved in the growth of malignant cells *in vitro*. Our findings carry therapeutic implications: pharmacologic intervention at the level of TCGF production or action may well provide new, more selective approaches to the therapy of leukemia.

## 2. TCGF PHYSIOLOGY: FUNCTIONAL ASPECTS OF TCGF IN THE GROWTH OF NORMAL T-CELLS

Antigen or lectin introduced into a mixed population of lymphocytes and macrophages gives rise to a series of reactions that ultimately culminate in T-cell proliferation [4, 7]. At least three functionally distinct cells are essential participants: macrophages, TCGF-producer T-cells, and TCGF responder T-cells (Figure 1). As a result of antigen/lectin binding to specific membrane receptors on these cells, all become 'activated.' Although the morphological and biochemical consequences of activation for each cell type still remain to be defined, it is evident that the initial triggering process is of itself insufficient for the initiation of mitosis. Subsequent to antigen/lectin triggering, activated macrophages secrete a product, aptly designated lymphocyte activating factor (LAF), that facilitates TCGF production by antigen/lectin-activated TCGF-producer T-cells [8–10]. Detailed studies with cloned T-cell lymphomas [10] and with T-T-cell hybridomas [11] have shown that LAF causes a concentration-dependent increase in TCGF release, provided that the cells are also activated by lectin/antigen. The kind

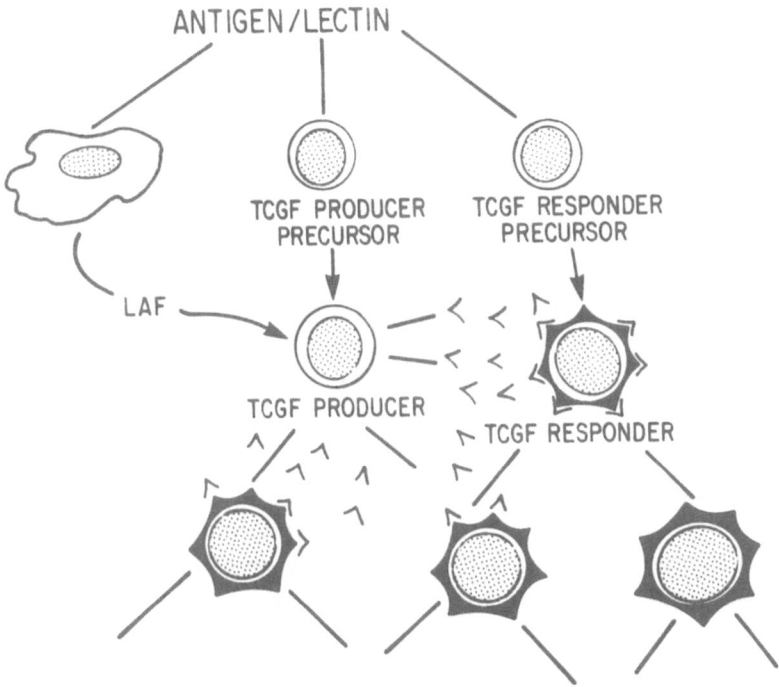

*Figure 1.* A model for T-cell activation. T-cell growth factor (TCGF) functions to provide the signal for T-cell mitosis rather than the antigen or lectin.

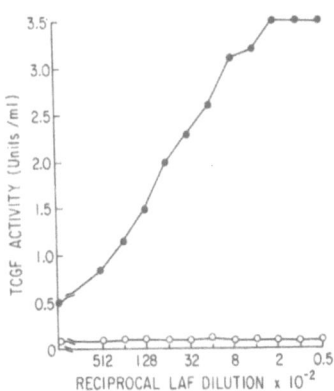

*Figure 2.* Lymphocyte activating factor (LAF) concentration-dependent enhancement of TCGF release from WEHI 7 clone 49 (•) and clone 8 (*w*). (From Smith *et al.* [10]). LAF functions to enhance the production of TCGF from murine lymphoma cells.

of evidence that attests to the concentration-dependency of the LAF effect is illustrated in Figure 2.

Studies by several groups have shown that the TCGF-producer T-cell expresses phenotypic markers of the classical T-helper cell required for antibody formation to T-dependent antigens [12–14]. Since this conclusion was derived from ablation experiments in which T-helper cells had been deleted by antibody plus complement, it remains uncertain whether *all* T-helper cells are potential TCGF-producer cells, or whether TCGF-producer cells constitute a specialized subset of T-helper cells. It is of interest, and especially significant, that cloned TCGF-dependent, antigen-specific T-helper cells are capable of elaborating a variety of growth-promoting factors including TCGF, B-cell growth factor, erythroid progenitor burst promoting activity, and myeloid-macrophage colony stimulating activity [15, 16].

A notable curious property of cloned T-helper cell lines is their propensity to elaborate and to respond to TCGF. The accumulated observations indicate that T-helper cells release TCGF only when stimulated with antigen or lectin in the presence of macrophages. If removed from antigen/lectin and macrophages, the cells cease to proliferate and eventually die. However, these cells supplied with exogenous TCGF can be maintained indefinitely without lectin/antigen or the presence of other cells [16]. This is in sharp contrast to cloned cytotoxic and suppressor T-cells, which comprise the third subset of cells involved in a T-cell proliferative response (i.e., TCGF-responder cells). Although cytolytic and suppressor T-cells have the capacity to respond to TCGF they do not appear capable of elaborating TCGF under any circumstances [4–7, 17].

Like macrophages and TCGF-producer cells, TCGF-responder cells must be activated before a proliferative response to TCGF is realized. The biologic economy of such a system is that *only* those cells that recognize the specific antigen become converted to active participants in the T-cell proliferative response. The consequence of the activation process is that TCGF-specific membrane binding sites appear only on activated T-cells. Detailed studies by several groups have shown that activated T-cells (but not activated B-cells, macrophages, or other cell types) absorb TCGF in a time-, temperature-, and cell concentration-dependent manner [18–20]. Furthermore, we have recently shown that radiolabeled TCGF binds specifically only to activated T-cells [21]. The binding of TCGF is concentration-dependent and saturable, which is in harmony with the observations that the mitogenic effect of TCGF is also concentration-dependent and saturable [4–7].

The ultimate consequence of the knowledge that two factors (i.e., LAF and TCGF) are essential for antigen/lectin-initiated T-cell proliferative responses is that normal T-cells rely on lymphocytotropic hormones for appropriate clonal expansion after antigen/lectin activation. Since the proliferation of T-cells is mediated by TCGF, it follows that TCGF-producer cells become the pivotal cells in the T-cell immune response. In situations where TCGF-producer cells are absent or deficient (e.g., as occurs in the athymic mouse) a T-cell proliferative response to antigen/lectin is precluded [22]. It follows also that physiological and/or pharmacological agents that operate as 'immunomodulators' either by suppressing or enhancing the T-cell immune response may function by modulating TCGF release from TCGF producer T-cells, or TCGF action on other T-cells.

## 3. THE EFFECTS OF GLUCOCORTICOIDS ON NORMAL T-CELL GROWTH: THE INHIBITION OF TCGF PRODUCTION

Glucocorticoid hormones, which are operative physiologically and also extensively utilized pharmacologically, have profound suppressive effects on T-cells. *In vitro,* glucocorticoids inhibit completely the T-cell proliferative response to lectin/antigen; they also appear to hasten lympholysis [23]. *In vivo,* glucocorticoids are known to exert a suppressive effect on the initial response to antigen, whereas their effects are considerably less dramatic with respect to an ongoing immune response [24, 25]. Additionally, early in the course of chemotherapeutic intervention in leukemia, it was noted that glucocorticoids effect a rapid lysis of leukemic cells, especially those thought to be of the lymphocyte lineage [26]. Combined with the demonstration of high affinity glucocorticoid-specific receptors in both normal and malignant lymphocytes [27, 28], the generally accepted notion derived from these observations was that glucocorticoids exerted their effects directly on lymphoid cells. However, the mechanism whereby glucocorticoids exert such inhibitory effects on lymphoid cells has remained obscure for more than two decades. Equally unclear has been the basis for the more marked cytolytic effects noted on malignant lymphoid cells as compared to normal lymphocytes.

In seeking to elucidate the mechanism of inhibition exerted by glucocorticoids on normal T-cell proliferative responses to lectin/antigen, our experimental strategy was based on the knowledge that the T-cell proliferative response is ultimately mediated by TCGF and that several steps are involved in the release and action of TCGF. By virtue of the fact that it is possible to study LAF release, LAF action, TCGF release, and TCGF action in isolated, cloned cell systems, we could test whether the inhibitory effects of glucocorticoids on T-cell proliferation occur as a result of the abrogation of the release or action of one of these essential hormones.

We first examined the effect of glucocorticoids on TCGF action. Since it is possible to culture TCGF-dependent cells in the absence of other cell

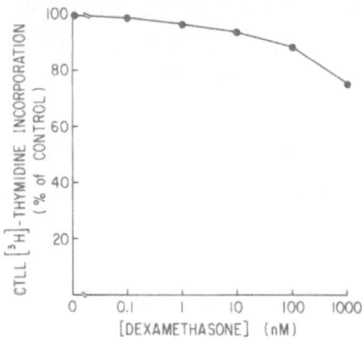

*Figure 3.* Dexamethasone concentration-dependent inhibition of TCGF activity. Murine cyto-lytic T-lymphocyte line clone 15H (Baker *et al.* [38]), cells were cultured (4 × 10⁴ cells/ml) with TCGF (1.0 μ/ml) and various concentrations of dexamethasone for 20 hours prior to a 4-hour incubation with (³H)-Tdr. Dexamethasone has a minimal effect on the proliferation-inducing activity of TCGF.

types, the effect of glucocorticoids on TCGF action could be evaluated inde-pendently of any effects on TCGF release. As shown in Figure 3, there is only a slight direct effect of glucocorticoids on TCGF-dependent T-cell pro-liferation. Concentrations as high as 1 μM exert only a 20–30% diminution of proliferation as monitored by tritiated thymidine (³H)-Tdr incorpora-tion [29, 30]. As these results could not account for the complete abrogation of T-cell proliferative responses to lectin/antigen, known to occur when glu-cocorticoids are present from the initiation of the response, it seemed a reasonable expectation that glucocorticoids inhibit the production of TCGF. Since LAF functions to markedly augment TCGF release, the effect of glu-

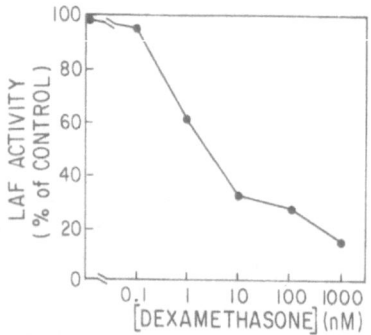

*Figure 4.* The effect of dexamethasone on LAF production by LPS (20 μg/ml)-induced BALB/c peritoneal macrophages. After dialysis to remove dexamethasone culture supernatants were tested for LAF activity on C3H/HeJ thymocytes. Control LAF activity at 100% = 119 471 cpm; 0% = 6 898 cpm. (From Smith [4]). Dexamethasone inhibits the production of LAF from macrophages.

cocorticoids on LAF release from isolated macrophages was next examined. As shown in Figure 4, glucocorticoids exert a concentration-dependent suppression of LAF release, such that 1 µM dexamethasone causes a 80–90% inhibition of this essential function [4].

Although these results suggested that the inhibitory effects of glucocorticoids on T-cell proliferation might well be explained entirely by an effect mediated via macrophages, it was nonetheless possible that glucocorticoids might also suppress the function of TCGF-producer T-cells. To approach this issue, LAF was supplied to macrophage-depleted T-cell populations and the effects of glucocorticoids on TCGF release tested. With this experimental protocol, glucocorticoids still exert a similar concentration-dependent inhibition of TCGF release, even when LAF is present in excess [4]. The end result of the inhibition of TCGF release is a parallel suppression of T-cell proliferation (Figure 5). It thus appeared that the profound inhibitory effect of glucocorticoids on T-cell proliferative responses to lectin/antigen was mediated by the suppression of the release of the two hormone-like factors that ultimately supply the mitogenic stimulus for T-cells. Were this the case, TCGF-supplementation of glucocorticoid-treated cultures could be expected to circumvent the cause for the block in proliferation. Confirming this prediction, and thus proving that the mechanism of glucocorticoid suppression of T-cell proliferation is mediated by the abrogation of TCGF release, the restoration of TCGF to lectin-stimulated T-cells overcomes completely the inhibitory effect of glucocorticoids [4, 8, 28, 30] (Figure 6). Additionally, confirming the results obtained with isolated TCGF-dependent T-cell lines (Figure 3), there is no glucocorticoid-mediated lysis of the T-cells providing TCGF is present. These observations contrast sharply with the

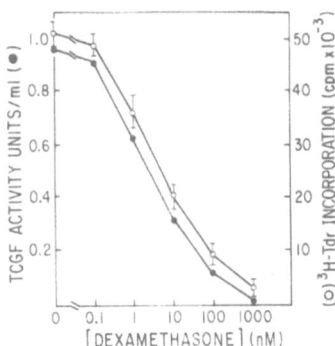

*Figure 5.* The effect of dexamethasone on Con-A (2.5 µg/ml)-stimulated rat splenocyte TCGF release (•), and resultant ($^3$H)-Tdr incorporation (w). From Smith [4]. Dexamethasone inhibits the production of TCGF by T-cells resulting in the inhibition of T-cell proliferation as determined by ($^3$H)-Tdr incorporation.

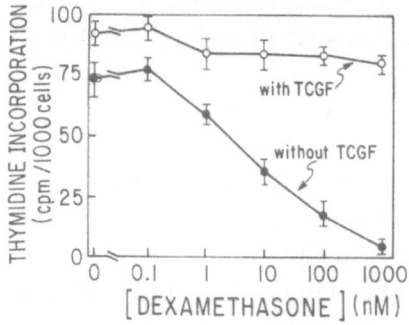

*Figure 6.* The effect of TCGF on the dexamethasone-induced suppression of human lymphocyte proliferation determined 72 hours after addition of PHA. (From Smith [4]). Exogenous TCGF supplementation circumvents the dexamethasone-induced block in TCGF production, thus permitting T-cell proliferation.

rapid cessation of proliferation and cell death observed when TCGF-dependent T-cells are deprived of TCGF, whether or not glucocorticoids are present. Further, these findings suggest that the lympholytic effects of glucocorticoids are mediated by the specific inhibition of a hormone-like entity (TCGF) essential for cellular proliferation.

## 4. TCGF AND MALIGNANT LYMPHOID CELLS

Once the striking effects of TCGF on normal T-cells were fully appreciated, malignant lymphoid cells were examined for evidence of TCGF dependency. Although these studies are still exploratory, the initial findings are provocative. Poiesz *et al.* [31] have successfully established TCGF-dependent T-cell lines from 12 of 14 patients with cutaneous T-cell lymphoma (CTCL), and 8 of 11 patients selected as having acute lymphocytic leukemia of T-cell origin (T-ALL). Several observations point toward a malignant cell origin of these cell lines. All of the lines were established using lectin-free, partially purified TCGF that was ineffective (in the absence of an activating signal supplied by lectin or antigen) in initiating T-cell growth from lymphocytes isolated from normal individuals [32]. Two cell lines originally dependent upon TCGF became independent of TCGF and were subsequently found to be constitutive low level TCGF-producers [31]. Additionally, more recent studies have shown that acid-glycine treatment of CTCL cells results in the release of membrane-associated TCGF-like activity [33]. Morphologically the cell lines derived from CTCL patients are markedly different from those derived from ALL patients or normal individuals. The cultured CTCL cell lines contain many giant multinucleated cells in addition to mono- and binucleated cells. Ultrastructural analysis revealed the presence of highly convoluted nuclei in three of the CTCL lines, very similar to the cells of the primary tumors of these patients, considered diagnostic for CTCL. Finally, the TCGF-dependent cells isolated from one CTCL patient have the same chromosomal aberrations found in freshly isolated tumor cells from this patient [31].

In contrast to these observations, similar studies performed with leukemia and lymphoma cell lines established without the aid of TCGF have been disappointing. We have examined more than 50 leukemia and lymphoma cell lines (15 terminal deoxyribonucleotidyl transferase-positive T-cell, 20 B-cell, 8 non-T-non-B-cell, and 8 non-lymphoid myeloid-macrophage) for constitutive TCGF production and have found all were negative [5]. Similar results were reported for murine cell lines of lymphocytic and macrophage origin [34]. Furthermore, we have obtained no evidence for TCGF absorption by established human malignant cell lines by means that easily detect TCGF absorption by TCGF-dependent T-cell lines derived from normal tissue. Finally, we have been unable to detect any growth-promoting effects by supplementing malignant T-cell lines with lectin-free partially purified TCGF. All in all, these results indicate that TCGF plays no role in the proliferation of the established cell lines that we have examined. Rather, these data suggest that establishment of these cell lines involved the selection of cells that either do not require TCGF or that depend upon some other growth factor beyond our present means of detection.

It bears emphasis that it is extremely difficult to initiate continuous neoplastic lymphoid cell lines (in the absence of Epstein-Barr virus) when cells are placed in conventional tissue culture media. Yet from the report of Poiesz et al. [31], by the simple expedient of supplementing the medium with TCGF, cell lines were derived in 85% of the cases of CTCL and 70% of the cases of T-ALL. If all of the cell lines that were derived in the presence of TCGF prove to be of neoplastic origin, the observations would support the view that at least some cells in the malignant population are likely to be TCGF-dependent. Should this prove to be so, one might then postulate that *in vivo* there is a source of TCGF sufficient to maintain growth of neoplastic T-cells to the point where the disease becomes clinically recognizable (e.g. at approximately $10^9$ to $10^{10}$ leukemic cells). This hypothesis is problematic in that considerable TCGF would have to be produced from *normal* TCGF producer cells to maintain such a large population of neoplastic, putatively TCGF-dependent cells. For the present it would seem more plausible if at least some of the neoplastic cells are capable of *both* releasing and responding to TCGF. In support of this interpretation is the finding that upon passage, two of the CTCL cell lines eventually

52

became TCGF independent; these cells were found to produce limited, but detectable amounts of TCGF activity [31, 33]. This observation strongly suggests that at least these cell lines are of neoplastic cell origin, inasmuch as normal TCGF-producer cells do not become self-replicating when they are cultured without antigen and macrophages; rather, they cease proliferating and eventually die out just as do TCGF-responder cells when deprived of TCGF. Tempering, but not disproving this line of reasoning, is the awareness that self-replicating murine or human neoplastic TCGF-producing T-cell lines have not yet been reported, with the notable exception of the CTCL cell lines.

## 5. THE MLA-144: A NEOPLASTIC TCGF-PRODUCER CELL THAT RESPONDS TO ITS OWN GROWTH FACTOR

A lymphoblastoid cell line with T-cell characteristics was established in 1972 from the peripheral blood of a gibbon ape suffering from a spontaneous lymphosarcoma [35]. Recently, Rabin *et al.* [36] reported that this cell line released TCGF-like activity that supported the continuous proliferation of human, mouse, and primate TCGF-dependent normal T-cell lines. Thus, this cell line appears to be unique and stands in contrast to all of the murine and human neoplastic cell lines established without the aid of TCGF. Although the quantity of TCGF activity released is rather low, it is readily detectable. A representative experiment is shown in Figure 7 where conditioned medium from MLA-144 was assayed for TCGF activity on a cloned murine TCGF-dependent cytolytic T-lymphocyte line (CTCL); a TCGF standard containing 1 unit/ml is included for comparison.

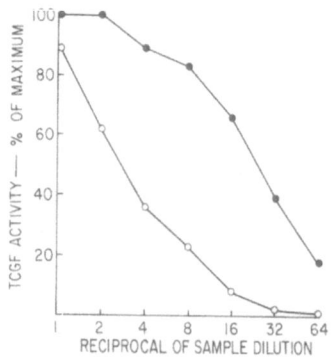

*Figure 7.* TCGF activity released by MLA-144 cells (w) compared to a standard TCGF preparation containing 1.0 μ/ml (●). MLA-144 cells produce TCGF spontaneously without inducing signals (e.g., lectin or LAF).

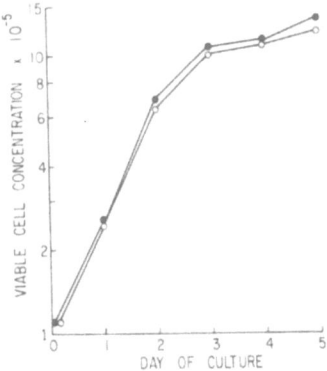

*Figure 8.* The proliferation of MLA-144 cells in the presence of medium (●) and 100 nM dexamethasone (○). Dexamethasone fails to block MLA-144 proliferation.

Once it was established that MLA-144 released TCGF activity, it was important to determine whether the released TCGF was in any way responsible for the growth of the cells *in vitro*. Since glucocorticoids were known to suppress TCGF release by normal T-cells, thus inhibiting T-cell proliferation, we sought to ascertain whether glucocorticoids had any effect on the proliferative rate of MLA-144. As shown in Figure 8, there was a slight but insignificant inhibition of MLA-144 proliferation in the presence of 100 nM dexamethasone. Thus, the glucocorticoid effect was not marked even at high concentrations of dexamethasone. We wondered, therefore, whether MLA-144 could be heterogeneous with respect to glucocorticoid sensitivity, i.e., whether it was comprised of a mixture of glucocorticoid-sensitive and glucocorticoid-resistant cells. To assess this possibility MLA-144 was cloned by limiting dilution (at 0.3 cells/well the Poisson calculated probability of cofertile wells was <0.05) in the presence of 1 μM dexamethasone, 1 unit/ml human TCGF, and unsupplemented culture medium. The results of these experiments suggested that MLA-144 might indeed be heterogeneous with respect to glucocorticoid sensitivity: the plating efficiency in the presence of 1 μM dexamethasone was only 7% whereas in either the presence of TCGF or medium alone, the plating efficiencies were 45% and 50% respectively. Upon testing of the clones for glucocorticoid sensitivity, a wide range of inhibition (from 8% to 70%) of cellular proliferation was noted in the presence of 100 nM dexamethasone, affirming that some clones were markedly sensitive to glucocorticoids whereas others appeared to be relatively resistant. To determine whether the heterogeneity of glucocorticoid effects among the clones involved the inhibition of TCGF release, cells were cultured in the absence and presence of 100 nM dexamethasone. After four days of culture, supernatants were removed for the determination of TCGF

54

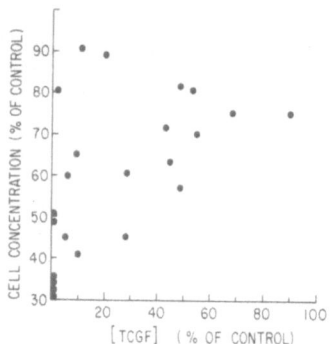

*Figure 9.* The effect of dexamethasone (100 nM) on MLA-144 clones as measured by inhibition of TCGF release and inhibition of cellular proliferation. Cells were cultured for 4 days in the absence and presence of dexamethasone prior to the assays. The response of isolated MLA-144 clones to dexamethasone is heterogeneous. There is a wide range in the degree of inhibition of TCGF production and cellular proliferation, and a significant correlation (r = 0.8, p = 0.003) between the magnitude of inhibition of TCGF production and the magnitude of inhibition of proliferation.

activity and viable cell concentrations were determined. The results (Figure 9) attest to a direct correlation between the magnitude of glucocorticoid-induced inhibition of cell proliferation and the magnitude of inhibition of TCGF release.

If the mechanism of glucocorticoid action was in fact based on the inhibition of TCGF release, then TCGF supplementation of glucocorticoid-

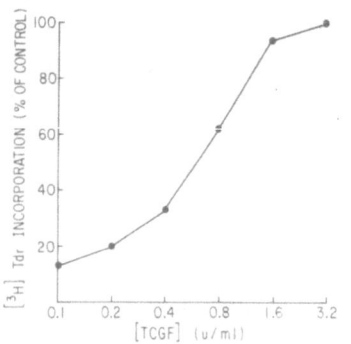 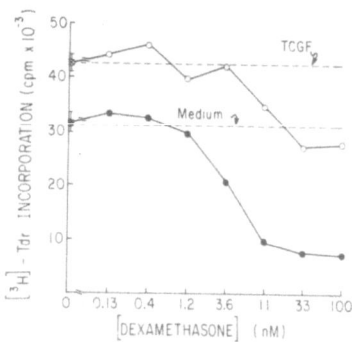

*Figure 10.* TCGF overcomes the dexamethasone-induced inhibition of proliferation. A: The effect of TCGF on MLA-144 clone 15T ($^3$H)-Tdr incorporation in the presence of 100 nM dexamethasone. Cells were cultured for 44 hours prior to a 4-hour incubation with ($^3$H)-Tdr. ($^3$H)-Tdr incorporation of control (without dexamethasone or TCGF) = 31 853±967 cpm. B: The effect of dexamethasone on MLA-144 clone 15T ($^3$H)-Tdr incorporation without (•) and with TCGF (1.4 μ/ml) (ω). The dashed lines depict the level of tritiated thymidine incorporation in the presence of medium (i.e., no TCGF) and TCGF without dexamethasone.

treated cells should overcome the steroid suppression of cellular proliferation. To test this hypothesis, one of the most glucocorticoid-sensitive clones was selected (clone 15T) and incubated overnight with 100 nM dexamethasone so as to maximally suppress ongoing TCGF release. The cells were then cultured with increasing concentrations of TCGF and 100 nM dexamethasone for an additional 48 hours. The results depicted in Figure 10a reveal that TCGF completely reverses the dexamethasone-induced block of cellular proliferation as measured by ($^3$H)-Tdr incorporation. The reciprocal experiment (Figure 10b) where the TCGF concentration was held constant (1.4 u/ml) and increasing concentrations of dexamethasone were included,

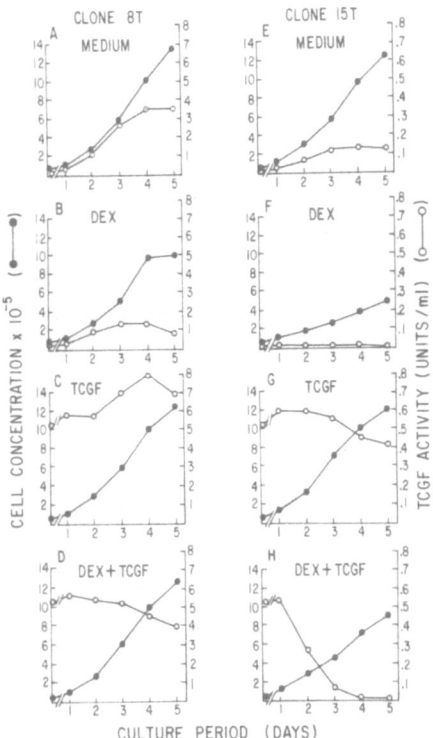

*Figure 11.* MLA-144 cells proliferate in response to the TCGF they produce and glucocorticoids inhibit their proliferation by suppressing TCGF production. The effect of dexamethasone and TCGF on MLA-144 clone 8T (a relatively glucocorticoid resistant clone) is shown in the left panels; and the effects of dexamethasone and TCGF on clone 15T (a glucocorticoid sensitive clone) are shown in the right panels. Cellular proliferation is depicted by the closed circles and TCGF production by the open circles. Panels A and E, medium control; B and F, dexamethasone (100 nM); C and G, TCGF (0.5 µ/ml); D and H, dexamethasone (100 nM) and TCGF (0.5 µ/ml).

similarly discloses that the concentration-dependent inhibition of cellular proliferation by dexamethasone is nullified by TCGF. It is also evident from Figure 10b that TCGF enhances the proliferation of clone 15T in the absence of glucocorticoid. These observations strongly suggest: 1) that the proliferation of the MLA-144 cells is dependent upon TCGF, and 2) that the mechanism of glucocorticoid-mediated suppression of proliferation is a consequence of the abrogation of TCGF release. Still other observations support these impressions: MLA-144 can be shown to deplete TCGF from the medium in a cell-concentration-dependent manner. Furthermore, radiolabeled TCGF binds specifically and saturably to MLA-144 cells. By analogy to the absorption and binding of TCGF mediated by normal activated T-cells, these results point towards MLA-144 cells expressing TCGF-specific membrane binding sites.

To provide definitive support for these impressions, two clones were selected for study: one clone (clone 15T) was very sensitive to glucocorticoid suppression whereas the other (clone 8T) was relatively glucocorticoid resistant. The cells were cultured in the absence and in the presence of both TCGF (2 u/ml) and dexamethasone (100 nM). After successive days of culture, aliquots of supernatant were removed for TCGF assay and viable cell concentrations were determined. The results depicted in Figure 11 reveal that: 1) the growth of the cells is dependent upon a source of TCGF (either endogenous or exogenous), 2) glucocorticoids inhibit TCGF production completely in the sensitive clone (15T) and less so in the resistant clone (8T), and 3) TCGF is consumed by the proliferating cells, especially when endogenous TCGF production is inhibited by dexamethasone.

### 6. CONCLUSIONS: THE POTENTIAL THERAPEUTIC SIGNIFICANCE OF TCGF IN LEUKEMIA

The conclusion drawn from these experimental probes is that some leukemic T-cells may produce their own growth factors and respond to them. The system described for the TCGF effect on normal and neoplastic T-cells may consequently serve as a model for leukemias and lymphomas of other cell lineages. The key to the observations on neoplastic T-cells has been a more complete understanding of the factors responsible for normal T-cell proliferation. It might be anticipated, therefore, that normal and neoplastic hematopoietic cells of all types may be found to depend on intrinsic hormone-like regulatory systems. As more is understood about the hormones that govern other hematopoietic cell types, and as sensitive specific assays are developed to detect these activities, our capacity to intervene and control leukemic cell growth should advance considerably.

The observations made with the gibbon ape MLA-144 cell line, in addition to those of Poiesz et al. [31] and Gootenberg et al. [33] on the TCGF-producing CTCL human cell lines, attest to the production of specific growth factors by neoplastic T-cells as a biologic reality. It remains to be determined whether this also occurs in vivo and, if so, the frequency of the phenomenon for different leukemias or among patient populations with a given type of leukemia. The understanding that at least some neoplastic cells require TCGF for growth in vitro, and that the rate of cell growth is dependent upon the concentration of TCGF available (Figure 10a), now helps to explain why it has been difficult to initiate leukemic cell growth in vitro in the absence of TCGF. It will be important to ascertain the frequency of leukemic T-cells capable of releasing TCGF. Additionally, the frequency of TCGF-responsive cells within a malignant clone may also determine the rapidity of onset and clinical course of the disease. Then too, either the lack of sufficient TCGF concentrations or the loss of TCGF-responsiveness (perhaps through the loss of TCGF receptors) could well account for the fact that many of the malignant cells are not in the proliferative cell cycle, but rather persist in $G_0$.

The observation that the anti-proliferative effects of glucocorticoids on MLA-144 are mediated by suppression of TCGF release, indicates that at least one mechanism responsible for glucocorticoid-mediated leukemic cell suppression is related to TCGF inhibition. Additionally, it is of interest that the glucocorticoid sensitivity of MLA-144 cells is markedly heterogeneous. Such heterogeneity offers an explanation for the emergence (selection) of glucocorticoid-resistance that often occurs after an initially successful therapeutic response to glucocorticoid therapy. This would be entirely analogous to antibiotic therapy giving rise to the selection of resistant variants. The specifity of glucocorticoid inhibitory effects on lymphoid malignancies as compared to myeloid leukemias also is understandable if leukemic T-cell growth is driven by TCGF, since one of the pharmacological actions of glucocorticoids on normal T-cell proliferation is an inhibition of TCGF release. It has been suggested that glucocorticoids exert little or no inhibition of normal myeloid proliferation and maturation [37]; they therefore, might be expected to have minimal effects on myeloid leukemias. Finally, an implication that could have considerable therapeutic importance can be drawn from the knowledge that glucocorticoids are inhibitory for MLA-144 cells because they inhibit TCGF release. Other, more specific therapeutic agents can now be envisioned that would function to inhibit neoplastic cell TCGF release, or prevent TCGF-mediated proliferation of neoplastic T-cells by an antagonistic competition at the level of TCGF or the TCGF receptor.

ACKNOWLEDGMENTS

The author thanks Ms. Margaret Favata for her invaluable technical assistance, Dr. Maurice Landy for his enthusiastic interest and excellent editorial suggestions, Dr. Allan Munck for his suggestions on experimental design, and Drs. Frank Ruscetti and Robert Gallo for the MLA-144 cell line.

REFERENCES

1. De Larco JE, Todaro FJ: Growth factors from murine sarcoma virus-transformed cells. Proc Natl Acad Sci 75: 4001, 1978.
2. Todaro GJ, Fryling C, de Larco JE: Transforming growth factors produced by certain human tumor cells: polypeptides that interact with epidermal growth factor receptors. Proc Natl Acad Sci 77(9):5258, 1980.
3. Mauer AM, Saunders EF, Lampkin BC: Possible significance of nonproliferating leukemic cells. Natl Cancer Inst Monogr 30:63–71, 1969.
4. Smith KA: T-cell growth factor. Immunol Rev 51:337, 1980.
5. Smith KA, Ruscetti FW: T-cell growth factor and the culture of cloned functional T-cells. In: Advances in immunology, vol 31, Kunkel H, Dixon F (eds). New York: Academic Press, 1981, p 137.
6. Smith KA, Gillis S, Baker PE: The role of soluble factors in the regulation of T-cell immune reactivity. In: The Molecular Basis of Immune Cell Function, Kaplan JG (ed). Amsterdam: Elsevier/North Holland Biomedical Press, 1979, p 223.
7. Smith KA, Baker PE, Gillis S, Ruscetti FW: Functional and molecular characteristics of T-cell growth factor. Mol Immunol 17:579, 1979.
8. Smith KA, Lachman LB, Oppenheim JJ, Favata MF: The functional relationship of the interleukins. J Exp Med 151:1551, 1980.
9. Larsson E-L, Iscove NN, Coutinho A: Two distinct factors are required for induction of T-cell growth. Nature 283:664, 1980.
10. Smith KA, Gilbride KJ, Favata MF: Lymphocyte activating factor promotes T-cell growth factor production by cloned murine lymphoma cells. Nature 287:853, 1980.
11. Skidmore BJ, White J, DeFreitas EC, Kappler J, Marrack P, Chiller JM: Exposing T-cells in vitro to antigen-pulsed, ultraviolet light-treated macrophages induces specific unresponsiveness. Fed. Proc. (Abstract) (3)40:1060, 1981.
12. Wagner H, Rollinghoff M: T–T-cell interactions during in vitro cytotoxic allograft responses. J Exp Med 148:1523, 1978.
13. Okada M, Klimpel Gr, Kuppers RC, Henney CS: The differentiation of cytotoxic T-cells in vitro. I. Amplifying factor(s) in the primary response is Lytl$^+$ cell dependent. J Immunol 122:2527, 1979.
14. Paetkau V, Shaw J, Mills G, Caplan B: Cellular origins and targets of Costimulator (IL2). Immunol Rev 51:155–175, 1980.
15. Schreier MH, Iscove NN: Haematopoietic growth factors are released in cultures of H-2-restricted helper T-cells, accessory cells and specific antigen. Nature 287:228, 1980.
16. Schreier MH, Iscove NN, Tees R, Aarden L, von Boehmer, H: Clones of killer and helper T-cells: Growth requirements, specificity and retention of function in long-term culture. Immunol. Rev. 51:315–336, 1980.

17. McVay-Boudreau L, Fresno M, Nabel G, Cantor H: Functional analysis of Ig-specific suppressor molecules synthesized by T-suppressor clones. 4th Int Congr Immunol (Abstract) 4.2.14, 1980.

18. Smith KA, Gillis S, Baker PE, McKenzie D, Ruscetti FW: T-cell growth factor-mediated T-cell proliferation. Ann NY Acad Sci, 332:423, 1979.

19. Bonnard GD, Yasaka D, Jacobson D: Ligand-activated T-cell growth factor-induced proliferation: absorption of T-cell growth factor by activated T-cells. J Immunol 123:2704, 1979.

20. Coutinho A, Larsson E-L, Gronvik KO, Anderson J: Studies on T-lymphocyte activation. II. The target cells for concanavalin A-induced growth factors. Eur J Immunol 9:587, 1979.

21. Robb RJ, Munek A, Smith KA: T-cell growth factor receptors: Quantitation, specifity and biological relevance. J Exp Med 154:1455, 1981.

22. Gillis S, Union NA, Baker PE, Smith KA: The in vitro generation and sustained culture of nude mouse cytolytic T-lymphocytes. J Exp Med 149:1460, 1979.

23. Nowell PC: Inhibition of human leukocyte mitosis by prednisolone in vitro. Cancer Res 12:1518, 1961.

24. Billingham RE, Krohn PL, Medawar PB: Effect of cortisone on survival of skin homografts in rabbits. Br J Med 2:1157–1163, 1951.

25. Medawar PB, Sparrow EM: The effects of adrenocortical hormones, adrenocorticotrophic hormone and pregnancy on skin transplantation immunity in mice. J Endocr 14:240–256, 1956.

26. Ranney HM, Gellhorn A: The effect of massive prednisone and prednisolone therapy on acute leukemia and malignant lymphomas. Am J Med 23:405–413, 1957.

27. Smith KA, Crabtree GR, Kennedy S, Munck A: Glucocorticoid receptors and glucocorticoid sensitivity of mitogen stimulated and unstimulated human lymphocytes. Nature 267:523, 1977.

28. Crabtree GR, Smith KA, Munck A: Glucocorticoid receptors and sensitivity of isolated human leukemia and lymphoma cells. Cancer Res 38:4268, 1978.

29. Gillis S, Crabtree GR, Smith KA: Glucocorticoid-induced inhibition of T-cell growth factor production. I. The effect on mitogen-induced lymphocyte proliferation. J Immunol 123:1624, 1979.

30. Gillis S, Crabtree CR, Smith KA: Glucocorticoid-induced inhibition of T-cell growth factor production. II. The effect on the in vitro generation of cytolytic T-cells. J Immunol 123:1632, 1979.

31. Poiesz BJ, Ruscetti FW, Mier JW, Woods AM, Gallo RC: T-cell lines established from human T-lymphocytic neoplasias by direct response to T-cell growth factor. Proc Nat Acad Sci 77:6815–1819, 1980.

32. Mier JW, Gallo RC: Purification and some characteristics of human T-cell growth factor (TCGF) from PHA-stimulated lymphocyte conditioned media. Proc Nat Acad Sci 77:6134–6138, 1980.

33. Gootenberg JE, Ruscetti FW, Mier JW, Gazdar A, Gallo RC: Human cutaneous T-cell lymphoma cell lines produce and respond to T-cell growth factor activity. J Exp Med 154:1403, 1981.

34. Gillis S, Scheid M, Watson J: Biochemical and biologic characterization of lymphocyte regulatory molecules. III. The isolation and phenotypic characterization of Interleukin-2 producing T-cell lymphomas. J Immunol 125(6):2570–2578, 1980.

35. Kawakami T, Huff S, Buckley P, Dungworth D, Synder S, Gilden R: C-type virus associated with gibbon lymphosarcoma. Nature New Biol 235:170–172, 1972.

36. Rabin H. Hopkins RF, Ruscetti FW, Neubauer RH, Brown RL, Kawakami TG: Sponta-

neous release of a factor with T-cell growth factor activity from a continuous line of primate tumor T-cells. J Immunol 127:1852, 1981.

37. Athens JW, Haab OP, Raab SO, Boggs DR, Cartwright GE, Wintrobe MM: The mechanism of steroid granulocytosis. J Clin Invest 41:1342, 1962.

38. Baker PE, Gillis S, Smith KA: Monoclonal cytolytic T-cell lines. J Exp Med 149:273, 1979.

# 3. Treatment related leukemia

CHARLES A. COLTMAN, JR.

CONTENTS

1. INTRODUCTION

The literature is replete with reports of the putative relationship of aggressive treatment of malignant, and even benign, disease and the development of acute myelogenous leukemia. Do these reports reflect an increased risk of developing acute leukemia? If so, is this simply a part of the natural history of the primary neoplasm, or benign disease, which is more recently becom-

*C.D. Bloomfield (ed.), Adult leukemias 1, 61–108. All rights reserved.*
*Copyright © 1982 Martinus Nijhoff Publishers, The Hague/Boston/London.*

ing manifest because of improvement in treatment and concomitant improvement in survival? On the other hand, is this risk of leukemia due to the more aggressive treatment programs themselves? The characteristic clinical picture and the refractory nature of the leukemia which occurs in the setting is clearly different from the spontaneous acute leukemia seen in otherwise normal patients and makes unlikely the alternative possibility of spontaneous leukemia occurring in long term survivors.

This chapter is a partial review of the English literature on the management of a number of benign and malignant diseases in which a fairly uniform acute leukemia picture supervenes as the terminal event. The review begins with a commentary on the potential factors which may contribute to its pathogenesis. The several disease entities with treatment related leukemia are reviewed to examine the relationship of the type and intensity of treatment to the leukemia. The characteristic features of the leukemia are detailed, as well as possible approaches to prevention.

## 2. MULTIPLE MALIGNANCIES

What is the risk of a patient with one primary cancer spontaneously developing a later second (metachronous) independent primary cancer in another organ? One needs an answer to this question in order to show that an intervening treatment enhances that risk. A basic problem with studies directed toward quantification of the risk is the question of how representative of the entire population of patients with a given primary malignancy is the population from which the cases of the second malignancy are drawn. Because the majority of secondary leukemias are anecdotal reports, little can be said about the populations from which they were drawn.

Moertel and Hagedorn [1] reviewed the literature and the Mayo Clinic experience between 1944 and 1953 to examine the risk of leukemia and lymphoma patients developing multiple primary neoplasms. One hundred and ninety-four of 4424 Mayo Clinic patients with leukemia and lymphoma had a coexistent primary neoplasm. They concluded that the presence of leukemia or lymphoma did not predispose to the development of any other specific type of malignancy. It is impossible, as the authors pointed out, to make a valid comparison between the incidence of malignant disease in their series and that in the general population because of the referral nature of the Mayo Clinic population.

Einhorn and Jakobsson [2] reviewed the 1681 patients with carcinoma of the lip, treated at the Radiumhemmet between 1910 and 1950, for the risk of developing a second malignancy of an organ other than the lip. All but six patients were followed until death. Two hundred and twenty-six of the 1675 developed a second primary. The data show that, among patients between the ages of 25 and 50, there was a 16-fold increased risk of a second malignancy, than expected by chance alone. The risk among older patients was that attributable to chance. Berg [3] could not demonstrate an increased risk of another malignancy occurring in the course of leukemia than that expected in the general population. They did note that the risk is relatively highest in middle-aged adults and decreases after sixty to that in the general population.

One might conclude, given one malignancy, that there may be an increased risk of a second simultaneous (synchronous) or subsequent (metachronous) malignancy among patients who have their first disease in middle age (30–60). Among those with synchronous malignancies, one must ask the question as to whether both malignancies are related to the same etiological factor. Among those with metachronous second malignancies the question is whether the second is induced and related to the treatment of the first. To prove treatment related leukemia, one must show clear evidence of an increased risk of leukemia above that which one would expect as a background level of risk in a population of second tumors.

## .3. PATHOGENESIS OF MULTIPLE METACHRONOUS MALIGNANCIES

There are a variety of factors which are potential influences on the development of metachronous malignancy related to treatment. Among them are immunological compromise of the host, immunosuppression related to treatment, chromosomal damage, and the carcinogenicity of both drugs and ionizing radiation.

### 3.1. Immunological Compromise

The incidence of malignancy in various immunodeficiency states is 10 000 times that of the general age matched population [4]. Kersey et al. [5] have found that children with congenital immunodeficiency have a 2–10% chance of developing cancer in their lifetime and that 75% of the cancers are leukemia or lymphoma. Good [6] has reviewed the association between immunity and malignancy and found not only a clear increase in malignancy among immunodeficient children, but evidence that carcinogenic chemicals, oncogenic viruses, nutritional deprivation, and aging each compromise the immune mechanism. The relationship of immunity and malignancy is clear and is brought into better focus during therapeutic immunosuppression.

Leibowitz and Schwartz [7] in 1971, reviewed the literature in support of malignancy as a complication of immunosuppressive therapy. At that time, the incidence of malignancy in the renal transplant patient was 33 times and lymphoma 4000 times that of the age corrected normal population. There is no question that agents such as cyclophosphamide, azathioprine, and prednisone, used in renal transplantation, compromise the humoral and cellular immune mechanism; but, immunosuppression in and of itself, should not lead to malignant transformation of cells. On the other hand, immunosuppressive chemotherapeutic agents may have a direct oncogenic effect, may potentiate other carcinogens in the environment, and may permit the growth of oncogenic viruses.

## 3.2. Chromosomal Damage

Some malignant diseases have a consistent chromosomal abnormality such as chronic myelogenous leukemia (CML) (22q-) and Burkitt's lymphoma (8q-). Others have variable patterns such as acute myelogenous leukemia and polycythemia vera. Rowley [8] hypothesized that those with a consistent cytogenetic pattern may have a form of the disease caused by specific etiological agent while those with variable changes might have diverse etiologies. While the etiology of CML is not clear, there is substantial data that the Epstein-Barr virus is related to the etiology of Burkitt's lymphoma.

Initial studies using banding techniques demonstrated 51% (46/70) of patients with spontaneous acute myelogenous leukemia (AML) to have cytogenetic abnormalities on admission to the hospital [9] (see chapter by Golomb). Except for acute promyelocytic leukemia ($\dagger$(15:17)), these were random abnormalities. Those patients with only abnormal karyotypes had no complete remissions and very short median survival (2 months). Based upon the Rowley hypothesis [8], patients with acute promyelocytic leukemia may have a common specific etiological agent, whereas patients with other forms of AML, those with both normal and abnormal karyotypes, may have diverse etiologies. Of particular relevance to this review is the observation of poor response and survival among those patients with AML whose metaphases are all abnormal [9].

Jensen [10] studied chromosomes in patients with autoimmune disease and psoriasis prior to, during, and after treatment with azathioprine and amethopterin. Both agents were shown to produce various types of chromosome breakages. Rowley et al. [11] reported on the ten patients, among 450 with malignant lymphoma and 250 with Hodgkin's disease, from the University of Chicago Hospital, who developed acute myelogenous leukemia following treatment (Hodgkin's — 7, non-Hodgkin's — 3). Six of the nine patients were evaluated on a continuing basis and were found to have a preleukemic syndrome [12] lasting from two to 20 months. None of the four patients treated with intensive chemotherapy for their acute leukemia responded. The time between the original diagnosis of malignant lymphoma and the diagnosis of leukemia ranged from 29 to 132 months with a median of 58 months. All 10 patients had chromosomal abnormalities in cells obtained from bone marrow and a consistent clonal pattern could be identified in every patient. The preleukemia phase in six of nine patients, who had serial evaluations, had a specific chromosomal abnormality. Cells from all but one patient were lacking a B chromosome, consisting of the loss of number five (8/9) and number seven (5/9). Loss of number five, the most common change in acute myelogenous leukemia occurring after treatment of malignant lymphoma, was only the third most frequent change (16%) among patients with leukemia *de novo* [9].

Chromosome abnormalities are associated with malignant disease and leukemia specifically. Chemotherapeutic agents can produce somatic chromosomal abnormalities and patients with Hodgkin's disease and malignant lymphoma who are treated and develop acute leukemia acquire a non-random hypodiploid pattern associated with deletions in group B, specifically chromosomes five and seven. Rowley *et al.* [11] found no relationship of the chromosome picture to the type of leukemia or the treatment and thus a common etiology for this non-random abnormality is unlikely. More likely is a common mechanism of transformation. Additional prospective banding studies in this setting are needed.

### 3.3. Leukemogenesis of Radiation

The first radiation induced cancer in man, as reviewed by Cade [13], was reported in 1902 by Frieben in a 33-year-old technician who developed epithelioma of the hand, with axillary metastases, while employed as a demonstrator of the roentgen ray. The first case of radiation related leukemia was reported by Emil-Weil and Lacassagne in 1925 [14]. In 1946 Ulrich [15] reported an eight-fold increase in leukemia among radiologists, when compared to other physicians. The Atomic Bomb Casualty Commission has demonstrated ample evidence of leukemia in survivors of a single large dose of ionizing radiation [16]. Court-Brown and Doll [17] studied 14 559 patients with ankylosing spondylitis treated with radiotherapy. At 9.5 times the expected number of deaths from leukemia, the peak mortality was passed by 15 years of follow-up.

Smith [18], in a pivotal study, examined the risk of leukemia induced by pelvic irradiation. He compared those treated with pelvic irradiation for the induction of menopause and other benign causes (marrow dose from 10 to 190 rads) with those treated for carcinoma of the cervix (marrow dose from 300 to 1500 rads). In contrast to an anticipated dose response relationship, there were no acute leukemias occurring among those treated to a high dose, in which marrow cells were totally destroyed. There was, however, an approximate two-fold increase in risk of leukemia among those treated with a lower sequential marrow dose which produced sublethal damage. Linos *et al.* [19], on the other hand, examined low dose (<300 rads) delivered over long periods of time for diagnostic and low level therapeutic radiation and found no significant increase in leukemia. The evidence for the leukemogenic effect on whole body radiation, though somewhat contradictory, appears related to a dose sufficient to produce sublethal damage to normal bone marrow.

## 3.4. Leukemogenesis of Chemotherapeutic Agents

It has been suggested that the majority of human cancers are caused by carcinogenic chemicals [20]. Tumor incidence is directly related to the dose of chemical carcinogen in man and animals. The risk of lung cancer is related to the dose of cigarettes [21] and that of bladder cancer to the length of exposure to aromatic amines [22]. Cocarcinogens and carcinogens interact to the increased risk. Lung cancer is increased eight-fold among smokers exposed to asbestos, when compared to smokers alone, and 92-fold when compared to non-smokers [23].

There is abundant evidence that chemotherapeutic agents produce structural and numerical damage to chromosomes. Alkylating agents, antimetabolites and anti-tumor antibiotics produce chromosomal damage *in vitro*. Sieber and Adamson [24] report on a variety of alkylating agents which exert an adverse effect on human chromosomes *in vitro* and *in vivo*. A nonspecific pattern of chromosomal rearrangements has been reported with human leukocytes incubated with nitrogen mustard for 48 hours. Cytoxan, thiotepa, busulfan, and chlorambucil produce similar changes.

O'Gara *et al.* [25] reported on the development of AML in two rhesus monkeys 17 months and 5½ years after treatment with procarbazine. Of 23 spontaneous hematopoietic malignancies reported in the animal literature of the past 50 years, only one was acute myeloid leukemia, supporting the leukemogenic potential of procarbazine.

The remainder of this chapter will deal with the evidence for treatment related leukemia in man. The use of carcinogens and leukemogens to treat malignant disease in man is clearly justified when one examines the great benefit of treatment (i.e., MOPP in Hodgkin's disease) with the relatively low risk of treatment related leukemia. There remains some question about their use in some of the more benign conditions. Under any circumstances, continued surveillance of chronic toxicity of treatment is clearly important.

4. BENZENE AND LEUKEMIA

Vigliani and Forni [26] recently reviewed the association of benzene and acute leukemia. Benzene's role as a marrow toxin has been known for over a century. More than 100 cases of leukemia attributed to benzene have been reported, mostly among workers exposed to benzene in rotogravure plants and shoe factories. Aksoy and Erdem [27], followed 44 pancytopenic patients with benzene exposure. Complete remission was seen in 23 patients and death due to pancytopenia occurred in 14. Six pancytopenic patients developed acute leukemia after six months to six years of aplasia and a mean exposure of 95 months. Cytogenetic abnormalities have been noted in benzene induced leukemia [28]. Van den Berghe *et al.* [29] studied two patients with putative benzene induced preleukemia through their course until the development of frank leukemia. Patient one developed karyotypic abnormalities in all marrow cells in the form of translocations (t(9; 10) and t(4; 15)). Patient two had a chromosome seven monosomy. This latter patient demonstrated the second most common abnormality among the non-random chromosomal abnormalities seen in leukemia among patients treated for Hodgkin's disease and non-Hodgkin's lymphoma as reported by Rowley *et al.* [11]. These are the only cases of benzene related leukemia studied by banding techniques.

In addition to the cytogenetic abnormalities, benzene exposure and treatment related leukemia share similarities. They have a similar latent period, a variable preleukemic phase, and a failure to respond to treatment for the leukemia. The two situations have in common a sub-lethal damage to bone marrow, with significant periods of pancytopenia (preleukemia) and the development of leukemia in a fraction of patients.

5. DISEASES ASSOCIATED WITH TREATMENT RELATED LEUKEMIA

The vast majority of reports on the putative relationship of the treatment of both malignant and benign disease to the development of acute myelogenous leukemia are anecdotal. In these reports it is impossible to assess risk. Among those few population-based studies, there are multiple methodological reasons to question the validity of the assessment of risk. There can be little doubt, however, that this is a phenomenon recognized at a time when aggressive treatment of these diseases has made a major impact on the survival of many. This partial review of the English literature on treatment related acute myelogenous leukemia will cover eight different disease categories (see Table 1).

Cases are included if the leukemia is clearly metachronous (>6 month

*Table 1.*

| Disease | Table no. | Cases of AML |
|---|---|---|
| Hodgkin's Disease | 2 | 159 |
| Multiple myeloma | 6 | 84 |
| Non-Hodgkin's lymphoma | 7 | 51 |
| Chronic lymphocytic leukemia | 8 | 7 |
| Ovarian cancer | 9 | 32 |
| Breast cancer | 10 | 34 |
| Other cancers | 11 | 22 |
| Non-malignant | 12 | 55 |
| | | —— |
| | | 444 |

interval between the disease and the leukemia) and where there is sufficient data to evaluate treatment, interval to the development of leukemia, and the type of leukemia. Pre-leukemic interval, treatment of the leukemia, and cytogenetics were also sought. Only cases of acute myelogenous leukemia and its variants are included.

## 5.1. Hodgkin's Disease

Table 2 reviews 159 reported cases of Hodgkin's disease in which a metachronous acute leukemia has developed [11, 30–76]. Occasional reports of acute leukemia developing in Hodgkin's disease preceded the report by Crosby [77] of his survey of 25 medical centers where Hodgkin's disease was treated, inquiring as to the incidence of acute granulocytic leukemia. Information was received from 23 of 25 institutions on 17 cases among an estimated 10 000 cases of Hodgkin's disease treated between 1950 and 1969. He estimated an excess of acute granulocytic leukemia which he attributed to radiation therapy. Arseneau and associates [78] reported on 19 second malignancies among 425 Hodgkin's disease patients treated between 1953 and 1971 at the National Cancer Institute. They found evidence that patients who received both intensive radiotherapy and intensive chemotherapy were at greatest risk for the development of a second malignancy with an observed rate 23 times that expected. Aggressive solid tumors, rather than leukemia, were most prevalent, and the patient's Hodgkin's disease was in relapse at the time of the development of the second malignancy. This inferred that the second malignancy was also related in some way to the aggressive nature of the patient's original Hodgkin's disease. Toland and Coltman [79, 66] confirmed a relationship between second malignancy and the intensity of treatment. Two major differences were noted, however. All but one of the patients (17/18) remained in complete remission of their

Table 2. Treatment related leukemia: Hodgkin's disease.

| Ref. | Age/Sex | Chemo-therapy | Radio-therapy | Interval to leuk. | Pre-leuk. | Type leuk. | Leukemia treatment | Resp. | Resp. dur. | Cyto-genetics |
|---|---|---|---|---|---|---|---|---|---|---|
| 30 | 19/F | None | IR | 16 | 8 | AML | — | — | — | — |
| 31 | -/- | None | IR | 51 | — | AML | — | — | — | — |
| 32 | 26/F | None | IR | 42 | 1 | AML | — | — | — | — |
| 33 | 37/M | IC (2nd) | IR (1st) | 87 | — | AML | — | — | — | — |
| 34 | 20/F | IC (1st) | IR (2nd) | 31 | 2 | AML | — | — | — | ABN |
| 35 | 37/M | IC | IR | 120 | 2 | ERY | — | — | — | ABN |
| 36 | 72/M | None | IR | 25 | 3 | AML | — | — | — | — |
|  | 26/F | IC (2nd) | IR (1st) | 87 | 0 | ERY | — | — | — | — |
| 37 | 28/M | SC | IR | 223 | — | AML | 6MP | NR | — | — |
|  | 26/M | None | IR | 19 | — | AMML | None | — | 1 | — |
|  | 38/M | SC | IR | 66 | 7 | AMML | None | — | 1 | — |
|  | 68/M | None | SR | 57 | — | AMML | Yes? | NR | — | — |
| 38 | 60/M | SC | IR | 9 | NO | AML | None | — | — | — |
| 39 | 36/F | IC (2nd) | IR (1st) | 96 | 1 | AML | — | — | — | ABN |
|  | 30/M | IC (2nd) | IR (1st) | 110 | 7 | AML | — | — | — | — |
| 40 | 23/M | IC (2nd) | IR (1st) | 126 | 15 | AML | — | — | — | — |
| 41 | 58/M | None | IR | 144 | 6 | AML | — | — | — | — |
|  | 28/F | IC(2nd) | IR (1st) | 60 | — | AML | — | — | — | — |
| 42 | 20/M | None | IR | 18 | 10 | AML | — | — | — | — |
| 43 | 13/F | IC (1st) | IR (2nd) | 80 | 9 | AML | — | — | — | — |
| 44 | -/- | IC | None | 38 | — | AML | — | — | — | — |
| 45 | 56/M | IC | None | 14 | — | AML | — | — | — | — |
| 46 | 8/M | IC (2nd) | IR (1st) | 178 | 48 | AML | — | — | — | ABN |
| 47 | 51/M | None | IR | 43 | 3 | AML | — | — | — | — |
|  | 23/M | IC | IR | 84 | 11 | AML | — | — | — | — |
|  | 28/M | None | IR | 23 | 4 | AML | — | — | — | — |
| 48 | 19/F | None | IR | 15 | 3 | AML | — | — | — | — |
| 49 | 27/F | IC (1st) | IR (2nd) | 57 | — | AML | — | — | — | — |

Table 2. (Continued).

| Ref. | Age/Sex | Chemo-therapy | Radio-therapy | Interval to leuk. | Pre-leuk. | Type leuk. | Leukemia treatment | Resp. | Resp. dur. | Cyto-genetics |
|---|---|---|---|---|---|---|---|---|---|---|
| 50 | 32/F | IC (1st) | IR (2nd) | 102 | 2 | AML | – | – | – | – |
| | 49/M | IC | None | 10 | 3 | AML | – | – | – | – |
| | 21/F | IC (2nd) | IR (1st) | 98 | 10 | AML | – | – | – | – |
| 51 | 38/M | IC (2nd) | IR (1st) | 26 | 0 | AML | Yes | NR | 0 | ABN |
| 52 | 17/F | IC (1st) | IR (2nd) | 31 | – | AML | – | – | – | ABN |
| | 23/M | IC (2nd) | IR (1st) | 40 | – | AML | – | – | – | – |
| 53 | 20/M | IC (1st) | IR (2nd) | 88 | 3 | AML | – | – | – | – |
| 54 | 23/F | IC (1st) | IR (2nd) | 98 | 6 | AML | – | – | – | – |
| 55 | 22/F | None | IR | 24 | 0 | AML | – | – | – | ABN |
| 56 | 57/M | IC (2nd) | IR (1st) | 56 | 0 | AML | – | – | – | – |
| | 30/F | IC (1st) | IR (2nd) | 140 | 0 | AML | – | – | – | – |
| | 37/M | IC (2nd) | IR (1st) | 33 | 6 | AML | – | – | – | – |
| | 33/F | IC (2nd) | IR (1st) | 67 | 1 | AML | – | – | – | – |
| | 22/F | IC (2nd) | IR (1st) | 40 | 0 | AML | – | – | – | – |
| | 74/M | IC (2nd) | IR (1st) | 64 | 2 | AML | – | – | – | – |
| | 49/M | IC (2nd) | IR (1st) | 64 | 6 | AML | – | – | – | – |
| | 40/M | IC (2nd) | IR (1st) | 8 | 0 | AML | – | – | – | – |
| | 19/F | IC (2nd) | IR (1st) | 110 | – | AML | – | – | – | – |
| 57 | –/– | IC (2nd) | IR (1st) | 23 | 0 | AML | – | – | – | – |
| | –/– | IC (2nd) | IR (1st) | 23 | 0 | AML | – | – | – | – |
| 58 | 9/F | IC | None | 20 | 5 | AML | – | – | – | – |
| 59 | 47/F | SC | SR | 94 | – | AML | – | – | 2 | – |
| | 66/F | IC | SR | 50 | – | AML | – | – | 2 | – |
| | 23/F | IC | None | 41 | – | AML | – | – | 7 | – |
| | 52/M | IC | None | 32 | – | AML | – | – | 4 | – |
| | 8/M | IC | IR | 168 | – | AML | – | – | 4 | – |
| | 43/M | IC | IR | 72 | – | AML | – | – | 8 | – |
| | 16/M | IC | IR | 59 | – | AML | – | – | 3 | – |

Table 2. (Continued).

| Ref. | Age/Sex | Chemo-therapy | Radio-therapy | Interval to leuk. | Pre-leuk. | Type leuk. | Leukemia treatment | Resp. | Resp. dur. | Cyto-genetics |
|---|---|---|---|---|---|---|---|---|---|---|
| | 25/F | IC | IR | 141 | — | AML | — | — | 1 | — |
| | 20/F | None | IR | 11 | — | AML | — | — | 10 | — |
| | 27/M | IC | IR | 60 | — | AML | — | — | 5 | — |
| | 27/F | None | IR | 17 | — | AMML | — | — | 7 | — |
| | 58/M | None | SR | 75 | — | AMML | — | — | 1 | — |
| | 25/F | SC | SR | 80 | — | AMOL | — | — | 18 | — |
| | 44/M | IC | None | 63 | — | ERY | — | — | 3 | — |
| | 57/M | IC | SR | 72 | — | ERY | — | — | 3 | — |
| | 44/M | IC | IR | 44 | — | ERY | — | — | 6 | — |
| | 39/F | IC | SR | 45 | — | UNDIFF | — | — | 10 | — |
| | 26/F | SC | SR | 132 | — | UNDIFF | — | — | 8 | — |
| | 42/F | IC | SR | 28 | — | UNDIFF | — | — | 3 | — |
| 60 | 28/F | IC | SR | 76 | 9 | AML | CYT, ARAC TG | NR | — | ABN |
| | 48/M | None | IR | 95 | 0 | AML | Yes? | NR | 6 | — |
| | 44/F | IC | IR | 68 | 1 | AML | MTX, ADR, CYT | NR | 1 | ABN |
| | 27/M | IC | IR | 55 | — | AML | ARAC, DNR | PR | 1 | ABN |
| 61 | 27/M | IC (2nd) | IR (1st) | 49 | 7 | AML | ARAC, DNR | NR | 0 | — |
| 62 | 39/M | IC | SR | 108 | — | AML | ARAC, DNR | NR | 2 | ABN |
| | 28/F | IC | SR | 120 | — | AML | None | NR | 0 | Extra C |
| | 28/M | SC | IR | 15 | — | AMOL | ARAC, ADR | NR | 0 | Normal |
| | 45/M | SC | SR | 132 | — | AMOL | ARAC, DNR | NR | 1 | Missing #7 |
| 63 | 55/M | IC (2nd) | IR (1st) | 27 | 0 | AMML | None | — | — | — |
| | 43/M | IC (2nd) | SR (1st) | 93 | 0 | ERY | None | — | — | — |
| | 23/M | IC (2nd) | IR (1st) | 78 | 0 | AMML | None | — | — | — |
| | 28/M | IC (2nd) | SR (1st) | 50 | 3 | AML | ARAC, TG | NR | 6 | ABN |

*Table 2.* (Continued).

| Ref. | Age/Sex | Chemo-therapy | Radio-therapy | Interval to leuk. | Pre-leuk. | Type leuk. | Leukemia treatment | Resp. | Resp. dur. | Cyto-genetics |
|---|---|---|---|---|---|---|---|---|---|---|
| 64 | 52/M | IC (2nd) | IR (1st) | 79 | 0 | AML | None | — | — | — |
|  | 27/M | SC (2nd) | IR (1st) | 26 | 3 | AML | Yes | NR | 1 | ABN |
| 65 | 26/M | IC (2nd) | IR (1st) | 36 | 3 | AML | None | — | 2 | — |
|  | 29/M | IC (2nd) | IR (1st) | 54 | 9 | AML | None | — | 5 | — |
|  | 19/F | SC (2nd) | IR (1st) | 14 | 1 | AML | None | — | 1 | — |
|  | 27/F | IC (2nd) | IR (1st) | 96 | 7 | AML | None | — | 6 | — |
|  | 32/M | IC (2nd) | IR (1st) | 32 | 0 | AML | None | — | 3 | — |
|  | 41/M | IC (2nd) | IR (1st) | 72 | 71 | AML | None | — | 3 | — |
|  | 56/M | IC (2nd) | IR (1st) | 54 | 0 | AML | None | — | 5 | — |
|  | 39/M | IC (2nd) | IR (1st) | 60 | 2 | AML | None | — | 3 | — |
| 11 | 37/F | SC | IR | 132 | — | AML | ARAC, TG | NR | — | ABN |
|  | 35/F | IC | None | 80 | — | AML | ARAC, TG | NR | — | ABN |
|  | 37/M | IC | IR | 41 | — | AML | None | — | — | ABN |
|  | 27/F | IC | IR | 76 | 6 | AML | Hydrea | PR | 3 | ABN |
|  | 50/F | IC | SR | 74 | — | APL | None | — | — | ABN |
|  | 68/F | None | SR | 29 | — | ERY | None | — | — | ABN |
|  | 31/M | IC | IR | 51 | — | AML | None | — | — | ABN |
| 66 | 39/M | SC (1st) | IR (2nd) | 49 | — | AMML | None | — | 2 | — |
|  | 24/M | SC (1st) | IR (2nd) | 30 | — | AML | COAP | NR | 2 | — |
|  | 39/F | SC (1st) | IR (2nd) | 32 | — | AML | None | — | 1 | — |
|  | 22/M | SC (1st) | IR (2nd) | 38 | — | AML | ARAC | NR | 1 | — |
|  | 23/M | SC (1st) | IR (2nd) | 33 | — | AML | ADOAP | NR | 1 | — |
|  | 41/M | SC (1st) | IR (2nd) | 82 | — | ALL | None | — | — | — |
|  | 48/M | SC (1st) | IR (2nd) | 65 | — | AML | ARAC | NR | — | — |
|  | 41/M | IC | SR | 53 | — | AMML | — | NR | — | — |
|  | 45/M | IC | SR | 34 | — | AMML | — | — | — | — |
|  | 40/M | IC | SR | 61 | — | SMOLDER | — | — | — | — |
|  | 20/F | IC | SR | 46 | — | AML | — | — | — | — |

*Table 2.* (Continued).

| Ref. | Age/Sex | Chemo-therapy | Radio-therapy | Interval to leuk. | Pre-leuk. | Type leuk. | Leukemia treatment | Resp. | Resp. dur. | Cyto-genetics |
|---|---|---|---|---|---|---|---|---|---|---|
| | 45/M | IC | SR | 14 | — | AML | — | — | — | — |
| | 63/F | IC | None | 45 | — | ERY | ADOAP | NR | 3 | — |
| | 28/M | IC | None | 29 | — | AMML | — | — | — | — |
| | 39/M | IC | None | 32 | — | AML | — | — | — | — |
| | 9/F | IC | None | 55 | — | AMML | — | — | — | — |
| 67 | 57/M | SC | IR | 48 | — | AMML | — | — | — | — |
| | 51/M | SC | IR | 37 | — | AML | — | — | — | — |
| 68 | 56/F | IC (2nd) | IR (1st) | 40 | 0 | IBL | CYT, P | NR | 1 | — |
| 69 | 31/M | IC | IR | 123 | — | AML | DNR, ARAC | NR | — | ABN |
| | 19/F | IC | IR | 35 | — | AML | DNR, ARAC | PR | — | ABN |
| | 35/M | IC | None | 14 | — | AML | — | — | — | — |
| | 52/F | IC | None | 85 | — | AML | — | — | — | — |
| 70 | 48/M | IC | IR | 57 | 8 | AML | None | — | — | — |
| | 36/M | IC | IR | 95 | 46 | AML | None | — | 1 | — |
| 71 | -/- | IC | IR (1st) | 30 | — | AML | — | — | — | — |
| | -/- | IC | IR (1st) | 31 | — | AML | — | — | — | — |
| | -/- | IC | IR (1st) | 56 | — | AML | — | — | — | — |
| | -/- | IC | IR (1st) | 32 | — | AML | — | — | — | — |
| | -/- | IC | IR (1st) | 65 | — | AML | — | — | — | — |
| | -/- | IC | IR (1st) | 34 | — | AML | — | — | — | — |
| | -/- | IC | IR (1st) | 127 | — | AML | — | — | — | — |
| | -/- | SC | SR (1st) | 102 | — | AML | — | — | — | — |
| | -/- | IC | None | 20 | — | AML | — | — | — | — |
| | -/- | IC | SR | 66 | — | AML | — | — | — | — |
| 72 | 9/F | SC (2nd) | IR (1st) | 125 | 0 | AML | — | — | 8 | ABN |
| 73 | 29/M | SC (2nd) | IR (1st) | 42 | 25 | AML | — | 1 | 1 | — |
| | 30/F | SC (2nd) | IR (1st) | 83 | 7 | ERY | — | 5 | — | — |
| | 43/M | IC (2nd) | IR (1st) | 53 | 14 | AMML | — | — | 1 | — |

*Table 2.* (Continued).

| Ref. | Age/Sex | Chemo-therapy | Radio-therapy | Interval to leuk. | Pre-leuk. | Type leuk. | Leukemia treatment | Resp. | Resp. dur. | Cyto-genetics |
|---|---|---|---|---|---|---|---|---|---|---|
|  | 47/M | IC | None | 59 | 3 | AML | – | – | 1 | – |
|  | 26/F | IC (2nd) | IR (1st) | 29 | 4 | AML | – | – | 1 | – |
|  | 40/M | SC (2nd) | IR (1st) | 36 | 24 | ERY | – | – | 12 | – |
|  | 63/M | SC | None | 12 | 10 | AML | – | – | 2 | – |
| 74 | 49/F | IC | SR | 72 | 2 | ERY | – | – | 1 | ABN |
|  | 60/F | IC | None | 62 | – | AMML | – | – | 4 | – |
|  | 50/M | IC | None | 32 | – | AMML | – | – | 4 | – |
|  | 49/M | IC | None | 50 | 2 | AMML | – | – | ½ | – |
|  | 23/F | IC | None | 72 | 2 | ERY | – | – | 3 | – |
| 75 | 47/M | IC (2nd) | IR (1st) | 34 | 6 | AML | None | – | – | – |
|  | 52/M | IC (2nd) | IR (1st) | 32 | 1 | AML | None | – | – | – |
|  | 51/M | IC (2nd) | IR (1st) | 32 | 0 | AML | Yes | – | 5 | – |
|  | 23/M | IC (2nd) | IR (1st) | 43 | 2 | AML | None | – | – | – |
|  | 62/F | IC (2nd) | IR (1st) | 88 | 0 | AML | None | – | 2 | – |
|  | 25/M | IC (2nd) | IR+GOLD | 74 | 1 | AML | None | – | 2 | – |
|  | 32/M | IC (2nd) | IR+GOLD | 98 | – | AML | Yes | NR | 2 | – |
|  | 53/M | IC | None | 52 | 4 | AML | None | – | 14 | – |
|  | 29/F | IC | None | 83 | 13 | AML | None | – | 1 | – |
|  | 27/F | – | – | 152 | – | AML | None | – | 0 | – |
|  | 23/F | IC (2nd) | IR (1st) | 106 | – | AML | – | – | 0 | – |
| 76 | –/– | IC (2nd) | SR (1st) | – | – | AML | – | – | – | – |
|  | –/– | IC (2nd) | SR (1st) | – | – | AML | – | – | – | – |

IR—intensive radiotherapy; SR—some radiotherapy; IC—intensive chemotherapy; SC—some chemotherapy; AML—acute myelogenous leukemia; AMML—acute myelomonocytic leukemia; AMOL—acute monocytic leukemia; ERY—erythroleukemia; UNDIFF—undifferentiated leukemia; SMOLDER—Smoldering leukemia; 6MP—6, mercaptopurine; CYT—cyclophosphamide; ARAC—arabinosyl cytosine; TG—6-thioguanine; MTX—methotrexate; ADR—adriamycin; DNR—daunorubicin; HYDREA—hydroxyurea; COAP—cyclophosphamide, oncovin, ARAC and prednisone; ADOAP—adriamycin, oncovin, ARAC, and prednisone.

Hodgkin's disease at the time of the second malignancy, and eleven of eighteen patients had acute myelogenous leukemia.

Table 2 reviews the treatment of the patient's Hodgkin's disease and its intensity. The criteria for intensity of treatment are those of Arseneau *et al.* [78]. Patients who received no chemotherapy or radiotherapy were listed as none. Those who had some chemotherapy (SC) received up to, but not including, six cycles of MOPP, whereas those with more treatment were considered to have received intensive chemotherapy (IC). Those who received up to, but not including, total nodal or extended field radiotherapy, are listed as some radiotherapy (SR) and those who received more as intensive radiotherapy. Sixteen of those on Table 2 had no chemotherapy and 23 no radiotherapy while 83/168 had intensive chemotherapy and intensive radiotherapy. Cadman and associates [60] examined the latent period from the diagnosis of Hodgkin's disease to the diagnosis of leukemia and found it to be significantly shorter ($p<0.0005$), among those who received intensive chemotherapy and intensive radiotherapy combined, than those who had less treatment. Further, that the median interval was shorter when chemotherapy was followed by radiotherapy than with the reverse order. Sixteen of the 159 reported leukemias (Table 2) occurred in patients who had radiotherapy alone and 14 of them had intensive radiotherapy. It is, however, of interest that among two large series, one from Stanford [65, 75] and the other from the Southwest Oncology Group [66], with a total population of 1764 patients, no cases of leukemia were seen following radiotherapy alone. It is likely that these patients received a marrow lethal dose to the areas of marrow treated and were at lower risk for the development of radiation induced leukemia [18].

Brody and Schottenfeld [80] reviewed the cumulative probabilities of multiple primary cancers among patients treated for Hodgkin's disease at Memorial Sloan-Kettering during 1950–1954, 1960–1964, and 1968–1972. The probabilities were 1.26%, 1.22% and 4.05% respectively, showing a clearly enhanced risk within the more recent time frame. A recent update of the Southwest Oncology Group data [81] shows 28 second malignancies (18 AML) among 687 patients treated for Hodgkin's disease of all stages. Table

*Table 3.* Actuarial risk of leukemia.

| Study group | No. of patients | No. at risk at 5 years | Risk (%) * at 5 years | P value |
|---|---|---|---|---|
| Stanford [65] | 680 | 340 | 1.5±0.6 | 0.10 |
| SWOG [81] | 687 | 149 | 3.5±0.7 | |

* Mean ±SEM.

3 shows the actuarial risk of leukemia in SWOG compared to that at Stanford [65].

Among those who received combined treatment at Stanford, the actuarial risk of leukemia was 2.58%±1.2 at five and 3.9±1.5 at seven years. In a recent review from Stanford [75] 20 leukemias, eleven more than previously reported [65], have appeared among 1086 patients treated for an actuarial risk of leukemia of 3.9%±1.0 for the entire group, and 7.1%±2.6% for the adjuvant MOPP chemotherapy subgroup at nine years. The data clearly show a relationship between the intensity of treatment and the risk of leukemia.

Although there may be subsets of patients with Hodgkin's disease who require initial combined modality treatment, in the vast majority of patients single modality therapy, followed by salvage treatment, with the same or another modality at the time of relapse, results in equivalent survival [57, 76]. A case in point is the Southwest Oncology Group protocol (SWOG 781) for stage I and II Hodgkin's disease in which patients were randomly assigned to treatment with extended field radiotherapy (EFXRT) or involved field radiotherapy plus six cycles of MOPP (IF+MOPP) [76]. Although at eight years follow-up relapse-free survival favored the combined modality (P = 0.048) because of salvage therapy, there was no difference in overall survival (P = 0.69). Table 4 shows the causes of death among the 230 patients in the two limbs of the study.

It comes as no surprise that the two acute leukemias occurred among those 116 patients treated with involved field radiotherapy plus MOPP. While the data are not significant at this point (P = 0.50), the expected trend is present and further follow-up is needed.

None of the studies have sufficient follow-up to determine whether there

*Table 4.* RAC No. 1 (SWOG 781): causes of death.

| Cause | EFXRT [114] | IF + MOPP [116] |
|---|---|---|
| Progressive disease | 4 | 6 |
| Acute leukemia | — | 2 * |
| Oat cell of lung | 1 | — |
| Infection | 2 | 1 |
| Cardiogenic shock | 1 | — |
| Trauma | 1 | — |
| Pulmonary embolus | 1 | — |
| Unknown | — | 1 |
| | 10 | 10 |

* P = 0.50 (Fisher Exact).

*Table 5.* Treatment related leukemia: Milan experience [71].

| Treatment | No. pts. | Median exposure (months) | % Incidence | | |
|-----------|----------|--------------------------|-------------|------|-------|
| | | | 3 yr | 5 yr | 10 yr |
| RT + MOPP | 147 | 40 | 2.9 | 5.4 | 5.4 |
| RT + ABVD | 55 | 45 | 0 | 0 | 0 |

RT—Radiotherapy.

is a plateau appearing in the risk of leukemia. Valagussa *et al.* [71] have reported on the second malignancies seen at the National Cancer Institute in Milan. In their combined modality studies they had 145 patients treated with total or subtotal nodal radiotherapy plus MOPP (XRT + MOPP), and 55 with comparable radiotherapy plus ABVD (Adriamycin, Bleomycin, Velban, and Dacarbazine) (XRT + ABVD). Table 5 shows the actuarial risk of leukemia among patients treated on the two regimens.

The risk for RT + MOPP is 5.4% at five years and the same at ten years, suggesting a plateau or a peak incidence at five years. It is of some interest that no leukemias have developed to date in the RT + ABVD group. While the group is small, two leukemias would have been seen, based on the MOPP data. The ABVD regimen does not include procarbazine or an alkylating agent. It is clear that procarbazine [25] is leukemogenic in animals and alkylating agents [24] such as nitrogen mustard, produce cytogenetic changes *in vitro* and *in vivo*. Further follow-up of this important lead from Milan will be necessary.

A preleukemic picture, similar to that described by Saarni and Linman [82], lasting from one to 71 months, has been reported in 64 cases (Table 2). It is said to be absent in 23 cases and not mentioned or not recognized in the other reports. This fairly consistent finding is, in many ways, similar to the cytopenia seen with benzene exposure. The total number of patients with Hodgkin's disease who have some degree of cytopenia, at some time remote from their treatment, is not known. It is likely that it would more commonly be identified among patients who ultimately go on to develop leukemia. The best review on the preleukemia picture is by Foucar *et al.* [69]. They report on a panmyelosis in 15 patients, which is common to treatment related leukemia in a variety of diseases, including Hodgkin's disease. Pancytopenia, anisopoikilocytosis, normoblastemia, large hypergranular platelets, hypogranular neutrophiles, pseudo-Pelger Huet nuclei, low myeloblast counts and basophilia were most commonly seen in the peripheral blood. Marrows were hypercellular, had increase numbers of myeloblasts (2–82%), peroxidase positive blasts, dysmyelopoiesis, dyserythropoiesis, ringed sideroblasts, PAS positive erythroblasts, and micromegakaryocytes with nuclear abnormalities.

The types of leukemia which are reported in Table 2 are of the acute myelogenous leukemia variety. The only group underrepresented is acute promyelocytic. Many of the reviews do not classify the leukemia beyond the designation of acute non-lymphocytic leukemia (ANLL). Parmley et al. [58] addressed the question as to whether the leukemia is simply a reflection of marrow involvement with the malignant cell of Hodgkin's disease, the Reed-Sternberg cell. They performed ultrastructural and immunocytochemical studies on the tumor and the leukemia which occurred in a young girl, and found that the evidence suggested that the AMML which she had was a second neoplasm. Although the evidence would suggest that treatment related leukemias are one of the variants of acute myelogenous leukemia, careful prospective classification of these leukemias, in accordance with the French-American-British (FAB) classification, is needed (see chapter by Bennett).

The vast majority of the patients who have been reported to develop treatment related leukemia have not been treated. Table 2 lists 30 patients treated for their leukemia and only two partial responses. This lends support for the refractory nature of the leukemia. Treatment varied from single agents to modern day combination chemotherapy regimens. This refractoriness may be related to the heavy prior treatment or to the cytogenetic aberrations commonly seen. Beltran and Stuckey [83], on the other hand, reported in abstract form, four patients with Hodgkin's disease and two with non-Hodgkin's lymphoma, and five of six achieved complete remission. How these patients differ from the literature experience is not known. Suffice it to say that while the outlook is grim, it may not be totally hopeless.

Cytogenetic abnormalities were reported in 26 of 27 patients in whom such studies were reported (Table 2). The vast majority of reports showed hypodiploidy. The most definite report is that by Rowley et al. [11], in which there appeared to be a consistent pattern with deletion of chromosomes five and seven predominantly. These changes are similar to those reported in acute leukemia [84]. The refractoriness of treatment related leukemia may correlate with the cytogenetic abnormalities. Golomb et al. [9] showed that, among patients with de novo AML, those with all abnormal metaphases respond poorly, with no complete remission, and die quickly (median survival−2 months).

## 5.2. Multiple Myeloma

Multiple myeloma is the second most common disease associated with the development of leukemia. Table 6 includes 84 cases reported from the

Table 6. Treatment related leukemia: multiple myeloma.

| Ref. | Age/Sex | Chemo-therapy | Radio-therapy | Interval to leuk. | Pre-leuk. | Type leuk. | Leukemia treatment | Resp. | Resp. dur. | Cyto-genetics |
|---|---|---|---|---|---|---|---|---|---|---|
| 85 | 62/M | MEL | None | 120 | — | AML | — | — | — | — |
| 86 | 41/M | MEL | None | 48 | — | AMML | — | — | — | — |
| 87 | 62/F | MEL | None | 41 | — | AML | — | — | — | — |
| | 71/F | MEL | Yes | 15 | — | AML | — | — | — | — |
| | 45/M | MEL | None | 60 | — | AML | — | — | — | — |
| | 61/F | CYT | Yes | 68 | — | AML | — | — | — | — |
| 88 | 55/M | MEL | Yes | 44 | — | AMML | — | — | — | — |
| | 59/M | MEL | None | 33 | — | AMML | — | — | — | — |
| | 67/M | MEL | Yes | 30 | — | AMML | — | — | — | — |
| 89 | –/– | MEL | Yes | — | — | AML | — | — | — | — |
| | –/– | MEL | Yes | — | — | AML | — | — | — | — |
| | –/– | MEL | Yes | — | — | AML | — | — | — | — |
| | –/– | MEL | Yes | — | — | AML | — | — | — | — |
| | –/– | MEL | Yes | — | — | AML | — | — | — | — |
| 90 | 40/M | MEL | Yes | 51 | — | AML | — | — | — | — |
| 91 | 59/M | MEL | None | 30 | — | AMML | — | — | — | — |
| 92 | 35/F | MEL | None | 72 | — | AMML | — | — | — | — |
| | 26/M | MEL | None | 84 | — | AMML | — | — | — | — |
| 93 | 63/M | MEL | None | 48 | — | AMML | — | — | — | — |
| 94 | ?/M | MEL | None | 36 | — | AMML | — | — | — | — |
| 95 | 61/F | MEL | None | 71 | — | AMML | — | — | — | — |
| | 68/F | MEL | Yes | 22 | — | AML | — | — | — | — |
| 96 | 64/F | MEL | None | 51 | — | APL | — | — | — | — |
| 97 | 48/M | MEL | None | 84 | — | AMML | — | — | — | — |
| 98 | 50/M | MEL | None | 108 | — | AMML | — | — | — | — |
| | 55/F | MEL | None | 54 | — | AMML | — | — | — | — |
| | 50/M | MEL | Yes | 40 | — | AMML | — | — | — | — |
| 99 | 52/F | MEL | None | 147 | — | AML | — | — | — | — |
| | 53/M | MEL | None | 98 | — | AML | — | — | — | — |
| 100 | 59/F | MEL | Yes | 107 | — | AMML | — | — | — | — |

*Table 6.* (Continued).

| Ref. | Age/Sex | Chemo-therapy | Radio-therapy | Interval to leuk. | Pre-leuk. | Type leuk. | Leukemia treatment | Resp. | Resp. dur. | Cyto-genetics |
|---|---|---|---|---|---|---|---|---|---|---|
| 101 | 57/M | MEL | None | 15 | — | AMOL | Supportive | NR | — | — |
| | 40/F | MEL, CYT | Yes | 54 | — | AML | None | — | 4 | None |
| | 54/F | MEL, CYT | Yes | 47 | 9 | AML | None | — | 4 | None |
| | 48/M | MEL | Yes | 45 | 3 | AML | None | — | 4 | None |
| | 78/F | CYT | None | 14 | 11 | AMML | Yes | NR | 3 | None |
| 102 | 55/F | MEL | Yes | 120 | — | AML | — | — | — | — |
| | 59/F | MEL | None | 79 | — | AMML | — | — | — | — |
| | 46/M | MEL | Yes | 48 | — | AML | — | — | — | — |
| | 56/M | MEL | None | 60 | — | AMML | — | — | — | — |
| | 37/M | MEL | Yes | 74 | — | AMML | — | — | — | — |
| | 66/M | MEL | None | 60 | — | AMML | — | — | — | — |
| | 54/M | MEL | None | 52 | — | AMML | — | — | — | — |
| | 62/M | MEL | None | 41 | — | AMML | — | — | — | — |
| | 74/M | MEL | None | 28 | — | AML | — | — | — | — |
| | –/M | MEL | Yes | 33 | — | AMML | — | — | — | — |
| 103 | 60/M | MEL | None | 68 | — | AML | — | — | — | — |
| | 54/M | MEL | None | 74 | — | AMOL | — | — | — | — |
| | 48/M | MEL | Yes | 65 | — | AMOL | — | — | — | — |
| 104 | 60/F | MEL | Yes | 60 | — | MEG | — | — | — | — |
| 105 | 55/M | MEL | Yes | 44 | — | AML | — | — | — | — |
| | 54/M | MEL | None | 33 | — | AML | 6MP, VCR, P | NR | — | — |
| | 67/M | MEL | Yes | 30 | 3 | AML | P | NR | — | — |
| | 54/M | MEL | Yes | 56 | — | AML | — | — | — | — |
| | 48/M | MEL | None | 30 | — | AML | — | — | — | — |
| 106 | 60/F | MEL | None | 32 | 10 | AML | — | — | — | — |
| | 57/M | MEL | None | 40 | 2 | AMML | — | — | — | ABN |
| | 69/F | MEL | Yes | 39 | — | AML | — | — | — | ABN |
| 107 | 64/M | MEL | None | 30 | — | AMML | — | — | — | ABN |
| 108 | 73/M | MFI | None | 42 | — | AML | — | — | — | — |

Table 6. (Continued).

| Ref. | Age/Sex | Chemo-therapy | Radio-therapy | Interval to leuk. | Pre-leuk. | Type leuk. | Leukemia treatment | Resp. | Resp. dur. | Cyto-genetics |
|---|---|---|---|---|---|---|---|---|---|---|
| 109 | 50/M | MEL | None | 26 | — | AML | — | — | — | — |
| | 61/F | MEL | None | 35 | — | AML | — | — | — | — |
| | 61/M | MEL | Yes | 73 | — | ERY | — | — | — | — |
| 110 | 55/M | MEL | Yes | 73 | — | ERY | — | — | — | — |
| | 59/M | CYT | None | 71 | — | ERY | — | — | — | — |
| 62 | 61/M | MEL | Yes | 36 | — | ERY | ARAC, TG | — | 3 | ABN |
| | 59/M | MEL | Yes | 228 | — | ERY | ADR, ARAC | — | 7 | ABN |
| 111 | 58/F | MEL | Yes | 32 | 2 | AML | — | — | — | — |
| | 65/M | MEL | None | 73 | 2 | AML | — | — | — | ABN |
| | 78/F | MEL | None | 73 | 2 | AML | — | — | — | ABN |
| | 59/M | MEL | Yes | 58 | 4 | AML | — | — | — | — |
| | 52/M | MEL | None | 27 | 2 | AML | — | — | — | — |
| | 67/M | MEL | Yes | 13 | 8 | AML | — | — | — | — |
| 112 | 59/M | MEL | Yes | 43 | — | AML | — | — | — | — |
| 113 | 45/M | MEL | Yes | 80 | — | AMML | — | — | — | — |
| | 37/M | MEL | Yes | 73 | — | AMML | — | — | — | — |
| | 66/F | MEL | None | 69 | — | ERY | — | — | — | — |
| 114 | 64/M | MEL | Yes | 12 | — | AML | — | — | — | — |
| 69 | 56/F | MEL | None | 60 | 2 | ANNL | — | — | — | — |
| | 69/F | MEL | Yes | 56 | 1 | ANNL | — | — | — | — |
| 115 | 37/M | MEL | — | 105 | — | AML | — | — | — | Normal |
| 116 | 56/M | MEL | None | 40 | 7 | AMML | — | — | — | ABN |
| 74 | 67/M | MEL | Yes | 21 | 0 | ERY | — | — | 5 | ABN |
| | 66/M | MEL | None | 60 | 0 | AML | — | — | 2 | ABN |
| | 65/M | MEL | None | 48 | 9 | AML | — | — | 5 | — |

MEL—melphalan; CYT—cyclophosphamide; AML—acute myelogenous leukemia; AMML—Acute myelomonocytic leukemia; AMOL—acute monocytic leukemia; APL—acute promyelocytic leukemia; ERY—erythroleukemia; MEG—megakaryocytic leukemia; ARAC-arabinosyl cytosine; TG—6-thioguanine; ADR-adriamycin; ABN—abnormal chromosomes; P—prednisone; VCR—vincristine.

*Table 7.* Treatment related leukemia: non-Hodgkin's lymphoma.

| Ref. | Age/Sex | Primary diagnosis | Chemo-therapy | Radio-therapy | Interval to leuk. | Pre-leuk. | Type leuk. | Leukemia treatment | Resp. | Resp. dur. | Cyto-genetics |
|---|---|---|---|---|---|---|---|---|---|---|---|
| 120 | 19/M | RCS | None | IR | 54 | – | AML | – | – | – | – |
| 121 | 43/F | GFL | None | IR | 36 | – | AML | – | – | – | – |
| 122 | 50/M | RCS | None | IR | 24 | – | AMML | – | – | – | – |
| 123 | 43/M | LSA | None | SR | 60 | – | AML | – | – | – | – |
| 123 | 53/M | LSA | CLB, P | IR | 120 | – | AML | – | – | – | – |
| 124 | 51/M | LSA | CLB, PRED | SR | 24 | – | ERY | – | – | – | – |
| 125 | 53/F | PDLL-N | CLB | None | – | – | ERY | – | – | – | – |
| 125 | 54/F | PDLL-N | CLB | None | 108 | – | AML | – | – | – | – |
| 104 | 68/F | WDLL-D | CLB | TBI | – | – | AML | ARAC, TG | PR | 4 | – |
| 126 | 66/F | WDLL-D | None | TBI | 42 | – | ERY | – | – | – | – |
| 11 | 57/F | NHL | None | IR | 38 | 20 | BLMPD | ARAC, TG | NR | 3 | ABN |
| 11 | 57/F | NHL | IC | IR | 61 | 2 | BLMPD | DNR | NR | 1 | ABN |
| 11 | 51/F | NHL | IC | None | 56 | 6 | BLMPD | None | – | 4 | ABN |
| 127 | –/– | LSA-N | CLB | TBI | 84 | – | AMML | Yes | NR | 2 | – |
| 128 | 37/M | POLL-N | CYT | SR | 68 | – | AML | – | – | 6 | – |
| 128 | 40/M | PDLL-N | COPP | SR | 156 | – | AML | DNR | NR | 6 | – |
| 128 | 43/F | PDLL-N | COP | SR | 108 | – | AML | 6MP, P | NR | 1 | – |
| 128 | 44/M | PDLL-N | COP | None | 66 | – | AML | COAP | CR | 13 | – |
| 62 | 62/F | LSA | CYT | SR | 108 | – | ERY | ARAC, TG | – | 8 | ABN |
| 62 | 75/M | RCS | CYT | SR | 60 | – | AMOL | ADR | – | 1 | ABN |
| 129 | 41/F | LYM | CLB | SR | 60 | – | AML | – | – | – | – |
| 129 | 66/M | LYM | None | IR | 36 | – | AML | – | – | – | – |
| 130 | 77/M | DHL | SC | IR | 51 | – | AML | – | – | – | – |
| 69 | 43/F | PDLL-N | CTX | IF | 160 | – | ANNL | DNR,ARAC | CR | 14 | – |
| 69 | 37/M | PDLL-N | CTX | SR | 70 | – | ANNL | DNR | NR | 4 | ABN |
| 69 | 40/M | PDLL-N | CTXMTX | IF | 157 | – | ANNL | ARAC | NR | 5 | ABN |
| 69 | 44/M | PDLL-N | CYT | None | – | 66 | ANNL | – | 0 | 6 | ABN |
| 69 | 60/M | PDLL-D | CTX | SR | 72 | – | ANNL | None | – | 1 | – |

*Table 7. (Continued).*

| Ref. | Age/Sex | Primary diagnosis | Chemo-therapy | Radio-therapy | Interval to leuk. | Pre-leuk. | Type leuk. | Leukemia treatment | Resp. | Resp. dur. | Cyto-genetics |
|---|---|---|---|---|---|---|---|---|---|---|---|
| 131 | 56/M | DHL | COPP | None | 8 | — | AMML | — | — | — | — |
| | 46/F | PDLL-N | CLB | SR | 60 | — | AMML | — | — | — | — |
| | 83/F | DML | COP | IR | 48 | — | ERY | — | — | — | — |
| | 25/M | DML | COPP | IR | 24 | — | AML | — | — | — | — |
| | 11/F | PDLL-N | COPP | SR | 8 | — | AML | — | — | — | — |
| | 17/M | PDLL-D | COPP | TBI | 36 | — | AML | Yes | CR | 6 | — |
| | 59/M | PDLL-D | CYT | TNI | 84 | — | AML | Yes | CR | 9+ | — |
| | 58/M | DHL | CHOP | None | 6 | — | AMML | — | — | — | — |
| | 77/M | DHL | COP | SR | 60 | — | AMML | — | — | — | — |
| | 53/M | PDLL-D | None | TNI | 60 | — | AMOL | — | — | — | — |
| | 56/M | PDLL-D | COP | TNI | 32 | — | AMOL | — | — | — | — |
| | 69/F | PDLL-D | None | SR | 6 | — | AML | — | — | — | — |
| 132 | 62/M | PDLL-N | None | TBI | — | — | ANNL | — | — | — | — |
| | 28/M | PDLL-N | COP | TBI | — | — | ANNL | — | — | — | — |
| | 62/M | NML | COP | TBI | — | — | ANNL | — | — | — | — |
| | 33/M | PDLL-N | COP | TBI | — | — | ANNL | — | — | — | — |
| | 61/F | PDLL-N | — | – | — | — | ANNL | — | — | — | — |
| | 24/M | PDLL-N | — | TBI | — | — | ANNL | — | — | — | — |
| | 48/M | PDLL-D | — | TBI | — | — | ANNL | — | — | — | — |
| 116 | 45/M | PDLL-D | CYT | None | 59 | — | ERY | — | — | 1 | ABN |
| 74 | 56/M | DHL | COP | None | 16 | — | AML | — | — | 1 | — |
| | 45/M | DHL | COP | SR | 12 | — | AMML | — | — | 1 | — |
| | 64/F | PDLL-D | THIO | SR | 120 | — | AML | — | — | 2 | — |

RCS—reticulum cell sarcoma; GFL—giant follicular lymphoma; LSA—lymphosarcoma; PDLL-N—poorly differentiated lymphocytic lymphoma, nodular; PDLL-D—poorly differentiated lymphocytic lymphoma, diffuse; WPLL-D—well differentiated lymphocytic lymphoma-diffuse; LYM—lymphoma; DML—diffuse mixed lymphoma; DHL—diffuse histiocytic lymphoma; NML—nodular mixed lymphoma; CLB—chlorambucil; P—prednisone; IC—intensive chemotherapy; CYT—cyclophosphamide; COPP—CYT, oncovin, procarbazine, prednisone; COP—CYT, oncovin, P; CHOP—CYT, adriamycin, oncovin, P; THIO—thiotepa; IR—intensive radiotherapy; SR—some radiotherapy; TBI—total body radiotherapy; TNI—total nodal radiotherapy. For abbreviations on type of leukemia and leukemia treatment see Tables 2 & 6.

English literature [62, 69, 74, 85–116] in which myeloma was followed by the development of metachronous acute leukemia. Tursz *et al.* [117] reported on the simultaneous occurrence of AML and myeloma. In their monumental review of multiple myeloma terminating in leukemia, Rosner and Grunwald [118] report 19 of 145 cases of leukemia from the world's literature who had the two diseases diagnosed simultaneously or within months. Simultaneous cases are not included in Table 6, but they do raise the question as to whether the two diseases have a common etiology. Bergsagel *et al.* [119] reported briefly on 14 acute leukemias among 364 patients (not on Table 6) entered into a cooperative group study in Canada between 1973 and 1977. This high relative risk of leukemia was 214 times that expected in a normal population and the actuarial risk of developing leukemia reached 17.4% at 50 months of observation and was still on the rise. The confidence limits of that figure are diminished by the fact that only 35 patients were at risk at 48 months. The only other incidence data from a large group are those of the Southwest Oncology Group [111] where six of 476 patients developed acute leukemia. No actuarial risk is reported and the relative risk is obscured by the inclusion in the calculation of five cases of sideroblastic anemia.

Melphalan is the compound most commonly used in the successful management of myeloma. It comes as no surprise that most of the leukemia patients have received it. While alkylating agents clearly cause chromosomal aberrations *in vivo* and *in vitro* [24] its role in this setting is unclear. Radiotherapy was given to some of the patients, generally locally for pain relief, and its role in leukemogenesis is even less clear. The median interval between diagnosis of myeloma and leukemia is 52 months (range 12 to 228). Thus it is necessary that patients survive for a long time to have the leukemia develop. This raises the question as to whether its occurrence is simply a part of the natural history of myeloma, which was not manifest until the development of successful treatment.

Preleukemia was reported in 16 patients (Table 6). This is associated with pancytopenia and frequently sideroblastic anemia. Gonzalez *et al.* [111] reported on five patients with myeloma who developed sideroblastic anemia but not acute leukemia. Marked cytogenetic abnormalities, with hypodiploidy as a common feature, were seen in four of five with preleukemia. Among those who developed leukemia, only one of ten had normal cytogenetics. The other nine had totally abnormal chromosomes. Hypodiploidy and random abnormalities were seen in most. None of the studies were done with banding techniques. Variants of acute myelogenous leukemia were noted in all. Acute promyelocytic leukemia was noted in one case [97]. Only two patients were treated for their leukemia and no responses were noted.

## 5.3. Non-Hodgkin's Lymphoma

Table 7 is a tabulation of 51 patients with a variant of non-Hodgkin's lymphoma who have developed a metachronous acute leukemia [11, 62, 69, 74, 116, 120–132]. Kapadia and Kaplan [133] and Youness *et al.* [134] have reported the simultaneous occurrence of acute myelogenous leukemia in nodular poorly differentiated lymphocytic lymphoma. These cases could represent a fortuitous association—one patient had chronic insecticide exposure [134]—or that both diseases could be etiologically related. Neither patient's leukemia responded to treatment. Table 7 lists the diagnoses of the subclassifications of lymphoma according to that used in the reference. All types of diffuse and nodular disease are represented. All of the patients were treated. Nine patients had no chemotherapy and seven of those nine had intensive radiotherapy (IR) or total body radiotherapy (TBI). Two patients had only localized radiotherapy (SR) in their treatment [123, 131]. Carabell *et al.* [135] report on the development of two acute leukemias among 58 patients with lymphoma treated with total body radiotherapy (TBI). Two cases of erythroleukemia are mentioned, and said to have occurred after combination chemotherapy was given for relapse following TBI. Young *et al.* [127] reported on another AML following TBI, but that patient also received chlorambucil. Rappaport *et al.* [126] and O'Donnell *et al.* [132] report four cases with TBI alone. The chemotherapy (Table 7) was variable from single agents to intensive combinations. Nine leukemias were seen with chemotherapy alone [11, 69, 74, 116, 125, 128, 131]. No specific pattern of treatment related to its intensity or form is evident.

Acute leukemia appeared from six to 160 months from the diagnosis of the lymphoma. This pattern is similar to that seen in Hodgkin's disease and multiple myeloma. The types of leukemia are similar to the other diseases as well. Again, there were four complete [69, 128, 131] and one partial [104] remission among the nine patients treated for their leukemias. Nothing about these cases sets them apart from the rest. One complete remission was achieved after a partial remission by marrow transplantation [131]. Cytogenetics were examined in nine cases and were abnormal in all. No specific abnormalities were noted. It would appear that metachronous acute leukemia occurring following treatment for lymphoma is more responsive to treatment than with other diseases.

## 5.4. Chronic Lymphocytic Leukemia (CLL)

Table 8 lists seven patients with chronic lymphocytic leukemia who developed a metachronous acute myelogenous leukemia [74, 104, 115, 131, 136, 137]. This is a relatively infrequent event. Zarrabi *et al.* [138] reported on 31 cases in which acute lymphoblastic or plasma cell leukemia devel-

*Table 8.* Treatment related leukemia: chronic lymphatic leukemia.

| Ref. | Age/Sex | Chemo-therapy | Radio-therapy | Interval to leuk. | Pre-leuk. | Type leuk. | Leukemia treatment | Resp. | Resp. dur. | Cyto-genetics |
|------|---------|---------------|---------------|-------------------|-----------|------------|--------------------|-------|------------|---------------|
| 136  | 75/F    | CLB           | SR            | 24                | –         | AML        | –                  | –     | –          | –             |
|      | 38/M    | CLB           | SR            | –                 | –         | AML        | –                  | –     | –          | –             |
| 137  | 54/M    | CLB           | None          | 48                | –         | AMML       | –                  | –     | –          | –             |
| 104  | 55/M    | URACIL-MUST.  | None          | 60                | –         | ERY        | –                  | –     | –          | –             |
| 115  | 70/M    | CLB           | None          | 88                | –         | AML        | –                  | –     | –          | –             |
| 131  | 74/F    | None          | TBI           | –                 | –         | ANNL       | –                  | –     | 1          | –             |
| 74   | 55/M    | CLB           | None          | 132               | –         | AMML       | –                  | –     | 4          | ABN           |

URACIL MUST. – uracil mustard.

oped. Eighteen of the patients had no chemotherapy, raising the important question as to whether terminal acute lymphoblastic or plasma cell leukemia was part of the natural history of CLL. The development of AML is more likely treatment related. All of the patients in Table 8 received chemotherapy or radiotherapy and two received both.

## 5.5. Ovarian Cancer

Table 9 lists the 32 cases of metachronous acute myelogenous leukemia which are associated with the treatment of ovarian cancer [69, 74, 139–152]. All of the patients were treated with chemotherapy (30/32) and/or radiotherapy. Zarrabi et al. [151] reported on seven patients in whom acute leukemia occurred in the absence of treatment. Alkylating agents (chlorambucil, melphalan and thiotepa) were most commonly used. Radiotherapy was predominately directed at the pelvis in the 14 patients in which it was used. Eighteen patients received chemotherapy alone. The interval to acute leukemia varied from 18 to 90 months. Preleukemia was rarely noted. Reimer et al. [147] reviewed 70 institutions and identified 13 cases of acute leukemia among 5455 patients treated for ovarian carcinoma and found a relative risk of 21.0. All 13 had received alkylating agents and nine also had radiotherapy. They compared this with an historical control group of 13 300 patients in the National Cancer Institute's End Results Program and found no excess of leukemia, even among 6596 patients who had received radiation. They concluded the leukemogenic effect was due to the alkylating agents alone. Einhorn [148] surveyed 474 patients with ovarian cancer treated with melphalan. Of these, 48 patients had received >300 mg of melphalan. Four cases of acute leukemia developed, and all were among 12 cases receiving 800 mg of melphalan. These data suggest a dose response relationship.

Table 9 lists 13 patients whose leukemia was treated. Two of them showed a response of unknown duration. Eleven patients had cytogenetic studies on the leukemic cells with all of them abnormal and no specific pattern.

## 5.6. Breast Cancer

Table 10 is a list of 34 metachronous acute leukemias which have been reported in the course of the treatment of breast cancer [74, 115, 153–157]. Rosner et al. [157] reported on eight cases of acute leukemia occurring simultaneously with the diagnosis of breast cancer. An additional seven cases (five listed in Table 10) had no post mastectomy radiotherapy or chemotherapy and developed acute leukemia between one and 23 years after the diagnosis. Clearly, the acute leukemias in these patients are not

Table 9. Treatment related leukemia: ovarian cancer.

| Ref. | Age/Sex | Chemo-therapy | Radio-therapy | Interval to leuk. | Pre-leuk. | Type leuk. | Leukemia treatment | Resp. | Resp. dur. | Cyto-genetics |
|---|---|---|---|---|---|---|---|---|---|---|
| 139 | 70/F | TT | None | 30 | – | AML | – | – | – | – |
| 140 | 32/F | CLB | None | 89 | – | AML | – | – | – | – |
| 141 | – | TT, CLB | None | 72 | 3 | AML | – | – | – | – |
| 142 | 38/F | TT, MTX | None | 18 | – | AML | – | – | – | – |
| 143 | 54/F | TT, MTX | None | 87 | 60 | AML | – | – | – | – |
| 144 | 44/F | CYT, TT | 9000R | 40 | – | AML | – | – | – | – |
| 145 | – | CLB | None | 91 | 3 | AML | – | – | – | – |
| 146 | 39/F | CLB | None | 40 | – | ERY | None | – | 2 | – |
| 147 | – | TT | None | 52 | – | AML | – | – | – | – |
| 62 | 48/F | MEL | Pelvis | 48 | – | ERY | DNR, ARAC | – | 10 | ABN |
| 148 | 68/F | MEP | None | 46 | – | AML | None | – | – | – |
| 149 | 51/F | TT | 4500R | 44 | – | AML | DNR, ARAC | NR | 1 | ABN |
| 150 | 56/F | MEL | None | 25 | – | – | – | – | – | – |
| | 47/F | CLB | 5000R | 33 | – | AML | ARAC, TG | Yes | – | – |
| | 45/F | CLB | None | 30 | – | AML | ARAC | Yes | – | – |
| 69 | 56/F | MEL | Pelvis-Abdomen | 42 | – | AML | None | – | 2 | ABN |
| | 37/F | MEL | Pelvis-Abdomen | 31 | – | AML | DNR, ARAC TG OP | NR | 4 | ABN |

*Table 9.* (Continued).

| Ref. | Age/Sex | Chemo-therapy | Radio-therapy | Interval to leuk. | Pre-leuk. | Type leuk. | Leukemia treatment | Resp. | Resp. dur. | Cyto-genetics |
|---|---|---|---|---|---|---|---|---|---|---|
| 151 | 33/F | MEL | Yes | 33 | – | AML | – | – | – | – |
| | 66/F | – | Yes | 90 | – | AML | – | – | – | – |
| | 40/F | FU | Yes | 60 | – | AMML | – | – | – | ABN |
| | 43/F | FU | Yes | 84 | – | AMML | – | – | – | – |
| | 49/F | TT, CYT | None | 92 | – | AMML | – | – | – | – |
| | 56/F | CLB | Yes | 72 | – | ERY | – | – | – | – |
| 152 | 39/F | TREO | None | 51 | – | AML | AODAP | NR | 2 | ABN |
| | 66/F | TREO | None | 53 | – | – | OP | NR | 1 | – |
| | 65/F | TREO | 5000R | 21 | – | AML | OP | NR | 2 | – |
| | 52/F | TREO | None | 56 | – | AML | P | NR | 6 | ABN |
| | 70/F | TREO | None | 48 | – | AML | O, P, TG | NR | 2+ | ABN |
| | 45/F | TREO | None | 48 | – | AML | P, OXY, MTX | NR | 1+ | ABN |
| | 65/F | TREO | None | 58 | – | AMML | P | NR | – | – |
| | 58/F | – | 5000R | 31 | – | AML | None | NR | 1+ | ABN |
| 74 | 47/F | MEL, CLB | 5000R | 56 | – | AML | – | – | 1 | ABN |

TT – thiotepa; FU – 5-fluorouracil; TREO – treosulfan; OP – oncovin, prednisone; OXY – oxymethalone.
For other abbreviations, see prior tables.

*Table 10.* Treatment related leukemia: breast cancer.

| Ref. | Age/Sex | Chemo-therapy | Radio-therapy | Interval to leuk. | Pre-leuk. | Type leuk. | Leukemia treatment | Resp. | Resp. dur. | Cyto-genetics |
|---|---|---|---|---|---|---|---|---|---|---|
| 153 | 56/F | None | Yes | 18 | – | AML | – | – | – | – |
| 154 | 37/F | CYT, CLB | 2500 RT Pelvis | 27 | 1 | AMML | 6MP+P | NR | 1 | 0 |
| 155 | 56/F | CYT, HEX, F | None | 40 | 4 | AML | Supportive | – | 4 | 0 |
| | –/F | None | Yes | – | – | AML | – | – | – | – |
| | –/F | None | Yes | – | – | AML | – | – | – | – |
| | 45/F | None | Yes | 36 | – | AML | – | – | – | – |
| | 65/F | None | None | 48 | – | ALL | – | – | – | – |
| | 67/F | CMF | None | 48 | – | APL | – | – | – | – |
| | 54/F | MFP | None | 96 | – | APL | – | – | – | – |
| | 42/F | None | 5850R | 60 | – | AML | – | – | – | – |
| | 51/F | None | 10,357R | 72 | – | AML | – | – | – | – |
| | 72/F | None | None | 48 | – | AML | – | – | – | – |
| | 62/F | MFV, CLB | 6500R | 72 | – | AML | – | – | – | – |
| | 63/F | None | None | 168 | – | AML | – | – | – | – |
| | 66/F | None | None | 60 | – | AMOL | – | – | – | – |
| | 61/F | None | Yes | 36 | – | AML | – | – | – | – |
| | 42/F | None | Yes | 108 | – | AML | – | – | – | – |

Table 10. (Continued).

| Ref. | Age/Sex | Chemo-therapy | Radio-therapy | Interval to leuk. | Pre-leuk. | Type leuk. | Leukemia treatment | Resp. | Resp. dur. | Cyto-genetics |
|---|---|---|---|---|---|---|---|---|---|---|
| | 31/F | None | 300R | 228 | 1 | AML | – | – | – | – |
| | 44/F | None | 7200 | 108 | – | AML | – | – | – | – |
| | 55/F | THIOTEPA | None | 84 | – | AML | – | – | – | – |
| | 56/F | THIOTEPA | None | 48 | – | AMML | – | – | – | – |
| | 56/F | None | 4600 | 276 | – | AML | – | – | – | – |
| | 67/– | None | | 92 | – | AML | – | – | – | – |
| | 50/F | None | 3500R | 192 | – | AML | – | – | – | – |
| | 51/F | None | 5000R | 24 | – | AMOL | – | – | – | – |
| | 45/F | None | Yes? | 12 | – | AMML | – | – | – | – |
| | 74/F | PAM | Yes? | 18 | – | AMML | – | – | – | – |
| | 24/F | CMFVP | None | 54 | – | AML | – | – | – | – |
| 115 | 57/F | None | Yes | 168 | – | AML | – | – | 2 | – |
| | 52/F | None | Yes | 120 | 48 | AML | – | – | 1 | – |
| | 64/F | None | Yes | 36 | – | AML | – | – | 3 | – |
| | 71/F | None | None | 60 | – | AMOL | – | – | 14 | – |
| 74 | 57/F | TT | ? | 168 | 2 | AML | – | – | 2 | ABN |
| | 67/F | TT | Yes | 120 | 2 | AML | – | – | 2 | – |

HEX – hexamethamelamine; MFV – methotrexate, fluorouracil, vincristine and prednisone. For other abbreviations, see prior tables.

*Table 11.* Treatment related leukemia: other cancers.

| Ref. | Age/Sex | Primary diagnosis | Chemo-therapy | Radio-therapy | Interval to leuk. | Pre-leuk. | Type leuk. | Leukemia treatment | Resp. | Resp. dur. | Cyto-genetics |
|---|---|---|---|---|---|---|---|---|---|---|---|
| 162 | 57/M | Lung | TT | Yes | 60 | – | AML | – | – | – | – |
| 163 | 44/F | Melanoma | Mel | None | 24 | – | AML | DNR, ARAC | NR | – | – |
| 32 | –/– | Brain | BCNU | Yes | 62 | – | AML | DNR, ARAC | CR | 1 | – |
| 62 | 63/M | Thyroid | None | Yes | 36 | – | AMML | – | – | 2 | ABN |
| 78 | 44/M | Seminoma | None | Yes | 24 | – | AMML | – | – | – | ABN |
| 164 | 56/F | Endometrial | Adriacytoxan | Pelvic | 28 | – | AML | ARAC | – | 0 | No |
| 165 | 16/M | Ewing | VCRCYTA | 5000 | 16 | – | AMML | ADR, ARAC | CR | 5 | – |
| 69 | 36/M | Seminoma | None | ABD | 182 | – | ANNL | DNR, ARAC | CR | 4 | – |
|  | 65/M | Lung | CTX, TT | 0 | 42 | – | ANNL | 6-MP | NR | 1 | – |
|  | 47/M | Undiffr. | CCNU | 0 | 48 | – | ANNL | None | – | 2 | – |
| 151 | 39/M | Testis | None | Yes | 264 | – | AML | POMP | NR | 5 | – |
|  | 29/M | Testis | Multiple | None | 27 | – | AML | ARAC, TG | CR | 29 | – |
|  | 24/M | Testis | None | Yes | 15 | – | AML | ARAC, TG | CR | Alive | – |
|  | 32/M | Testis | None | Yes | 192 | – | AMML | ARAC, CYT | NR | 1 | – |
|  | 45/F | Cervix | None | Yes | 9 | – | AVL | 6MP, DNR | PR | 5 | – |
|  | 62/F | Endometrial | None | Yes | 12 | – | AMML | ARAC, DNR | NR | 1 | – |
|  | 57/F | Colon | None | Yes | 42 | – | AML | ARAC, DNR | NR | 1 | – |
|  | 37/F | Colon | TT, CYT | None | 30 | – | AMML | ARAC, DNR, TG | NR | 1 | – |
|  | 66/M | Colon | CYT, VCR | Yes | 36 | – | ERY | None | – | 1 | – |
|  | 75/M | Bladder | TT | None | 72 | – | AML | PRED | NR | 1 | – |
|  | 60/M | Larynx | None | None | 84 | – | AML | ARAC, TG | PR | 9 | – |
| 116 | 42/M | Tonsil | DTIC | Yes | 64 | 18 | AMML | – | – | 1 | – |

ADRIA—adriamycin; VCR—vincristine; POMP—6 mercaptopurine, oncovin, methotrexate and prednisone. For other abbreviations, see prior tables.

treatment related. There appears to be a disproportionately high percentage of breast cancer with simultaneous or non-treatment related metachronous acute leukemia. Both breast cancer [158] and acute leukemia [159] have been shown to have reverse transcriptase; thus, a common viral etiology is possible.

Ten of 36 patients listed in Table 10 received chemotherapy and six of those had no radiotherapy. Nineteen of 36 received radiotherapy, four of them received concomitant chemotherapy. Thus, only four of the listed leukemia patients received both modalities. The interval prior to the development of leukemia ranged from 12 to 276 months. Only six patients (Table 10) had a documented preleukemic phase. Only one patient was treated and that was unsuccessful. There are scant data on cytogenetics. Robins *et al.* [160] have suggested that there may be two syndromes of leukemia, therapy related, with abnormal cytogenetics and resistance to therapy, versus *de novo* leukemia, which may potentially be more responsive. Detailed prospective studies are needed to sort out these patients.

Of particular importance in evaluating this problem is the virtual uniform use of adjuvant chemotherapy in stage II breast cancer patients in the community today. Lerner [161] reported on 13 patients with positive axillary nodes who were placed on long-term adjuvant chemotherapy with chlorambucil at a dose of 0.2 mg/kg daily to a white count of 3000/µl and then maintained between 0.03 and 0.1 mg/kg. Three patients, ages 49, 52 and 64, developed acute myelogenous leukemia. All had chlorambucil continuously for five years and two of three had radiotherapy. The patients had sudden onset of leukemia with no preleukemic phase. All patients failed to respond to treatment of their leukemia. It comes as no surprise that this large cumulative dose of an alkylating agent would net this result. These are clearly treatment related leukemias.

## 5.7. Other Cancers

Table 11 lists 22 patients with a variety of malignant diseases [32, 62, 69, 78, 116, 158, 162–165] who developed metachronous acute myelogenous leukemia in the course of treatment of their primary tumor. One patient [79] received no chemotherapy or radiotherapy. Twelve of 22 patients had chemotherapy, 15 of 22 patients had radiotherapy, and only six had both. Alkylating agents were the predominant form of chemotherapy. The interval to the development of leukemia ranged from nine to 264 months. Only one patient was noted to have preleukemia. The AML variant was treated in 16 of the 22 patients. There were an unprecedented five complete and two partial remissions among these 22 cases. Two of the patients were long-term survivors of their leukemia treatment. Cytogenetics were not performed in any of those cases where a remission was achieved.

This astonishing response rate sets these cases apart from the usual poor responses seen with putative therapy related leukemia. Some of them may be cases of *de novo* metachronous acute myelogenous leukemia. This is yet another justification for careful prospective study of acute leukemia in this setting.

Just as we have seen acute leukemia develop with the use of adjuvant chemotherapy of breast cancer [161], so also does the specter of therapy related leukemia raise its head in the major cooperative group adjuvant studies of other tumors. The use of nitrosoureas in the adjuvant therapy of Dukes' C colon cancer and in Clark's level III melanoma, as part of large scale cooperative clinical trials, will, in the years to come, potentially bring us yet another rash of treatment related leukemia.

## 5.8. Non-malignant Diseases

Table 12 is a list of 55 patients with a wide variety of non-malignant conditions who have developed a metachronous acute myelogenous leukemia [69, 88, 115, 116–186]. Most of these non-malignant diseases have in common a proported immunological mechanism as their basis. The drugs, predominantly alkylating agents and antipurines, are used for their immunosuppressive activity and anticipated positive effect on the disease process. Radiation plays little or no role in this setting. Only three of the 54 patients received any radiation, one received an intraarticular isotope, and two received long wave ultraviolet light (puva) for their psoriasis. The interval prior to the development of leukemia varied from 9 to 132 months. Preleukemia was rarely mentioned. Tulliez *et al.* [174] characterized a 13-month preleukemic phase in a patient treated with chlorambucil for scleroderma for three years. Serial bone marrow examinations showed a gradual decrease in erythroid activity and an increase in myeloblasts. Treatment of the leukemia was sporadic with the expected absence of responses. Chromosome studies were abnormal in seven of eight cases in which they were studied. Tolchin *et al.* [196] studied chromosomes in patients with rheumatoid arthritis and scleroderma before and after the administration of cyclophosphamide, in a dose of 0.5–2.0 mg/kg/day. Chromosome abnormalities were appreciably increased (greater frequency of hypodiploid cells and chromosome breaks) with long-term cyclophosphamide.

The question of whether patients with so-called autoimmune disease are predisposed to the development of malignant disease remains unanswered. Talal *et al.* [197] presented evidence that patients with Sjögren's syndrome, in the absence of immunosuppressive chemotherapeutic agents, are predisposed to develop extra salivary lymphoid abnormalities, including reticulum cell sarcoma. Oleinick [198], on the other hand, found no support for the hypothesis of undue susceptibility to leukemia or lymphoma in individ-

Table 12. Treatment related leukemia: non-malignant diseases.

| Ref. | Age/Sex | Primary diagnosis | Chemo-therapy | Radio-therapy | Interval to leuk. | Pre-leuk. | Type leuk. | Leukemia treatment | Resp. | Resp. dur. | Cyto-genetics |
|---|---|---|---|---|---|---|---|---|---|---|---|
| 166 | –/– | Psoriasis | MTX | None | 84 | – | – | – | – | – | – |
| 167 | 7/M | Pyodermal gangrene | MP | None | 18 | 0 | AML | – | – | – | – |
| 88 | 63/M | Amyloid | MEL | None | 60 | – | AML | – | – | – | – |
| 168 | 54/M | Cold agg. disease | MEL | None | 36 | – | ERY | – | – | – | – |
| 169 | 55/M | RA | CYT, HN2 AZT, MTX | None | 60 | – | AML | – | – | – | – |
| 170 | –/– | Renal disease | CYT | None | – | – | – | – | – | – | – |
| 171 | 31/M | Psoriasis | Bus | None | 42 | – | AML | – | – | – | – |
| 172 | 60/M | Amyloid | MEL | None | 60 | – | AML | – | – | – | – |
| 173 | 29/M | Renal transplant | DAC, AZT | None | 48 | – | AML | – | – | – | – |
| | 18/M | Chronic hepatitis | AZT | None | 48 | – | AML | – | – | – | – |
| 174 | 34/F | Scleroderma | CLB | None | 60 | 13 | AML | Yes | NR | – | – |
| 175 | –/F | Psoriasis | MTX | None | 60 | – | AML | – | – | – | – |
| 176 | 58/F | RA | CYT | None | 72 | – | AMML | – | – | – | – |
| 177 | 49/M | Wegner's | CLB | None | 30 | – | AML | – | – | – | – |
| | 54/M | Wegner's | CYT, CLB | None | 72 | – | AML | – | – | – | – |
| 178 | 32/M | Nephritis | CYT | None | 30 | – | AML | – | – | – | – |
| | 21/M | Nephrotic | AZT, CYT | None | 90 | – | AMML | – | – | – | – |
| | 58/M | Nephritis | CYT | None | 96 | – | AML | – | – | – | – |
| 179 | 42/F | RA | CYT, AZT | None | 54 | – | ERY | – | – | – | – |
| | 47/M | RA | AZT, MEL | None | 72 | – | AML | – | – | – | – |

*Table 12.* (Continued).

| Ref. | Age/Sex | Primary diagnosis | Chemo-therapy | Radio-therapy | Interval to leuk. | Pre-leuk. | Type leuk. | Leukemia treatment | Resp. | Resp. dur. | Cyto-genetics |
|---|---|---|---|---|---|---|---|---|---|---|---|
| 180 | 46/M | RA | CYT | None | 42 | Yes | AML | – | – | – | ABN |
| | 46/F | MS | CLB | None | 96 | Yes | AML | – | – | – | NL |
| | 57/F | RA | CLB | Isotope | 60 | Yes | AML | – | – | – | – |
| 181 | 23/M | SLE | AZT | None | 9 | – | AMML | – | – | – | – |
| 182 | –/– | RA | – | – | – | – | AML | – | – | – | – |
| | –/– | RA | – | – | – | – | AML | – | – | – | – |
| | –/– | RA | – | – | – | – | AML | – | – | – | – |
| | –/– | RA | – | – | – | – | AML | – | – | – | – |
| | –/– | RA | – | – | – | – | AML | – | – | – | – |
| | –/– | RA | – | – | – | – | AML | – | – | – | – |
| | –/– | Scleroderma | – | – | – | – | AML | – | – | – | – |
| | –/– | Temporal | – | – | – | – | AML | – | – | – | – |
| | –/– | Nephritis | – | – | – | – | AML | – | – | – | – |
| 183 | 48/M | Wegner's | CYT | None | 57 | – | AML | – | – | – | – |
| 184 | 45/F | Scleromyxede-ma | MEL | None | 120 | – | ERY | – | – | – | – |
| 185 | 73/F | RA | AZT | None | 39 | – | AML | – | – | – | – |
| 186 | 33/M | Renal trans-plant | AZT | None | 57 | – | AML | – | – | – | – |
| 187 | 44/M | Renal trans-plant | AZT | None | 21 | – | AML | – | – | – | – |
| 188 | 44/F | Sjögrens | CYT | None | 42 | – | AML | – | – | – | – |
| 189 | 51/F | RA | CYT | None | 48 | – | AML | Yes | NR | 1 | ABN |
| 190 | –/– | Psoriasis | NONE | PUVA | – | Yes | PRE | – | – | – | ABN |
| 69 | 34/F | Behçet's | CLB | None | 53 | – | AML | None | – | 5 | – |

*Table 12.* (Continued).

| Ref. | Age/Sex | Primary diagnosis | Chemo-therapy | Radio-therapy | Interval to leuk. | Pre-leuk. | Type leuk. | Leukemia treatment | Resp. | Resp. dur. | Cyto-genetics |
|---|---|---|---|---|---|---|---|---|---|---|---|
| 115 | 52/F | RA | CLB | None | 24 | 2 | AML | — | — | 1 | — |
| | 52/F | Nephrotic | AZT, CLB | None | 60 | — | AML | — | — | 1 | — |
| 191 | 73/F | Psoriasis | 8-METHOX-YPSORLN | PUVA | 35 | — | AML | 6TG, ARAC | NR | 1 | — |
| 192 | -/- | Scleroderma | CLB | None | 26 | — | AMML | OAP | — | 1 | ABN |
| | -/- | Arteritis | CYT, AZT | None | 61 | — | AMML | None | — | 1 | — |
| | -/- | RA | MTX | None | 30 | — | AML | OAP | — | 4 | ABN |
| | -/- | RA | TT, MTX | None | 130 | — | AML | AdOP | — | 1 | ABN |
| | -/- | RA | CLB | None | 24 | — | AMML | COAP | — | 1 | — |
| | -/- | RA | CLB | None | 36 | — | AML | AdOAP | — | 1 | — |
| | -/- | RA | CLB, MTX | None | 56 | — | AMML | COAP | — | 2 | — |
| | -/- | RA | AZT, 6MP | None | 132 | — | ERY | COAP | — | 1 | ABN |
| 193 | 60/M | Sarcoid | MTX | None | 54 | — | AML | — | — | — | — |
| 194 | 1/M | RA | CLB | None | 24 | — | AML | RUB, ARAC | — | — | — |
| 195 | 20/F | MS | CLB | None | 72 | — | AML | DNR, ARAC | — | NR | — |

RA—rheumatoid arthritis; SLE—systemic lupus erythematosis; MS—multiple sclerosis; PUVA—long wave ultraviolet light. For other abbreviations, see prior tables.

uals with autoimmune disease. Clearly, there is a risk of developing acute leukemia when alkylating agents are used in this setting. They should not be used in an indiscriminate fashion, but rather reserved for those life-threatening or truly 'malignant' forms of autoimmune disease.

## 6. DISCUSSION

This review of the English literature on treatment related leukemia does not uniformly or unambiguously answer the question as to whether there is an increased risk of acute myelogenous leukemia following aggressive treatment for malignant and some benign disease. The data concerning the risk of a second malignancy of any kind, given the first, are at best confusing [1–3]. One cannot help but suspect, however, that these predominantly anecdotal reports of treatment related leukemia dating from 1936 to the present may be trying to tell us something.

The pathogenesis of these leukemias is not clear but immunological compromise [4–7], both congenital and acquired, chromosomal damage [8–12] and direct leukemogenic effects of radiation [13–19] and drugs [20–25] undoubtedly play a role. The relationship of benzene exposure [26–28] and acute leukemia represents an interesting model for treatment related leukemia. The pancytopenia, preleukemic phase, latent period for the development of leukemia, cytogenetic abnormalities, and the refractory nature of the acute leukemia, are all features common to treatment related leukemia.

Hodgkin's disease has been most commonly associated with treatment related leukemia. The data from Memorial [80] clearly show an enhanced risk of second malignancy comparing the 1950s with the 1970s. There are two large studies which show that there is an increased actuarial risk of leukemia with intensive combined modality treatment [65, 66, 75]. That risk in one study is now $7.1 \pm 2.6\%$, at nine years [75]. While some cases occur with chemotherapy or radiotherapy alone, the real hazard is with combined modality treatment.

Multiple myeloma is also commonly associated with metachronous acute myelogenous leukemia, but the picture is obscured by 19 reported cases of simultaneous acute leukemia [118], raising the question as to the role of therapy in the metachronous cases. In the only real population study [119] the relative risk of leukemia was 214 times expected, with an actuarial risk of 17.4% at 50 months. This still does not establish cause and effect, in light of the 19 simultaneous cases [118]. This could just be a reflection of myeloma patients at longer risk to develop an acute leukemia, as part of their natural history.

Ovarian cancer has been associated with acute leukemia in the absence of therapy in seven cases [151]. Reimer *et al.* [147], in a survey, have clearly shown a relative risk of acute leukemia in ovarian cancer of 21.0 among 5455 patients treated. They compared this to a historical control of 13 300 patients and found no excess of leukemia. They conclude that alkylating agents were leukemogenic.

Breast cancer presents an unusual problem. Carey *et al.* [199] have found that cancer of the breast treated with surgery alone is associated with a risk of developing acute myelogenous leukemia, which is 30 times that in the general population. The attribution of leukemia to treatment, with chemotherapy and/or radiotherapy, in this setting is clearly a difficult one in the absence of a prospective controlled clinical trial. The definitive answer will come from the national surgical adjuvant breast project (NSABP) comparing L-PAM with placebo (NSABP protocol no. B-05) in stage II breast cancer [200]. The spontaneous leukemias will occur in the placebo group.

The prevention of treatment related leukemia is a complex issue. In Hodgkin's disease there is strong evidence for a relationship with combined modality therapy. Thus, its use as a routine in primary treatment should be avoided. The evidence that combined modality up front enhances survival may be limited to only a few presentations of Hodgkin's disease [57, 76], and only in those cases should treatment begin with combined modality. Another prospect is the use of less leukemogenic combinations of drugs such as ABVD [71]. Careful attention must be given to adjuvant clinical trials in breast, colon cancer, and melanoma. Protracted use of alkylating agents in this setting will inevitably result in the emergence of acute myelogenous leukemia. This is of considerable concern because some of these patients have been cured by their surgical procedure alone. Finally, while the use of leukemogenic agents in advanced malignancy may result in a small percentage of cases of treatment related leukemia, the cost benefit ratio is quite clearly in favor of treatment. Such cannot be said for non-malignant diseases. In these cases, immunosuppressive drugs should be reserved for those truly lifesaving situations with 'malignant' progression of disease.

The future understanding of this problem requires a prospective clinical evaluation of patients in this setting. It should include monitoring for the preleukemic phase, careful cytogenetics, detailed study of the leukemia with surface markers, FAB classification and tissue culture, as well as a careful evaluation of therapy. Only then will we have the tools to manage this perplexing problem, if it cannot be prevented.

REFERENCES

1. Moertel OG, Hagedorn AB: Leukemia or lymphoma and coexistent primary malignant lesions: a review of the literature and a study of 120 cases. Blood 12:788–802, 1957.

2. Einhorn J, Jakobsson P: Multiple primary malignant tumors. Cancer 17:1437–1444, 1964.

3. Berg JW: The incidence of multiple primary cancers. I. Development of further cancers in patients with lymphomas, leukemias, and myeloma. J Natl Cancer Inst 38:741–752, 1967.

4. Gatti RA, Good RA: Occurrence of malignancy in immunodeficiency diseases. Cancer 28:89–98, 1971.

5. Kersey JH, Spector BD, Good RA: Primary immunodeficiency diseases and cancer. The immunodeficiency-cancer registry. Int J Cancer 12:333–347, 1973.

6. Good RA: Relations between immunity and malignancy. Proc Nat Acad Sci 69:1026–1032, 1972.

7. Leibowitz S, Schwartz RS: Malignancy as a complication of immunosuppressive therapy. Adv Intern Med 17:95–123, 1971.

8. Rowley JD: Do human tumors show a chromosome pattern specific for each etiologic agent? J Natl Cancer Inst 52:315–320, 1974.

9. Golomb HM, Vardiman JW, Rowley JD, Testa JR, Mintz V: Correlation of clinical findings with quinicrine-banded chromosomes in 90 adults with acute non-lymphocytic leukemia. An eight year study (1970–1977). N Engl J Med 299:613–619, 1978.

10. Jensen MK: Chromosome studies in patients treated with azathioprine and amethopterin. Acta Med Scand 182:445–455, 1967.

11. Rowley JD, Golomb HM, Vardiman J: Non-random chromosomal abnormalities in acute nonlymphocytic leukemia in patients treated for Hodgkin's disease and non-Hodgkin's lymphomas. Blood 50:759–770, 1977.

12. Pierre RV: Preleukemic states. Sem Hematol 11:73–92, 1974.

13. Cade SS: Radiation induced cancer in man. Br J Radiol 30:393–404, 1957.

14. Emile-Weil P, Lacassagne A: Anémie pernicieuse et leucémie myéloide mortelles provaquées par la manipulation de substances radio-actives. Bull Acad Med 93:237–241, 1925.

15. Ulrich H: The incidence of leukemia in radiologists. N Engl J Med 234:45–46, 1946.

16. Brill AB, Tomonaga M, Heissel RM: Leukemia in man following exposure to ionizing radiation: and a comparison with other human experience. Ann Intern Med 56:590–609, 1962.

17. Court-Brown WM, Doll R: Mortality from cancer and other causes after radiotherapy for ankylosing spondilitis. Br Med J 2:1327–1332, 1965.

18. Smith PG: Leukemia and other cancers following radiation treatment of pelvic disease. Cancer 39:1901–1906, 1977.

19. Linos A, Gray JE, Orvis AL, Kyle RA, O'Fallow WM, Kurland LT: Low-dose radiation and leukemia. N Engl J Med 302:1101–1105, 1980.

20. Harris CC: The carcinogenicity of anticancer drugs: a cancer in man. Cancer 37:1014–1023, 1976.

21. Wydner E: Etiology of lung cancer. Cancer 30:1332–1339, 1970.

22. Hoover R, Cole P: Temporal aspects of bladder carcinogenesis. N Engl J Med 288:1040–1043, 1973.

23. Selikoff I, Hammond E: Environmental cancer in the year 2000. In: Proc 7th National Cancer Conference. Philadelphia: JP Lippencott, 1973, pp 687–696.

24. Sieber SM, Adamson RH: Toxicity of antineoplastic agents in a man: chromosomal aberrations, antifertility effects, congenital malformations, and carcinogenic potential. Adv Cancer Res 22:57–155, 1975.

25. O'Gara RW, Adamson RH, Kelly MG, et al.: Neoplasms of the hematopoietic system in nonhuman primates: report of one spontaneous tumor and two leukemias induced by procarbazine. J Natl Cancer Inst 46:1121–1130, 1970.

26. Vigliani EC, Forni A: Benzene and leukemia. Environ Res 11:122–127, 1976.
27. Askoy M, Erdem S: Followup study in the mortality and development of leukemia in 44 pancytopenic patients with chromic exposure to benzene. Blood 52:285–292, 1978.
28. Forni A, Moreo L: Chromosome studies in a case of benzene-induced erythro-leukemia. Eur J Cancer 5:459–463, 1969.
29. Van den Berghe H, Louwagie A, Broechaert-Van Orshoven A, et al.: Chromosomal analysis in two unusual malignant blood disorders presumably induced by benzene. Blood 53:558–566, 1979.
30. Craver LF: Clinical manifestations and treatment of leukemia. Am J Cancer 26:124–136, 1936.
31. Peters MJ, Middlemiss KCH: A study of Hodgkin's disease treated by irradiation. Am J Roentgen Radium Ther Nuc Med 79:114–121, 1958.
32. Cohen RJ, Wiernik PH, Walker MD: Acute nonlymphatic leukemia associated with nitrosourea chemotherapy: report of two cases. Cancer Treat Rep 60:1257–1261, 1976.
33. Greenberg LH, Cohen M: Histiomonocytic leukemia occurring in a patient with Hodgkin's disease. NY J Med 62:3817–3821, 1962.
34. Lacher MJ, Sussman LN: Leukemia and Hodgkin's disease. Ann Intern Med 59:369–378, 1963.
35. Durant JR: Coexistent DiGuglielmo's leukemia and Hodgkin's disease: a case report with cytogenetic studies. Am J Med Sci 254:824–830, 1967.
36. Ezdinili EZ, Sokal JE, Aungst CW, et al.: Myeloid leukemia in Hodgkin's disease: chromosomal abnormalities. Ann Intern Med 71:1097–1104, 1969.
37. Newman DR, Maldonado JF, Harrison EG, et al.: Myelomonocytic leukemia in Hodgkin's disease. Cancer 25:128–134, 1970.
38. Osta S, Wells M, Viamonte M, Harkness D: Hodgkin's disease terminating in acute leukemia. Cancer 26:795–799, 1970.
39. Steinberg MH, Geary CG, Crosby WH: Acute granulocytic leukemia complicating Hodgkin's disease. Arch Intern Med 125:496–498, 1970.
40. Bergevin PR, Bloom J: Hodgkin's disease terminating in acute erythromyeloblastic leukemia with diabetes insipidus: a case report and review. Med Ann DC 41:625–629, 1972.
41. Chan BWB, McBride JA: Hodgkin's disease and leukemia. Can Med Assoc J 106:558–561, 1972.
42. Kim L, Harley JB: Hodgkin's disease terminating in acute leukemia. W Va Med J 68:23–26, 1972.
43. Wakem CJ, Bennett JM: Hodgkin's disease terminating as acute leukemia. Case report and review of the literature. N Z Med J 76:187–194, 1972.
44. Bonadonna G, DeLena M, Banfi A, et al.: Secondary neoplasms in malignant lymphomas after intensive therapy. N Engl J Med 288:1242–1243, 1973.
45. Castro GAM, Church A, Pechet L, Snyder LM: Leukemia after chemotherapy of Hodgkin's disease. N Engl J Med 289:103–104, 1973.
46. Veenhof CHN, van der Meer J, Gousdmit R: Successfully treated pripism in acute myeloblastic leukemia complicating Hodgkin's disease. Acta Med Scand 194:349–352, 1973.
47. Weiden PL, Lerner KG, Gerdes A, et al.: Pancytopenia and leukemia in Hodgkin's disease: report of three cases. Blood 42:571–577, 1973.
48. Zwann FE, Speck B: Acute myelomonocytic leukemia in a patient with Hodgkin's disease. Acta Haematol 49:291–299, 1973.
49. Kardinal GC, Barnes A, Pugh RP: Acute leukemia: a disease of medical progress? Mo Med 71:683–684, 689, 1974.
50. Sahakian GJ, Al-Mondhiry H, Lacher MJ, et al.: Acute leukemia in Hodgkin's disease. Cancer 33:1369–1375, 1974.

51. Lundh B, Mittkeman F, Milsson DG, Stenstam M, Soderstrom N: Chromosome abnormalities identified by banding technique in a patient with acute myeloid leukemia complicating Hodgkin's disease. Scand J Haematol 14:303-307, 1975.

52. Canellos GP, Arseneau JC, DeVita VT, Wang-Peng J, Johnson REC: Second malignancy complicating Hodgkin's disease in remission. Lancet i:1294-1297, 1975.

53. Canellos GP, DeVita VT, Arseneau JC, et al.: Second malignancies complicating Hodgkin's disease in remission. Lancet i:947-949, 1975.

54. Connolly E: Hodgkin's disease complicated by acute leukemia. Ir Med J 68:6-8, 1975.

55. Raich PC, Carr RM, Meisner LF, et al.: Acute granulocytic leukemia in Hodgkin's disease. Am J Med Sci 269:237-241, 1975.

56. Rosner F, Grunwald H: Multiple myeloma terminating in acute leukemia: report of 12 cases and review of the literature. Am J Med 57:927-939, 1974.

57. Rosenberg SA, Kaplan HS: The management of stages I, II, and III Hodgkin's disease with combined radiotherapy and chemotherapy. Cancer 35:55-63, 1975.

58. Parmley RT, Spicer SS, Morgan SK, et al.: Hodgkin's disease and myelomonocytic leukemia. Cancer 38:1188-1198, 1976.

59. Kroese WFS, Sizoo W, Somers R: Leukemia of the myeloid series in patients with Hodgkin's disease. Neth J Med 19:234-238, 1976.

60. Cadman EC, Capizzi RL, Bertino JR: Acute nonlymphocytic leukemia. A delayed complication of Hodgkin's disease therapy. Analysis of 109 cases. Cancer 40:1280-1296, 1977.

61. Trump DL, Cowall DE: Acute myelogenous leukemia as a late complication of the multimodality therapy for Hodgkin's disease. Johns Hopkins Med J 141:249-251, 1977.

62. Preisler HD, Lyman GH: Acute myelogenous leukemia subsequent to therapy for a different neoplasm: clinical features and response to therapy. Am J Hematol 3:209-218, 1977.

63. Larsen J, Brincker H: The incidence and characteristics of acute myeloid leukemia arising in Hodgkin's disease. Scand J Hematol 18:197-206, 1977.

64. Cavillin-Stahl E, Landberg T, Ottow A, Mitelman F: Hodgkin's disease and acute leukemia. A clinical and cytogenetic study. Scand J Haematol 19:273-280, 1977.

65. Coleman CN, Williams CJ, Flint A, et al.: Hematologic neoplasia in patients treated for Hodgkin's disease. N Engl J Med 297:1249-1252, 1977.

66. Toland DM, Coltman CA Jr., Moon TE: Second malignancies complicating Hodgkin's disease: the Southwest Oncology Group experience. Cancer Clin Trials 1:21-33, 1978.

67. Neufeld H, Weinerman BH, Kamel S: Second malignant neoplasms in patients with Hodgkin's disease. JAMA 239:2470-2471, 1978.

68. Dick FR, Maca RD, Hankenson R: Hodgkin's disease terminating in a T-cell immunoblastic leukemia. Cancer 42:1325-1329, 1978.

69. Foucar K, McKenna RW, Bloomfield CD, et al.: Therapy-related leukemia. A pannmyelosis. Cancer 43:1285-1296, 1979.

70. Kitahara M et al.: Sideroblastic anemia pre-leukemic event in patients treated for Hodgkin's disease. Ann Int Med 92:625-7, 1980.

71. Valagussa P, Santoro A, Kenda RE, Fossati Bellani F, Franchi F, Banfi A, Rilke F, Bonadonna G: Second malignancies in Hodgkin's disease: a complication of certain forms of treatment. Br Med J 1:216-226, 1980.

72. Chan KW, Miller DR, Tan CT: Osteosarcoma and acute myeloblastic leukemia after therapy for childhood Hodgkin's disease – a case report. Med Pediatr Oncol 8:143-149, 1980.

73. Baccarani M, Bosi A, Papa G: Secondary malignancy in patients treated for Hodgkin's disease. Cancer 46:1735-1740, 1980.

74. Kapadia SB, Krause JR, Ellis LD, Dan SF, Wlad N: Induced acute nonlymphocytic leukemia following long-term chemotherapy. A study of 20 cases. Cancer 45:1315-1321,

1980.

75. Coleman CN, Burke JS, Varghese A, Rosenberg SA, Kaplan HS: Secondary leukemia and non-Hodgkin's lymphoma in patients treated for Hodgkin's disease. In: Advances in malignant lymphomas: etiology, immunology, pathology and treatment, Kaplan HS, Rosenberg SA (eds). Academic Press (in press).

76. Coltman CA Jr, Myers JW, Montague E, Fuller LA, Grozea PN, DePersio EJ, Dixon DO: Combined radiotherapy and chemotherapy in the primary management of Hodgkin's disease. A Southwest Oncology Group (SWOG) study. In: Advances in malignant lymphomas: etiology, immunology, pathology and treatment, Kaplan HB, Rosenberg SA (eds). Academic Press (in press).

77. Crosby WH: Acute granulocytic leukemia, a complication of therapy in Hodgkin's disease. Clin Res 17:463, 1969.

78. Arseneau JC, Sponzo RW, Levin DL, *et al.*: Nonlymphomatous malignant tumors complicating Hodgkin's disease. N Engl J Med 287:1119–1122, 1972.

79. Toland DM, Coltman CA Jr: Second malignancies complicating Hodgkin's disease. Proc Am Soc Hematol 18:59, 1975.

80. Brody RS, Schottenfeld D: Multiple primary cancers in Hodgkin's disease. Seminars in Oncology 7:187–201, 1980.

81. Coltman CA Jr: Unpublished SWOG data.

82. Saarni ML, Linman JW: Preleukemia: the hematologic syndrome preceding acute leukemia. Am J Med 55:38-48, 1973.

83. Beltran G, Stuckey WJ: Successful therapy of acute myelogenous leukemia in patients with malignant lymphomas. Blood 52:239 (Supplement), 1978, Abstract 493.

84. Rowley JD, Potter D: Chromosomal banding patterns in acute non lymphocytic leukemia. Blood 47:705–721, 1976.

85. Edwards GA, Zawadzki ZA: Extraosseous lesions in plasma cell myeloma. Am J Med 43:194–205, 1967.

86. Osserman EF: The association between plasmacytic and monocytic dyscrasias in man-clinical and biochemical studies. In: Gamma globulins structure and control of biosynthesis. Proc Nobel Symposium, Killander J (ed). New York: Interscience 1967, pp 573–583.

87. Anderson E, Videback A: Stem cell leukemia in myelomatosis. Scand J Hematol 7:201–201, 1970.

88. Kyle RA, Pierre RV, Bayrd ED: Primary amyloidosis and acute leukemia associated with melphalan therapy. Blood 44:333–337, 1974.

89. Holland JF: Epidemic acute leukemia. N Engl J Med 283:1165–1166, 1970.

90. Cohen SL, Dodsworth H, Whitelaw AGL: Leukemia on myeloma. Br Med J 4:490, 1971.

91. Mills RC, Cornwell GG III, McIntyre OR: Remission of leukemia associated with multiple myeloma. N Engl J Med 285:920–921, 1971.

92. Osserman EF: Monocytic and monomyelocytic leukemia with increased serum and urine lysozyme as a late complication in plasma cell myeloma. Br Med J 2:327, 1971.

93. Scamps RA, O'Neil BJ, Newland RC: A case of multiple myeloma terminating with acute myelomonocytic leukaemia. Med J Aust 2:1129–1130, 1971.

94. Videbaek A: Unusual cases of myelomatosis. Br Med J 2:326, 1971.

95. Webb JAW, Bateman CJT, Davies JD: Leukaemia on myeloma. Br Med J 4:231, 1971.

96. Quirt IC, Hart GD, Soots M: Leukemia on myeloma. Br Med J 1:248, 1972.

97. Holt JM, Robb-Smith AHT, Callender ST, Spriggs AL: Multiple myeloma – development of an alternative malignancy following second malignancy. Br J Haematol 22:633, 1972.

98. Khaleeli M, Keane WM, Lee GR: Sideroblastic anemia in multiple myeloma: a preleukemic change. Blood 41:17–25, 1973.

99. Van Hove W, Hamers J, Demeulenaere L: Acute leukemia in myeloma. Lancet ii:570, 1973.

100. Meytes D, Katz DR: Breast cancer and acute leukemia in a patient with multiple myeloma treated with melphalan. Isr J Med Sci 9:1044–1045, 1047, 1973.

101. Karchmer RK, Amare M, Larsen WE, Mallouk AG, Caldwell G: Alkylating agents as leukemogens in multiple myeloma. Cancer 33:1103–1107, 1974.

102. Rosner F, Grunwal H: Hodgkin's disease and acute leukemia. Report of eight cases and review of the literature. Am J Med 58:339–353, 1975.

103. Marcovic N, Hansson B, Hallen J: Myelomatosis and acute monocytic leukemia. Scand J Haematol 12:32–36, 1974.

104. Cardamone JM, Kimmerle RI, Marshall EY: Development of acute erythroleukemia in B-cell immuno-proliferative disorders after prolonged therapy with alkylating drugs. Am J Med 57:836–844, 1974.

105. Kyle RA, Pierre RV, Bayrd ED: Multiple myeloma and acute leukemia associated with alkylating agents. Arch Intern Med 135:185–192, 1975.

106. Hossfeld DK, Holland JF, Cooper RG, Ellison RR: Chromosome studies in acute leukemias developing in patients with multiple myeloma. Cancer Res 35:2808–2813, 1975.

107. Ligorsky RD, Baker LH, Carmel R: Letter: Multiple myeloma. JAMA 231:347, 1975.

108. Skinnider LF, Ghadially FN: Ultrastructure of acute myeloid leukemia arising in multiple myeloma. Hum Path 6:379–384, 1975.

109. Dahlke MB, Nowell PC: Chromosomal abnormalities and dyserythrpoesis in the preleukemic phase of multiple myeloma. Br J Haemat 31:111–116, 1975.

110. West WO: Acute erythroid leukemia after cyclophosphamide therapy for multiple myeloma: report of two cases. South Med J 69:1331–1332, 1976.

111. Gonzalez F, Trujillo JM, Alexanian R: Acute leukemia in myeloma. Ann Int Med 86:440–443, 1977.

112. Daeshvar-Alavi B, Lutcher CL, Welter D: Multiple myeloma terminating in acute myelogenous leukemia with the presence of a Philadephia (Phl) chromosome. South Med J 70:1477–1479, 1977.

113. Law P, Blom J: Second malignancies in patients with multiple myeloma. Oncology 34:20–24, 1977.

114. Jaeger S: Myelomatosis terminating in acute myelogenic leukemia. Scand J Haemat 20:410–412, 1978.

115. Auclerc G, Jacquillat C, Auclerc MF, Weil M, Bernard J: Post-therapeutic acute leukemia. Cancer 44:2017–2025, 1979.

116. Casciato DA, Scott JL: Acute leukemia following prolonged cytotoxic agent therapy. Medicine 58:32–47, 1979.

117. Tursz T, Flandrin G, Brouet J, et al.: Simultaneous occurrence of acute myeloblastic leukemia and multiple myeloma without previous chemotherapy. Br Med J 2:642–643, 1974.

118. Rosner F, Grunwald H: Multiple myeloma and waldenstrom's macroglobulinemia terminating in acute leukemia: a review with emphasis on karyotypic and ultrastructural abnormalities. NY State J Med 80:558–570, 1980.

119. Bergsagel DE, Bailey AJ, Langley GR, et al.: The chemotherapy on plasmacell myeloma and the incidence of acute leukemia. N Engl J Med 301:743–748, 1979.

120. Beutler F: The development of acute myelogenous leukemia in a patient with reticulum-cell lymphoma. Ann Intern Med 40:1217–1222, 1954.

121. Hornbaker JH: Giant follicular lymphoblastoma terminating in acute myelogenous leukemia. Ann Intern Med 53:221–227, 1960.

122. Zeffren JL, Ultmann JE: Reticulum cell sarcoma terminating in acute leukemia. Blood 15:277–284, 1960.

123. Poth JL, George RP, Creger WP, *et al.*: Acute myelogenous leukemia following localized radiotherapy. Arch Intern Med 128:802–805, 1971.

124. Gunz FW, Levi JA, Lind DE, *et al.*: Development of acute leukemia in a patient with lymphosarcoma. NZ Med J 78:71–75, 1973.

125. Steighbigel RT, Kim H, Potolsky A, Schrier SL: Acute myeloproliferative disorder following long term chlorambucil therapy. Arch Intern Med 134:728–731, 1974.

126. Rappaport AH, Cohen RJ, Castro JM: Erythroleukemia following total body irradiation for advanced lymphocytic lymphoma. Radiology 115:179–180, 1975.

127. Young RC, Johnson RE, Canellos GP, Chabner BA, Brereton HD, Berard CW, DeVita VT: Advanced lymphocytic lymphoma: randomized comparisons of chemotherapy and radiotherapy alone and in combination. Cancer Treat Rep 61:1153–1159, 1977.

128. Collins AJ, Bloomfield CD, Peterson BA, McKenna RW: Acute nonlymphocytic leukemia in patients with nodular lymphoma. Cancer 40:1748–1754, 1977.

129. Goh K, Bauman A, Barsmeier R, Lee H, Woll JE: Leukemia in radiation treated patients: cytogenetic studies in eight cases. Am J Med Sci 276:189–195, 1978.

130. Cavalli F, Sonntag RW, Zimmerman A, Deubelbeiss K, Ryssel HJ: Non-Hodgkin's lymphoma forminating in acute myelogenous leukemia. Acta Haematol 60:250–256, 1978.

131. Zarrabi MH, Rosner F, Bennett JM: Non-Hodgkin's lymphoma and acute myeloblastic leukemia: report of 12 cases and a review of the literature. Cancer 44:1070–1080, 1979.

132. O'Donnell JF, Brerton HD, Greco FA, Gralnick HR, Johnson RE: Acute nonlymphocytic leukemia and acute myeloproliferative syndrome following radiation therapy for non-Hodgkin's lymphoma and chronic lymphocytic leukemia: clinical studies. Cancer 44:1930–1938, 1979.

133. Kapadia SB, Kaplan SS: Simultaneous occurrence on non-Hodgkin's lymphoma and acute myelomonocytic leukemia. Cancer 38:2557–2560, 1976.

134. Youness E, Ahern MJ, Drewinko B: Simultaneous occurrence on non-Hodgkin's lymphoma and spontaneous acute granulocytic leukemia. Am J Clin Path 70:415–420, 1978.

135. Carabell SC, Chaffey JT, Rosenthal DS, Maloney WC, Helman S: Results of total body irradiation in the treatment of advanced non-Hodgkin's lymphomas. Cancer 43:499–1000, 1979.

136. McPhedran P, Health CW: Acute leukemia occurring during chronic lymphocytic leukemia. Blood 35:7–11, 1970.

137. Catovsky D, Galton DAG: Myelomonocytic leukemia supervening on chronic lymphocytic leukemia. Lancet i:478–479, 1971.

138. Zarrabi MH, Grunwald HR, Rosner F: Chronic lymphocytic leukemia terminating in acute leukemia. Arch Intern Med 137:1059–1064, 1977.

139. Allan, WSA: Acute myeloid leukemia after treatment by cytostatic agents. Lancet ii:775, 1970.

140. Smit CGS, Meyler L: Acute myeloid leukemia after treatment with cytostatic agents. Lancet ii:671–672, 1970.

141. Haque T, Lutcher C, Faquet G, Telledo O: Chemotherapy-associated acute myelogenous leukemia and ovarian carcinoma. Am J Med Sci 272:225–228, 1976.

142. Kaslow RA, Wisch N, Glass JL: Acute leukemia following cytotoxic chemotherapy. JAMA 219:75–76, 1972.

143. Greenspan E, Tung B: Acute myeloblastic leukemia after cure of ovarian cancer. J Am Med Assoc 230:418–423, 1974.

144. Rosner F: Acute leukemia as delayed consequences of cancer chemotherapy. Cancer 37:1033–1036, 1976.

145. Sotrel G, Jafari K, Lash A, Stepto E: Acute leukemia in advanced ovarian carcinoma after treatment with alkylating agents. Obstet Gynecol 47, No. 1 (Suppl):67s–71s, 1976.

146. Khandekar JD, Kurtides ES, Stalzer C: Acute erythroleukemia complicating prolonged chemotherapy for ovarian carcinoma. Arch Intern Med 137:355–356, 1977.

147. Reimer RR, Hoover R, Fraumeni JF Jr, *et al.*: Second primary neoplasms following ovarian cancer. J Natl Cancer Inst 61:1195–1197, 1978.

148. Einhorn N: Acute leukemia after chemotherapy (melphalan). Cancer 41:444–447, 1978.

149. Kapadia SB, Krause JR: Ovarian carcinoma terminating in acute nonlymphocytic leukemia following alkylating agent therapy. Cancer 41:1676–1679, 1978.

150. Morrison J, Yon JL: Case Report. Acute leukemia following chlorambucil therapy of advanced ovarian and fallopian tube carcinoma. Gynecol Oncol 6:115–120, 1978.

151. Zarrabi MH, Rosner F: Acute myeloblastic leukemia following treatment for non-hematopoietic cancers. Report of 19 cases and a review of the literature. Am J Haematol 7:357–367, 1979.

152. Pedersen-Bjergaard J, Nissen NI, Sorensen HM, *et al.*: Acute non-lymphocytic leukemia in patients with ovarian carcinoma following long-term treatment with Treosulfan (= Dihydroxbusulfan). Cancer 45:19–20, 1980.

153. Maloney WC: Leukemia and exposure to X-ray: a report of 6 cases. Blood 14:1137–1142, 1959.

154. Davis HL Jr, Prout MN, McKenna PJ, *et al.*: Acute leukemia complicating metastatic breast cancer. Cancer 31:543–546,1973.

155. Rodriguez V, Bodey GP, Trijillo JM, Freireich EJ: Previous radiation exposure in patients with leukemia. Arch Intern Med 132:874–877, 1973.

156. Gardais J: Acute myeloid leukemia complicating a breast cancer after mastectomy and radiotherapy. Scand J Hematol 16:353–356, 1976.

157. Rosner F, Carey RW, Zarrabi MH: Breast cancer and acute leukemia: report of 24 cases and review of the literature. Am J Hematol 4:151–172, 1978.

158. Axiel R, Gulati SC, Spiegelman: Particles containing RNA-instructed DNA polymerase and virus related RNA in human breast cancer. Proc Natl Acad Sci 69:3133–3137, 1972.

159. Gallo RC, Yang SS, Ting RC: RNA dependent DNA polymerase or human acute leukemic cells. Nature 128:927–929, 1970.

160. Robins HI, Ershler WB, Hafez GR, Dohlberg S, Arndt C: Acute non-lymphocytic leukemia in breast cancer: therapy related or de novo? Lancet i:91–92, 1980.

161. Lerner H: Acute myelogenous leukemia in patients receiving chlorambucil as long term therapy in breast cancer at the Pennsylvania Hospital. Cancer Treat Rep 62:1135–1138, 1978.

162. Solomon RB and Firat D: Acute leukemia following treatment with irradiation and alkylating agents. NY State J Med 71:2422–2425, 1971.

163. Burton IE, Abbott CR, Roberts, BE, Antonis AH: Acute leukemia after four years of melphalan treatment for melanoma. Br Med J 2:20, 1976.

164. Reimer RR, Hoover R, Fraumeni JF, Young RC: Acute leukemia after alkylating-agent therapy of ovarian cancer. N Engl J Med 297:177–181, 1977.

165. Smithson WA, Burgert E Jr, Childs DS, *et al.*: Acute myelomonocytic leukemia after irradiation and chemotherapy for Ewing's sarcoma. Mayo Clin Proc 53:757–759, 1978.

166. Rees RB, Bennett JH, Maibach HI, *et al.*: Methotrexate for psoriasis. Arch Dermatol 95:2–11, 1967.

167. Maldonado N, Dorres VM, Mendez-Cashion D, *et al.*: Pyo-derma gangrenosum treated with 6-mercaptopurine and followed by acute leukemia. J Pediatr 72:409–414, 1968.

168. Stavem P, Harboe M: Acute erythroleukemia in a patient treated with melphalan for the cold agglutnin syndrome. Scand J Haematol 8:375–379, 1971.

169. Cobau CD, Sheon RP, Kirsner AB: Immunosuppressive drugs and acute leukemia. Ann Intern Med 79:131–132, 1973.

170. Marshal VC: Skin tumours in immunosuppressed patients. Aus NZJ Surg 43:214–222, 1973.

171. Moller H, Waldenstrom J: ׀Bone marrow damage during treatment of psoriasis with busulfan. Acta Derm Venereol 53:515–516, 1973.

172. Kyle RA, Pierre RV, Bayrd ED: Multiple myeloma and myelomonocytic leukemia. N Engl J Med 283:1121–1125, 1970.

173. Silvergleid AJ, Schrier SL: Acute myelogenous leukemia in two patients treated with azathiprine for non-malignant diseases. Am J Med 57:885–888, 1974.

174. Tulliez M, Richard MF, Jan F, Sultan C: Preleukemaemic abnormal myelopoiesis induced by chlorambucil: a case study. Scand J Haematol 13:179–193, 1974.

175. Bailin PL, Tindall JP, Roenigk HH Jr, et al.: Is methotraxate therapy for psoriasis carcinogenic? A modified retrospective–prospective analysis. JAMA 232:359–362, 1975.

176. Love R, Sowa JM: Myelomonocytic leukemia following cyclophosphamide therapy of rheumatoid disease – a case report. Ann Rheum Dis 34:534–535, 1975.

177. Westberg NG, Swolin B: Acute myeloid leukemia appearing in two patients after prolonged continuous chlorambucil treatment for Wegener's granulomatosis. Acta Med Scand 199:373–377, 1976.

178. Roberts MM, Bell R: Acute leukemia after immunosuppressive therapy. Lancet ii:768–770, 1976.

179. Seidenfeld AM, Smythe HA, Ogryzlo, Dotten DA: Acute leukemia in rheumatoid arthritis treated with cytotoxic agents. J Rheumatol 3:295–304, 1976.

180. Tchernia G, Mielot F, Subtil E, Parmentier C: Acute myeloblastic leukemia after immunodepressive therapy for primary nonmalignant disease. Blood Cells 2:67–80, 1976.

181. Alexson E, Brandt LD: Acute leukemia after azothiodrine treatment of connective tissue disease. Am J Med Sci 273:335–340, 1977.

182. Bukowski RM, Weick JK, Reimer RR, et al.: Characteristics of acute leukemia in patients with non-malignant disease receiving alkylating agent therapy. Blood 50 (suppl):185, 1977.

183. Chang J, Geary GC: Therapy linked leukemia. Lancet i:97, 1977.

184. DeBock RFK, Peetermans ME: Leukemia after prolonged use of melphalan for non-malignant disease. Lancet i:1208–1209, 1977.

185. Gilmore IT, Holgen G, Rodan KS: Acute leukemia during azathioprine therapy. Postgrad Med J 53:173–174, 1977.

186. Sheil AGR: Cancer in renal allograft recipients in Australia and New Zealand. Transplant Proc 9:113–1136, 1977.

187. Sloan GM, Cole P, Wilson RE: Risk indicators of de novo malignancy in renal transplant recipients. Transplant Proc 9:1129–1132, 1977.

188. Hochberg MC, Shulman LE: Acute leukemia following cyclophosphamide therapy for Sjogren's syndrome. Johns Hopkins Med J 142:211–214, 1978.

189. Kapadia SB, Kaplan SS: Acute myelogenous leukemia following immunosuppressive therapy for rheumatoid arthritis. AJCP:301–302, 1978.

190. Wagner J, Manthorper, Philip P, et al.: Preleukemia (haematopoietic dysplasia) developing in a patient with psoriasis treated with 8-methoxypsoralen and haematol. Scand J Haematol 21:299–304, 1978.

191. Hansen NE: Development of acute myeloid leukemia in a patient with psoriasis treated with oral 8-methoxypsoralen and long wave ultraviolet light. Scand J Haematol 22:57–60, 1979.

192. Sheibani K, Bukowski RM, Tubbs RR, Savage RA, Sebek BA, Hoffman GC: Acute non-lymphocytic leukemia in patients receiving chemotherapy for non malignant diseases. Human Pathol 11:175–179, 1980.

108

193. Hermann C, Andersen E, Videbaek A: Acute myeloblastic leukemia in sarcoidosis treated with methotrexate. Scand J Haematol 24:234–236, 1980.
194. Lebranchu Y, Drucker J, Niuet H, Rolland JC, Grenier B, Lejars O, Lampagner JP, Buriot: Acute myeloblastic leukemia in child receiving chlorambucil for juvenile rheumatoid arthritis. Lancet i:649, 1980.
195. Aymard JP, Frustin J, Witz F, Colomb JN, Lederlin D, Herbeuac R: Acute leukemia after prolonged chlorambucil treatment for non-malignant disease: report of a new case and literature survey. Acta Haematol 63:283–285, 1980.
196. Tolchin SF, Winkelstein A, Rodnan GP, Pan SF, Nankin HR: Chromosome abnormalities from cyclophosphamide therapy in rheumatoid arthritis and progressive systemic sclerosis (scleroderma). Arth Rheum 17:375–382, 1974.
197. Talal N, Sokolof L, Barth WF: Extra salivary lymphoid abnormalities in Sjogren's syndrome (reticulum cell sarcoma, pseudolymphoma, macroglobulinemia). Am J Med 43:50–65, 1967.
198. Oleinick A: Leukemia or lymphoma occurring subsequent to an autoimmune disease. Blood 29:144–153, 1967.
199. Carey RW, Holland JF, Sheehe PR, Grahams S: Association of cancer of the breast and acute myelocytic leukemia. Cancer 20:1080–1088, 1967.
200. Fisher B, Redmond C: Breast cancer studies on the national surgical adjuvant breast and colon project (NSABP). In: Adjuvant therapy of cancer, Jones SE, Salmon SE (eds). New York: Grune and Stratton, 1979, pp 215–226.

# 4. The French-American-British Classification of the Acute Adult Myeloid Leukemias: Its Clinical Relevance

JOHN M. BENNETT *

CONTENTS

1.. INTRODUCTION

The acute myeloid leukemias result from the neoplastic transformation of a single pluripotential hematopoietic stem cell. The evidence that all four major morphologic cell lines (myelogenous, monocytic, megakaryocytic, and erythroid) are a part of the malignant process is both morphologic [1] and cytochemical [2]. Moreover, the development of sophisticated methods

* Supported in part by grants CA 11083 and 11198 from the National Cancer Institute, USPHS.

C. D. Bloomfield (ed.), Adult leukemias 1, 109–125. All rights reserved.
Copyright © 1982 Martinus Nijhoff Publishers, The Hague/Boston/London.

that allow for the separation and *in vitro* cloning of leukemic cells provides another piece of evidence supporting the abnormal growth characteristics of leukemic cells. Morphologically abnormal clusters of leukemia blasts can be identified in such cultures and those that have monocytic differentiation can even elaborate colony stimulating activity [3]. Maturation occurs rarely and the cluster (less than 30 colonies) to colony ratio is increased. In addition *in vitro* studies have helped to clarify and further define the important balance between granulocytes and monocytes in the regulation of myelomonopoiesis.

## 2. CLASSIFICATION

Traditionally, the classification of the acute leukemias has been morphologic, usually reflecting the predominant cell type present. The term 'acute' represents an undifferentiated or poorly differentiated blast cell and also refers to a short-term illness that is invariably fatal unless effective chemotherapy is offered to the patient.

The simplicity and ease of having both peripheral blood and bone marrow readily available for the preparation of air-dried films that fix and preserve enzymes, lipids, and glycogen has led to the introduction of both panoptic (Romanowsky stains) and a battery of cytochemical stains. The latter including peroxidase, Sudan black B, periodic acid–Schiff (PAS), esterases and acid phosphatase permit confirmation of the predominant cell type in the acute myeloid leukemias (myelogenous, myelomonocytic, monocytic, and erythroid). Despite the recognition of several subtypes of acute myeloid leukemia, the only neoplastic marker that has been identified with routine staining techniques has been the Auer rod [4]. The proof that these azurophil crystalline-like granules represent the coalescence of primary lysosomal granules of granulocytes has been documented by both histochemical and ultrastructural studies [5, 6].

As long as therapy for the acute myeloid leukemias remained essentially supportive, with complete remissions occurring in less than 10% of patients until the 1960s, attempts to provide uniform classification schemas were a futile exercise in nosology. However, with the advent of combination chemotherapy with cytosine arabinoside, daunorubicin, and 6-thioguanine, complete remissions of greater than 50% are readily achievable. In addition, a significant minority of patients are still in remission beyond two years (see chapter by Keating). It becomes important to include morphologic subtyping among the other known prognostic variables such as age, total leukocyte count and degree of thrombopenia. A uniform classification of the acute myeloid leukemias that is reproducible among different cooperative groups in the United States as well as other major European nations could be of considerable benefit in comparing response rates with similar drug regimens, in identifying geographic differences in subtype composition and in establishing whether favorable or unfavorable subtypes exist and respond differently to various drug regimens.

In 1976 after an intensive review of a large number of cases of various forms of acute myeloid leukemias (AML) a working party consisting of French, American, and British (FAB) morphologists proposed a classification of AML into six subtypes [7]. The proliferation of blast cells of a committed stem cell capable of granulocytic, monocytic, erythroid, and megakaryocytic differentiation can produce a myriad of morphologic variations. The task of the FAB group was to reduce the number of variations to the most commonly recognized subtypes and assign some characteristic features.

The problem that faced the group was to determine how easily the distinction could be made between so-called 'recognized cell types' and with what confidence or concordance among the observers. The role of cytochemistry, electron microscopy, and immunologic markers was also examined and specific recommendations were made.

The clinical features of certain of the myeloid variants have been recognized for many years. Thus the presence of gum hypertrophy and skin infiltrates is associated with a monocytic preponderance (either myelomonocytic or monocytic leukemia) [8, 9] and the occurrence of disseminated intravascular coagulation in acute promyelocytic leukemia is so well recognized that many authorities recommend various preventive measures, including heparin treatment [10].

The minimum requirements for morphologic specifications of each case of acute myeloid leukemia are well made Romanowsky marrow smears and the myeloperoxidase reactions [11]. The cytochemical identification of nonspecific cytoplasmic esterases utilizing sodium fluoride as a potent inhibitor of monocytic esterase is also useful. Utilizing naphthol-ASD acetate as a substrate and fast blue BBN as the diazo dye, acute monocytic leukemia cells invariably give an intense reaction that is strikingly reduced by sodium fluoride incubation. In those myeloid leukemias without a significant monocytic component (usually less than 20%), inhibition is not apparent. In acute myelomonocytic leukemia one can identify either an admixture of blast cells with both myeloid and monocytic features or both cell lines occurring together or combinations of either. There is usually inhibition of at least 25% of the leukemic cell esterase reaction by sodium fluoride [12] and often inhibition of an even larger fraction of the blast cell population. In acute monocytic leukemia virtually all of the blast cells show intense nonspecific esterase activity (either NASDA, alpha naphthyl acetate, or alpha naphthyl butyrate utilized as the substrate) with marked inhibition by sodium fluoride [13].

Other laboratory tests that may be of value in separating the myeloid leukemias include measurement of serum lysozyme, with high levels indicative of a predominant monocytic component, usually above 80 μg/ml [14]. Chromosome analysis, including banding studies, can reveal differences in the pattern of abnormalities as well as degree of aneuploidy [15] and may also have prognostic value [16] (see chapter by Golomb). *In vitro* studies utilizing soft agar gel or semisolid liquid cultures, in addition to providing information on response to colony stimulating factor, cloning efficiency, and colony/cluster ratios, can also provide morphologic evidence of the stem cell origin of the leukemic cells. Romanowsky stains and cytochemical reactions can be applied to the individual colonies [17, 6].

Before discussing the classification proposed by the FAB group for the myeloid leukemias, another problem must be discussed and placed into proper perspective. The FAB group's proposals should be applied only to overt leukemia. The lower limit established for the combined percentage of morphologically abnormal cells was 50%. This was deliberately set somewhat high to minimize the likelihood of a wrong diagnosis being made in the so-called dysmyelopoietic states (refractory anemia with excess blasts, chronic myelomonocytic syndrome, preleukemias) since these conditions may remain static for long periods of time.

## 3. DYSMYELOPOIETIC SYNDROMES (DMS)

DMS are characterized by various degrees of pancytopenia (anemia, thrombopenia, granulocytopenia) associated with normo- to hypercellular bone marrows [18]. Ineffective erythropoiesis is present and is a consequence of the intramedullary destruction of abnormal erythroid precursors. The morphologic expression includes megaloblastic changes, nuclear karyorrhexis, and multinucleation. The reticulocyte count is low, and there is iron accumulation in the bone marrow [19].

In the granulocyte:monocyte series morphologic and enzyme abnormalities are apparent also. Poorly granulated cytoplasm, pseudo-Pelger-Huet-like anomalies, low leukocyte alkaline phosphatase, and myeloperoxidase reactivity are noteworthy. Abnormal maturation in the bone marrow results in a variable increase in blasts and promyelocytes that may equal up to 30% of the total myeloid elements [20]. Similarly the degree of thrombocytopenia is variable with large platelets with prominent granules visible in the peripheral blood. The bleeding time and qualitative platelet studies may be abnormal [21]. Megakaryocytes are found in the bone marrow examination but often are atypical and small [22].

The major difference between refractory anemia with excess blasts (RAEB) and chronic myelomonocytic syndrome (CMMS) is the presence of an absolute monocytosis (greater than $2 \times 10^9$ cells/l) and monocytic precursors visible on bone marrow preparations or demonstrated by the esterase reaction [23]. Increased serum and urinary lysozyme is present invariably. In all of the DMS the disease usually affects patients older than 50 years, although rarely cases can be seen in younger patients.

In addition to the morphologic evidence, cell kinetic and chromosome studies suggest very strongly that DMS is a result of a neoplastic transformation of the committed hematopoietic stem cell [24–26].

The paradox has been the inability up to the present to predict accurately the survival outcome of this large group of patients that probably is equivalent to the number of overt leukemias diagnosed each year. The presence of increased numbers of blasts, promyelocytes, and/or monocytes implies that progression to leukemia should be a regular occurrence. However, a review of 102 patients with RAEB demonstrated that only 28% developed overt leukemias, with a median survival of approximately 2½ years and some patients lived without blastic progression for more than 4 years [18]. In my own experience patients who present with either severe granulocytopenia (below $5 \times 10^8$/l), severe thrombopenia (below $5 \times 10^{10}$/l) or circulating blast cells in the peripheral blood progress rapidly to overt leukemia, usually within a few months. The presence of unequivocal Auer rods in the blast cells is also an ominous sign and most authorities reject such cases from DMS.

Unfortunately the diagnosis of DMS signifies a fatal outcome in the majority of patients, certainly within five years, often from the consequences of marrow failure with death secondary to infection and/or hemorrhage. The introduction of aggressive combination chemotherapy in DMS is rarely effective [27], and patients usually expire with an aplastic marrow. Attempts to use 'gentle treatment' with corticosteroids or male hormones have had only limited success [28, 29]. General hematemics including folic acid, vitamin $B_{12}$, and pyridoxine have been tried without any benefit.

In order to allow for some leeway in the diagnosis and management of DMS and the diagnosis and treatment of the acute myeloid leukemias, the FAB group determined that a 'safety zone' of approximately 20% additional blasts and promyelocytes should exist between the two entities. Whenever the upper limit of 30% is identified in a patient with DMS, frequent bone marrows are necessary (usually every 2–3 months) to assess carefully progression toward overt leukemia. Unfortunately there is no current national trial that has addressed the question of conservative treatment with blood transfusion, platelets and antibiotics where indicated versus aggressive combination chemotherapy taken to marrow aplasia. Until this study is carried out, each patient with DMS should receive individualized treatment based on sound clinical judgment.

## 4. TREATMENT RELATED ACUTE LEUKEMIA

This topic is described fully in another chapter by Dr. Coltman. However, one issue should be addressed within the framework of classification of the acute leukemias and the dysmyelopoietic syndromes. In addition to the documentation of several hundred treatment related overt leukemias [30], evidence is accumulating that preleukemic states including refractory anemia with excess blasts can be induced by both alkylating agents, particularly chlorambucil [31] and other chemotherapeutic drugs, often with irradiation [32].

Few authors have addressed the specific cell type of the treatment related acute leukemias. Such terms as 'acute myeloid leukemia,' 'acute myeloblastic leukemia,' 'histiomonocytic leukemia,' 'acute myelogenous leukemia,' 'erythromegakaryocytic leukemia,' 'myelomonocytic leukemia,' 'acute non-lymphocytic leukemia,' 'erythroleukemia,' 'acute granulocytic leukemia,' and 'acute leukemia' have been introduced into the titles of articles written on this subject. Only a few authors [33, 34] have addressed the issue of subclassification of the myeloid leukemias in their articles. What can be said with certainty is that the vast majority of the induced leukemias are morphologically similar to the acute myeloid leukemias. When cytochemical studies have been carried out, confirmation of this class of leukemias has been found (peroxidase positive, elevated muramidase levels, high nonspecific esterase). Only a small number of lymphocytic induced leukemias have been reported. The specific subtype of acute lymphocytic leukemia has usually not been described. A recent article describes two cases of Burkitt's cell leukemia occurring in two adults with Hodgkin's disease treated with radiation therapy and nitrosourea-containing drug combinations [35].

The prevalence of the various subtypes and whether the induced leukemias have a different incidence when classified according to the FAB classification will require the establishment of a referral or repository center where all investigators can send material for confirmation of diagnosis. For the present the minimal requirements prior to publication of induced leukemia cases should be a cytochemical battery including peroxidase staining and nonspecific esterase. Until sufficient information is accrued on this important aspect of the treatment of induced leukemias, statements regarding the poor response to therapy should be viewed with some reservation, since certain cell types within the FAB classification may not respond as well as others.

5. THE ACUTE MYELOID LEUKEMIAS

Utilizing selected cytochemical stains and morphologic criteria the FAB group defined six variants of acute myeloid leukemia: three subtypes (labeled as M1, M2, and M3) are predominantly of granulocytic origin; two subtypes are predominantly or exclusively monocytic (M4, M5) with greater than 20% monocytic precursors recognized in the bone marrow morphologically or cytochemically or by an absolute peripheral blood monocytosis $(5 \times 10^9$ cells/l), and one type (M6) that has a higher proportion of erythroblasts.

## 5.1. Myeloblastic Leukemia without Maturation (M1)

This type consists of poorly differentiated blasts with rare azurophil granules and even some cells with Auer rods. In the total absence of granules, a diagnosis of acute undifferentiated leukemia would be a consideration of acute lymphocytic leukemia. Confirmatory cytochemical stains revealing greater than 3% positive peroxidase blast cells are necessary to establish a granulocytic origin.

## 5.2. Myeloblastic Leukemia with Maturation (M2, M3)

Both of these types require that greater than 50% of the abnormal cells have matured to the promyelocyte stage or beyond. In M2 the promyelocytes appear normal and Auer rods may be present in a moderate number of the cells. Eosinophilic myelocytes are often a prominent feature and pseudo-Pelger cells can be identified in the peripheral blood.

The special variant (M3), or hypergranular promyelocytic leukemia [36], reveals highly abnormal and bizarre blast cells with twisted and bilobed nuclei and cytoplasm packed with azurophil granules and at least a few cells with bundles of thin rods resembling Auer rods ('faggots'). An atypical form with minimal granulation has been described [37] with an emphasis on the bilobed or uniform nucleus. This variant of M3 is often associated with high leukocyte counts (up to $200 \times 10^9$ cells/l). As discussed in more detail in the chapter by Golomb, with both types a particular chromosomal translocation, t(15; 17) has been reported [38]. If the distinctive nuclear features of the variant cells are overlooked then a diagnosis of either M2 or myelomonocytic leukemia (M4) would be entertained. The distinction is of the utmost importance because of the regular association between M3 and disseminated intravascular coagulation.

## 5.3. Myelomonocytic Leukemia (M4)

In this form both monocytic and granulocytic components coexist in varying proportions but with a minimum of 20% monocytic precursors in the bone marrow. A well-recognized variant is characterized by a significant peripheral blood monocytosis. The monocytic component may be difficult to recognize on bone marrow aspirates, and therefore the nonspecific esterase stain with and without sodium fluoride is recommended, particularly when there is leukopenia present.

### 5.4. Acute Monocytic Leukemia (M5)

Acute monocytic leukemia exists in two forms. The absolute number of granulocytic precursors is below 20% and usually not a recognizable feature. In one type, referred to as $M5_A$, the blast cells are so poorly differentiated that most of the monocytic features are missing. The nuclear:cytoplasmic ratio is low and the cells are very large (up to 30 μm or larger). The nucleus is round to oval with a delicate or reticulated chromatin pattern. There are usually one or two prominent nucleoli. The cytoplasm is basophilic with rare azurophil granules or none. Auer rods are distinctly uncommon. $M5_A$ can be confused with acute lymphocytic leukemia and may resemble Burkitt's cell leukemia.

The second form of acute monocytic leukemia ($M5_B$) closely resembles that described by Schilling in 1913 [39]. The cells are more differentiated with twisted or folded nuclei. The cytoplasm is abundant with gray-blue color and scattered azurophil granules. The term 'promonocytes' can be applied to many of these leukemic blast cells. As a morphologic entity both forms of acute monocytic leukemia are very homogeneous and represent between 5 and 10% of cases in most series of acute myeloid leukemias.

*5.4.1. Cytochemistry of Acute Monocytic Leukemia ($M5_A/M5_B$).* The peroxidase reaction is usually weakly positive or can be negative. At least 50% of cases have no recognizable peroxidase activity. Occasionally the sudan black B reaction will be positive when the peroxidase stain is negative. The cells consistently have a strongly positive nonspecific esterase reaction which is sodium fluoride inhibited. Cells with monocytic differentiation at an early stage of maturation as described above ($M5_A$ and $M4_B$) may express on the cytoplasmic membrane receptors for 'cytophilic antibody' (the $F_c$ fragment of IgG). This receptor can be demonstrated utilizing the rosette formation with human erythrocytes that have been coated with anti-D. Correlations with cytochemistry and immunologic markers can be made successfully [40].

### 5.5. Acute Erythroleukemia (M6)

The diagnosis of acute erythroleukemia is clear when the majority of the bone marrow precursors are erythroblasts with megaloblastoid features. At least 30% of the nucleated marrow cells should be of erythroid origin with about equal numbers of blast cells of either granulocytic, myelomonocytic, or monocytic cell type. Usually the erythroid cells have striking nuclear: cytoplasmic asynchrony with bizarre nuclear outlines, nuclear karyorrhexis, and bi and tri nucleation. Howell-Jolly bodies are frequent. It is important to distinguish M6 from florid megaloblastic marrows (secondary to vitamin $B_{12}$ or folate deficiency, for example) and from the dysmyelopoietic syndromes (DMS) previously discussed. A trial of vitamin therapy or observation for several weeks if one suspects DMS is probably worthwhile when some doubt exists in establishing the diagnosis. Chromosome analysis may be of some help in separating M6 and DMS from benign megaloblastic marrow status [41]. The use of iron stains to demonstrate abnormal ringed sideroblasts and PAS stains that reveal, on occasion, diffuse or block staining, although positive in some cases of M6, can be demonstrated in megaloblastic marrows as well as in DMS.

## 6. REPRODUCIBILITY OF THE MYELOID LEUKEMIA CLASSIFICATION

There is virtually no literature available on the ability of one group to reproduce accurately the classification proposed by another group. In developing the FAB myeloid classification the morphologists were able to agree on about 85% of the cases examined. At a workshop sponsored by the Southwest Oncology Group in Phoenix, Arizona (Sept. 1, 1980), a series of slides were circulated by the pathologists representing the Hematology Committee. There was 100% concordance between the members of the committee and a representative from the FAB workers group (JMB) utilizing the FAB subtypes (M1–M6). A complete cytochemical profile was available in each case, including the esterase stains. We had demonstrated previously that consistent employment of cytochemistry enables the investigator to predict the correct FAB diagnosis in over 80% of cases [11].

Until recently the selection of patients for national leukemia trials was left to the discretion of the institutional hematologist or oncologist. The 'on study' diagnosis so recorded became the diagnosis of record. In 1973 the Eastern Cooperative Oncology Group initiated its first group-wide study of acute 'adult nonlymphocytic leukemia.' The results of this program will be discussed later [42]. A mandatory requirement for protocol eligibility in this program and all subsequent ECOG leukemia studies was the prompt submission of at least 6 unstained marrow slides for confirmatory cytochemical studies.

Since this study was begun prior to the publication of the FAB classification, only the major forms of ANLL were employed in subtyping: AML (peroxidase positive; NASDA positive and not inhibited by NaF); AMML (peroxidase positive; NASDA positive and inhibited by NaF); AMoL (usually peroxidase negative or weakly positive; NASDA strongly positive with marked inhibition by NaF) and erythroleukemia. There was complete agreement on only 48% of the cases studied. Only 2% of cases submitted were excluded because of a diagnosis of acute lymphocytic leukemia, the remainder representing minor disagreements among myeloid subtypes. There was no difference between subtypes in regard to the percentage agreement. The final distribution of subtypes established in the reference laboratory was: AML, 46%; AMML, 47%; AMol, 5%; erythroleukemia, 2%. Only one patient with acute promyelocytic leukemia was identified.

Considering the response rates based on the reference laboratory diagnosis, no significant differences were observed among the various morphologic subtypes. The complete remission rate (CR%) was 29% for the entire study (111 patients). Significant prognostic factors that favored a higher response included age (over 60 years having a CR% of 16%, under age 60 years, a CR% of 38%), performance status (nonambulatory, a CR% of 16%; ambulatory status, a CR% of 44%) and percentage of marrow blasts prior to therapy (>50% having a CR% of 24%, with <50% having a CR% of 48%). Response duration was significantly greater for AML (49 weeks) than for AMML (31 weeks) with a P value of 0.02. This did not translate into a survival advantage, however. All of the patients with acute monocytic leukemia have expired. At three years after entry of the last patient onto the protocol 10% of patients were still alive and 5.4% were still in their first complete remission.

In 1976 a successor study for adults with acute myeloid leukemia was launched by the ECOG [43]. Once again mandatory submission of unstained air-dried bone marrow smears was required. A cytochemical battery was performed and the cases were classified according to the FAB criteria. Of the 332 adults registered on this program, which compared the effectiveness of two induction schedules utilizing daunorubicin and cytosine arabinoside primarily, consolidation with the induction program, and maintenance with either BCG or BCG plus cytosine arabinoside and 6-thioguanine, 280 were eligible for response, response duration and survival.

The single most important disagreement in assessing the pretreatment bone marrow was the reclassification of cases as acute lymphocytic leukemia (ALL). This occurred in only 15 patients, representing 5.3% of the series. The diagnosis of ALL was made on the basis of a negative peroxidase reaction, low NASDA, and appropriate morphology (FAB types L1, L2, or L3). Most of the cases fell into the L2 category in which the cells are more pleomorphic and contain visible nucleoli. Of interest was the finding of three L3 cases ('Burkitt's cell leukemia').

Within the myeloid cell types according to the FAB criteria, the distribution revealed 10% as M1, 30% as M2, 11% as M3, 37% as M4, 9% as M5, and 3% as M6. The overall agreement percentage was 61% between the investigators' morphologic diagnosis and the repository center, with the highest concordance being with hypergranular promyelocytic leukemia, namely 88%. A major problem was in the overcalling of cases of M4 as M5 (4/17 cases) and the failure to recognize 18 cases of M5, classified by the investigators as M4. In virtually all of these instances there was no evidence that cytochemical stains were performed.

Yet, there was an improvement of 27% from the first ECOG leukemia study to this program in the agreement ratio. Of the 27 institutions contributing cases six carried out cytochemical staining on a routine basis. These programs contributed a significant minority of the cases and the agreement of their diagnoses was much closer to the repository center. It is likely that improved accuracy of subtype classification will occur when all institutions carry out routine cytochemical evaluation of their pretreatment bone marrow preparations.

Certain prognostic variables were examined among the M1–M6 cytologic types to determine if any imbalances had occurred that might impact on either response or survival. Patients with hypergranular promyelocytic leukemia tended to be younger (37% under age 30 years) compared to an average of 20% for the other types. Moreover, when a comparison of total leukocyte counts was made, 56% of patients with M3 had counts below 5000/µl compared to 21% of the other types. Therefore, in contrast to the other forms of acute myeloid leukemia, patients with M3 should have a more favorable outcome, if one views age and blast count as important prognostic parameters [44].

The overall complete remission rate was 51% from the first day of treatment [45]. Examination of the individual FAB subtypes revealed the following complete remission rates: M1 and M2, 53%; M3, 53%; M4, 61;; M5, 32%; and M6, 43%. The only statistically significant difference existed between M5 (acute monocytic leukemia) and all other cell types ($p<0.05$, $>0.01$).

The longest response duration occurred in patients with M3 (median of 47 weeks) and the shortest was in both cell types M5 and M6 (7 weeks). These latter two cell types were significantly lower than the others. All patients with acute monocytic leukemia and erythroleukemia have relapsed, whereas between 22 and 40% of the other myeloid cell types who entered complete remission had not relapsed 3½ years after the study was initiated.

## 7. SURVIVAL DATA

The median survival of all patients entered into this recent program was 28 weeks. However, patients treated with one of the two induction regimens

*Table 1.* Hypergranular promyelocytic leukemia.

|           | Heparin+   | Heparin−  | Total      |
|-----------|------------|-----------|------------|
| CR        | 11 (61 %)  | 5 (45 %)  | 16 (55 %)  |
| NC/PROG   | 7          | 6         | 13         |
| Total PTS | 18         | 11        | 29         |

(daunomycin and cytosine arabinoside) fared much better than the other (38 weeks vs. 9 weeks). Despite the longer remission duration of patients with M3, this was not reflected by a longer survival (28 weeks). This was due to a large number of early deaths, within the first five weeks of treatment, secondary to either massive pulmonary or intracranial hemorrhage (17 % of patients). Intravascular coagulopathy was present in 77 % of cases. The prophylactic administration of heparin to the majority of patients (Table 1) was associated with a higher though not statistically significant percentage of responses. More emphasis on adequate blood product replacement (platelets, fibrinogen, cryoprecipitate, etc.) is probably the single most important consideration during induction therapy.

There were 22 patients diagnosed as having acute monocytic leukemia (M5). Associated with the lower response rate of 32 % was a very poor median survival of 1 month, a short median survival of the responders (6.5 months) and an absence of any survivors beyond two years.

## 8. CENTRAL NERVOUS SYSTEM (CNS) RELAPSE

CNS relapse has been an uncommon event in this program to date. There have been 9 cases identified out of the 280 eligible for analysis (3.2 %). The onset of CNS leukemia ranged from presentation (one case) to two years after diagnosis. Six of the patients had a predominant monocytic component (four with M4 and two with M5). A recent prospective study of 39 patients with acute granulocytic leukemia [46] reported only positive CSF fluid for blast cells in patients with AMML (7 of 39 patients). The authors suggest that the leukemia cells in patients with AMML may have a higher tendency to penetrate the blood brain barrier. Support for this concept has been provided by Lichtman and Weed [47] and our own observations in which two-thirds of the relapses in CSF were observed in patients with either M4 or M5. If these observations can be repeated, then serious consideration for intrathecal treatment with methotrexate must be given for such patients.

The FAB classification of the acute myeloid leukemias was introduced in 1976. Since its publication few articles have appeared relating cell type to survival. Foon and co-workers [48] did not find significant differences between the FAB cell types. However, in their series, the complete remission rate was very high (86%) and extraordinary compared to most published studies [49] and the numbers of patients with the rarer cell types very low. Therefore there are insufficient patients with at least three FAB cell types (M3, M5, M6) to provide a valid comparison with the major cell types (M1, M2, and M4).

The literature on response rates and survival comparison between the major myeloid subtypes (M1 and M2) and myelomonocytic leukemia (M4) as well as our own data from the two studies discussed in detail does not support significant differences at the present time. However, several groups have confirmed the unfavorable prognosis of M5 [50, 13].

Cuttner and co-workers [51] reported that patients with either M4 or M5 were more likely to have leukocyte counts above 100 000/µl than patients with M1–M3. Cytochemical stains (peroxidase, NASDA, NASDA-F) were utilized to separate M1–M3 from M4–M5. Serum lysozyme levels were significantly higher in patients with M4 and M5 (mean 59.7 µg/ml) compared to M1–M3 (mean 18.9 µg/ml). Response rates were not significantly different between the two groups but patients with counts over 100 000/µl had lower response rates than those with lower counts (47% vs. 70%). The authors fail to separate the acute monocytic leukemias (M5) from the AMMLs (M4). Since this group of patients in our experience fares very poorly, it is difficult to appreciate what impact the M5 patients might have had in this study.

Patients with hypergranular promyelocytic leukemia (M3) are at significant risk from fatal hemorrhage early in the induction program. Our data demonstrate that appropriate vigorous support of such patients with or without heparin allows an identical response and durable remissions once achieved for over 50% of patients with M3. Similar results have been observed by Collins and co-workers [52] and by Bernard [35]. The latter group reported that there were six long-term survivors representing 24% of all patients treated between 1973 and 1976. Whether these impressive results can be duplicated elsewhere remains to be seen.

The final subtype of interest are the small numbers of patients with erythroleukemia (FAB M6). In our recent series the complete remission rate was 37% with a median survival of 42 days. As with acute monocytic leukemia, no patients remained in long-term remission and all patients have expired within 1 year of diagnosis.

Because of the paucity of cases of M6, there is very little literature available for comparison. Utilizing single drug therapy, Scott, Ellison, and Ley had no responses in 20 patients, but the series represented patients treated in the early 1960s [54]. More recently Bloomfield et al. treated nine patients with M6 and had four complete remissions. The median survival was 12 months, and two patients were still alive at 17 and 23 months, respectively, after treatment [55]. It is not apparent from a careful review of the data of this latter series and our own, what factors resulted in a better response duration in the Minnesota study. Nevertheless it is clear that remissions can be obtained in patients with acute erythroleukemia, but the long-term survival is probably inferior to the other subtypes with the exception of acute monocytic leukemia.

## 9. CONCLUSIONS

Well-prepared Romanowsky stained smears supplemented by appropriate staining procedures (peroxidase, nonspecific, and specific esterases) have become established as important aids in classifying the acute leukemias. Utilizing cytochemical criteria, the myeloid leukemias can be classified into six morphologic subtypes (M1–M6). Specific clinical and laboratory features are well-correlated with certain cell types such as M3 and M5. Recognition of these morphologic variants is important because of the catastrophic events that may occur following treatment (M3) or extramedullary relapses (M5) that impact adversely on survival. The increasing frequency of treatment induced leukemias provides another area for cytochemical investigations. Important clues as to etiology and causation may result from an analysis of distribution of cell types of induced acute myeloid leukemias compared to spontaneous cases.

Over the past decade treatment strategies for the acute myeloid leukemias have resulted in a steady improvement in complete remissions and the percentage of patients who survive for two years or longer. As the percentage of complete remissions increases, the ability to detect differences between morphologic subtypes becomes more difficult statistically. Consistency and reproducibility in the identification of morphologic variants becomes, then, increasingly important as well as large numbers of patients treated with identical regimens. The national and international cooperative groups, sponsored by the National Cancer Institute and other cooperating nations, provides such a mechanism. The establishment of sophisticated cytochemical and immunologic laboratories in support of these programs should allow for appropriate evaluation of the impressive results that have been reported in clinical trials of the acute myeloid leukemias.

REFERENCES

1. Morley A, Higgs D: Abnormal differentiation of leukemic cells in vitro. Cancer 33:716–720, 1974.

2. Jensen MK, Killman S-A: Additional incidence for chromosome abnormalities in the erythroid precursors in acute leukemia. Acta Med Scand 189:97–100, 1971.

3. Brennan JK, DiPerson JF, Abboud CN, Lichtman MA: The exceptional responsiveness of certain myeloid leukemic cells to colony stimulating activity. Blood 7:1230–1239, 1979.

4. Auer J: Some hitherto undescribed structures found in large lymphocytes of a case of acute leukemia. Am J Med Sci 131:1002–1015, 1906.

5. Ackerman GA: Microscopic and histochemical studies on the Auer bodies in leukemic cells. Blood 5:847–863, 1950.

6. Bainton DF, Friedlander LM, Shohet SB: Abnormalities in granule formations in acute myelogenous leukemia. Blood 49:639–704, 1977.

7. Bennett JM, Catovsky D, Daneil M-T, Flandrin G, Galton DAG, Gralnick HR, Sultan C: Proposals for the classification of the acute leukemias. Br J Haematol 33:451–458, 1976.

8. Forkner CE: Clinical and pathologic differentiation of the acute leukemias. Arch Intern Med 53:1–34, 1934.

9. Mercer ST: Dermatosis of monocytic leukemia. Arch Dermatol Syphil 31:615–635, 1935.

10. Gralnick HR, Sultan C: Annotation: acute promyelocytic leukemia, hemorrhagic manifestation and morphologic criteria. Br J Haematol 29:373–376, 1975.

11. Bennett JM, Reed CE: Acute leukemia cytochemical profile: diagnostic and clinical implications. Blood Cells 1:101–108, 1975.

12. Daniel M-T, Flandrin G, LeJeune F, Lisio P, Lortholary P: Les estérases, spécifiques monocytaire. Utilization des leucémies aiguës. Nouv Rev Fr Hématol 11:233–239, 1971.

13. Sultan C, Imbert M, Richard ME et al.: Pure acute monocytic leukemia. Am J Clin Pathol 68:752–757, 1977.

14. Currie G: Prognostic significance of serum lysozyme in adult acute myelogenous leukemia. Lancet i:835–837, 1976.

15. Rowley JD, Potter D: Chromosome banding patterns in acute nonlymphocytic leukemia. Blood 47:705–721, 1976.

16. Golomb HM, Vardiman JW, Rowley JD, et al.: Correlation of clinical findings with quinacrine-banded chromosomes in 90 adults with acute nonlymphocytic leukemia. N Engl J Med 299:613–619, 1978.

17. Spitzer G, Verma DS, Dicke KA, McCredie KB: Culture studies in vitro in human leukemia. Semin Hematol 15:352–378, 1978.

18. Dreyfus B: Preleukemic status: I. Definition and classification: II. Refractory anemia with excess of myeloblasts in the bone marrow (smouldering acute leukemia). Blood Cells 2:33–55, 1976.

19. Valentine WN, Konrad PN, Paglia DE: Dyserythropoiesis refractory anemia and 'preleukemia' metabolic features of the erythrocytes. Blood 41:857–875, 1973.

20. Sultan C: Dysmyelopoietic syndromes. In: Classification of acute leukemia, pp 749–752, Gralnick HR (moderator). Ann Intern Med 87:740–753, 1977.

21. Sultan Y, Cane JP: Platelet dysfunction in preleukemic states and various types of leukemia. Ann NY Acad Sci 201:300–306, 1972.

22. MacDonald JE, Pintado T: Ultrastructure of the megakaryocytes in refractory anemia and myelomonocytic leukemia. In: Platelet production, function, transfusion and storage, Baldini MG, Ebbe S (eds). New York: Grune and Stratton, 1974, p 105.

23. Zittoun R: Subacute and chronic myelomonocytic leukemia: a distinct hemotologic entity (annotation). Br. J Haematol 32:1–7, 1976.

24. Pierre RV: Preleukemic states. Semin Hematol 11:73–92, 1974.

25. Nowell PC, Finan J: Chromosome studies in preleukemic states. Cancer 42:2254–2261, 1978.

26. Koeffler HP, Golde DW: Cellular maturation in human preleukemia. Blood 52:355–361, 1978.

27. Cohen JR, Creger WP, Greenberg Pl, Schrier SL: Subacute myeloid leukemia. A clinical review. Am J Med 66:959–966, 1979.

28. Bagby CG Jr, Gabourel JD, Linman JW: Glucocorticoid therapy in the preleukemic syndrome: identification of responsive patients using in vitro techniques. Ann Intern Med 92:55–58, 1980.

29. Najean Y, Pecking A: Refractory anemia with excess of myeloblasts in the bone marrow: a clinical trial of androgens in 90 patients. Br J Haematol 37:25–33, 1977.

30. Toland DM, Coltman CA, Moon TE: Second malignancies complicating Hodgkin's disease: The Southwest Oncology Group experience. Cancer Clin Trials 1:21–33, 1978.

31. Tulliez M, Richard MF, Jan F, Sultan C: Preleukemic abnormal myelopoiesis induced by chlorambucil: A case study. Scand J Haematol 13:179–193, 1974.

32. Foucar K, McKenna RW, Bloomfield CD et al.: Therapy-related leukemia. A panmyelosis. Cancer 43:1285–1296, 1979.

33. Grunwald HW, Rosner F: Acute leukemia and immunosuppressive drug use. Arch Intern Med 139:641–466, 1979.

34. Zarrabi MH, Rosner F, Bennett JM: Non-Hodgkin's lymphoma and acute myeloblastic leukemia: report of the cases and review of the literature. Cancer 44:1070–1080, 1979.

35. Nassar VH, Jacobs J, Mirra SS, Pandya KJ, Bennett JM: Burkitt cell leukemia following therapy for Hodgkin's disease (unpublished observations).

36. Stavem P: Hypergranular acute promyelocytic leukaemia with intravascular coagulation. Scand J Haematol 2:249–252, 1973.

37. Bennett JM, Catovsky D, Daniel M-T, Flandrin G, Galton DAG, Gralnick HR, Sultan C: A variant form of hypergranular promyelocytic leukemia. Ann Intern Med 92:261, 1980.

38. Van Den Berghe H, Louwagie A, Boeckaert-Van Orshoven A, David G, Ver Wilghen R, Michaux JL, Sokal G: Chromosome abnormalities in acute promyelocytic leukemia. Cancer 43:558–562, 1979.

39. Forkner CE: Leukemia and allied disorders. New York: Macmillan, 1938, pp 5–8.

40. Abramson N, Deluca J, Bennett JM: Immune markers in adult leukemia. Am J Clin Pathol 66:111–116, 1976.

41. Jensen MK, Killman S-A: Additional evidence for chromosome abnormalities in the erythroid precursors in acute leukemia. Acta Med Scand 189:97–100, 1971.

42. Skeel RT, Costello W, Bennett JM, et al.: Cyclophosphamide, cytosine arabinoside and methotrexate versus cytosine arabinoside and thioguanine for acute non-lymphocytic leukemia in adults. Cancer 45:224–231, 1980.

43. Bennett JM, Begg CB: The cytochemistry of adult acute myeloid leukemia: correlation of subtypes with response and survival: an Eastern Cooperative Oncology Group Study. Cancer Res 41:4833–4839, 1981.

44. Gehan EA, Smith TL, Freireich EJ, et al.: Prognostic factors in acute leukemia. Semin in Oncol 3:271–283, 1976.

45. Bennett JM, Begg CB, Sartiano GC, Tartaglia A, Carbone PP: The chemotherapy of adult acute myeloid leukemia. Proc Am Soc Clin Oncol 21:434, 1980.

46. Meyer RI, Ferreira PPC, Cuttner J, et al.: Central nervous system involvement and presentation in acute granulocytic leukemia. Am J Med 68:691–694, 1980.

47. Lichtman MA, Weed RI: Peripheral cytoplasmic characteristics of leukocytes in monocytic leukemia. Blood 40:52–60, 1972.

48. Foon KA, Naiem F, Yale C, Gace RP: Acute myelogenous leukemia: morphologic classifications and response to therapy. Leukemia Res 3:171–173, 1979.

49. Wiernik PH, Glidewell OJ, Hoagland HC, et al.: A comparative trial of daunorubicin, cytosine arabinoside, and thioguanine, and a combination of the three agents for the treatment of acute myelocytic leukemia. Med Ped Oncol 6:261–277, 1979.

50. Straus DJ, Mertelsmann R, Koziner B, *et al.*: The acute monocytic leukemias: multidisciplinary studies in 45 patients. Medicine (in press).
51. Cuttner J, Conjalka MS, Reilly M, *et al.*: Association of monocytic leukemia in patients with extreme leukocytosis. Am J Med 69:555–558, 1980.
52. Collins AJ, Bloomfield CD, Peterson BA, *et al.*: Acute promyelocytic leukemia. Arch Intern Med 138:1677–1680, 1979.
53. Bernard J, Weil M, Jacquillant C: Acute promyelocytic leukemia. In: Therapy of acute leukemias, Mandelli E (ed.) 1977, pp 456–460.
54. Scott RB, Ellison RR, Ley AB: A clinical study of 20 cases of erythroleukemia. Am J Med 37:162–171, 1964.
55. Bloomfield CD, Brunning RD, Kennedy BJ: Daunorubicin prednisone treatment of erythroleukemia. Ann Intern Med 81:746–750, 1974.

# 5. Chromosome Abnormalities in Adult Acute Leukemia: Biologic and Therapeutic Significance

HARVEY M. GOLOMB*

CONTENTS

## 1. INTRODUCTION

Chromosome abnormalities in human disease could not be ascertained until the normal human complement was determined in 1956, to be 44 autosomes and two sex chromosomes. In 1960, the first chromosome abnormality in a human malignancy was described: the Philadelphia chromosome and its association with chronic myelogenous leukemia. Approximately 10 years later, banding techniques were introduced, which made possible

* Supported in part by NIH Grant No. CA-25568.

the identification of each individual chromosome. The specific patterns of banding could be correlated with the distribution of chromatin along the chromatid, and the short- and long-arm portions could be identified. Thus, balanced translocations could now be observed, and additional chromosome abnormalities associated with malignant diseases could be ascertained. In the mid-1970s, two specific chromosome translocations were found to be associated with acute leukemia: the 8/21 translocation with acute myelogenous leukemia, and the 15/17 translocation with acute promyelocytic leukemia. Not only were specific associations discovered but it was suggested and confirmed that the chromosome abnormalities had prognostic importance. It is our goal in this review to examine the biological and therapeutic significance of chromosome abnormalities in adults with acute leukemia as they have been studied during the past decade with the use of banding techniques.

## 2. CHROMOSOME IDENTIFICATION METHODS

An analysis of chromosome patterns, to be relevant to a malignant disease, must be based on a study of the karyotype of the tumor cells themselves. In the case of leukemia, the tumor specimen is usually a bone marrow aspirate that is either processed immediately or cultured for a short time. In patients with a white blood cell count higher than 15 500, with about 10% immature myeloid cells, a sample of peripheral blood can be cultured for 24 or 48 hours without addition of phytohemagglutinin (PHA). The karyotype of the dividing cells will usually be similar to that of cells obtained from the bone marrow.

When an abnormal karyotype is found in a tumor, it is important to analyze cells from normal tissues, such as skin fibroblasts or peripheral blood lymphocytes stimulated to divide by addition of PHA. In most instances, cells from these unaffected tissues will have a normal karyotype. The chromosome abnormalities observed in the tumor cells thus represent somatic mutations in an otherwise chromosomally normal individual.

Chromosomes obtained from bone marrow cells, particularly from patients with leukemia, frequently are very fuzzy, and the bands may be indistinct. For chromosomal analysis, one of several pretreatment methods may be used prior to staining with Giemsa, or the slides can be stained with quinacrine mustard for fluorescence. In patients with complex chromosome changes, multiple staining techniques are required for correct identification of the chromosomes involved in the rearrangements, and for accurate definition of the chromosome bands affected by the breaks. Experienced laboratories should be able to obtain a precise identification of the chromosome abnormalities in more than 90% of leukemic patients. Unused cell material can be stored in fixative in a freezer; usable quinacrine-fluorescent bands can be obtained from such material even after storage for more than a decade.

The observation of at least two 'pseudodiploid' (chromosome number of 46) or hyperdiploid (chromosome number >46) cells, or of three hypodiploid (chromosome number <46) cells, each showing the same abnormality, is considered evidence for the presence of an abnormal clone. Patients whose cells show no alterations, or in whom the alterations involve different chromosomes in different cells, are considered to be normal. Isolated changes may be due to technical artifacts or to random mitotic errors. In malignant cells with a very low mitotic index, however, only a single abnormal cell may undergo mitosis.

In the following discussion, the chromosomes are identified according to the Paris Nomenclature (1971), and the karyotypes are expressed as recommended under this system. The total chromosome number is indicated first, followed by the sex chromosomes and then by the gains, losses, or rearrangements of the autosomes. A + sign or − sign before a number indicates a gain or loss, respectively, of a whole chromosome; a + or − after a number indicates a gain or loss of part of a chromosome. The letters 'p' and 'q' refer to the short and long arms of the chromosome, respectively; 'i' and 'r' stand for 'isochromosome' and 'ring chromosome.' 'Mar' is marker, 'del' is deletion, 'ins' is insertion, and 'inv' is inversion. Translocations are identified by 't' followed by the chromosomes involved in the first set of brackets; the chromosome bands in which the breaks occurred are indicated in the second brackets. Uncertainty about the chromosome or band involved is signified by '?'.

## 3. ACUTE LEUKEMIAS IN ADULTS

In order to discuss the biologic and therapeutic significance of chromosome abnormalities in acute leukemia, one must define the diseases to be considered. In 1976, the French-American-British Co-operative Group published a study entitled 'Proposals for the classification of the acute leukemias' [1] (see chapter by Bennett). Since there had been no general agreement on nomenclature or classification or even on the methods for distinguishing myeloid from lymphoblastic leukemias prior to the first meeting in 1974, the group attempted to establish a uniform system for the classification and nomenclature of the acute leukemias. The proposal offered was based on conventional morphologic and cytochemical methods which they utilized to review peripheral blood and bone marrow films from some 200

*Table 1.* Abbreviated FAB classification of acute leukemias [1].

| | |
|---|---|
| Myeloid * | |
| M1 | Myeloblastic leukemia without maturation |
| M2 | Myeblastic leukemia with maturation |
| M3 | Hypergranular promyelocytic leukemia |
| M3 Variant † | 'Microgranular' promyelocytic leukemia |
| M4 | Myelomonocytic leukemia |
| M5 | Monocytic leukemia |
| M6 | Erythroleukemia |
| Lymphoblastic ‡ | |
| L1 | Small cells; homogeneous |
| L2 | Large cells; heterogeneous |
| L3 | Large cells; homogeneous |

* See chapter by Bennett for details.
† 1980 addition.
‡ Although seven features are considered, the listing only reflects cell size (see Table 1 in chapter by Esterhay and Wiernik).

patients with acute leukemia. Two groups of acute leukemias, 'lymphoblastic' and 'myeloid,' were further subdivided into three and six groups, respectively. Myeloid leukemias predominate in the adult population with a ratio of about 5:1, whereas lymphoblastic leukemia predominates in children in approximately the same ratio. We will examine in-depth chromosome abnormalities in the six categories of myeloid leukemia and deal only briefly with the three categories of lymphoblastic leukemias.

The six main types of myeloid leukemias (M1 to M6) are described according to 1) the direction of differentiation along one or more cell lines and 2) the degree of maturation of the cells. Thus, M1, M2, and M3 undergo predominantly granulocytic differentiation and differ from one another in the extent and nature of granulocytic maturation; M4 shows both granulocytic and monocytic differentiation; M5, predominantly monocytic differentiation; and M6, predominantly erythroblastic differentiation (Table 1).

For the 'lymphoblastic' leukemias, three types (L1, L2, L3) were defined according to the occurrence of individual cytologic features and the degree of heterogeneity in the distribution of some or all of these features among the leukemic-cell population. The features considered were cell size, distribution of nuclear chromatin, nuclear shape, number of nucleoli, and amount and basophilia of cytoplasm. Up to 10% of the cells could depart from any of the features considered characteristic of the type. In L1, the cells are usually small and homogeneous; in L2, they are usually large and heterogeneous; and in L3 (Burkitt type), they are usually large and homogeneous, with a high mitotic index (about 5%).

The FAB group regarded L1 as representing the type of acute leukemia common in childhood, but stated that L2, less common in children, requires differentiation from myeloblastic leukemia without maturation (M1) and is sometimes designated 'undifferentiated leukemia.'

Since this review is designed to consolidate and elucidate general trends and principles, the attempt by various authors to use the FAB classification system will be clearly noted for uniformity.

### 4. CHROMOSOMAL ABNORMALITIES IN POPULATIONS OF PATIENTS WITH ACUTE NON-LYMPHOCYTIC LEUKEMIA (ANLL)

Mitelman and Brandt reported in 1974 on ten untreated patients with AML whose cells were studied by Giemsa-banding techniques [2]. They found that one of five patients who had karyotypic abnormalities was pseudodiploid. It was not until 1976, however, that larger series of banding studies on adults with ANLL began to be published (Table 2).

Oshimura et al. [3] studied chromosomes from 38 patients with acute myeloblastic leukemia (the FAB classification was not specified). Sixteen of these patients had abnormal karyotypes. Three of the 16 patients had developed AML as a second malignancy. In three cases, there was a common translocation between the long arm of No. 8 and No. 21, i.e., [t(8; 21) (q22; q22)]; two patients had a 45,XX,-21 karyotype; and three had trisomy of the long arm of No. 1. Three patients had trisomy of No. 8, one of No. 9, and one patient had partial monosomy for No. 7; however, all these patients had additional chromosomal abnormalities.

Table 2. Percentage of normal and abnormal karyotypes in banding studies on adults with ANLL.

| Authors | Year | Country | No. of patients | Normal karyotype | Abnormal karyotype |
|---------|------|---------|-----------------|------------------|--------------------|
| Oshimura et al. [3] | 1976 | U.S.A. | 38 | 22 (58) * | 16 (42) |
| Golomb et al. [4] | 1976 | U.S.A. | 50 | 25 (50) | 25 (50) |
| Mitelman et al. [6] | 1976 | Sweden | 30 | 13 (43) | 17 (57) |
| Alimena et al. [7] | 1977 | Italy | 30 | 14 (43) | 16 (57) |
| Golomb et al. [8] | 1978 | U.S.A. | 40 | 19 (47) | 21 (53) |
| Philip et al. [9] | 1978 | Denmark | 88 | 51 (58) | 37 (42) |
| Hossfield et al. [10] | 1979 | Germany | 48 | 22 (46) | 26 (54) |
| Hagemeijer et al. [11] | 1980 | Holland | 86 | 39 (45) | 47 (55) |
| | | Total | 410 | 205 (50) | 205 (50) |

* ( ): percentages.

Golomb *et al.* [4] reported chromosome banding patterns in 50 of 55 consecutive adult patients with ANLL. According to the FAB classification, 22 of the 50 cases were diagnosed as AML (M1 and M2), two as APL (M3), 24 as AMMoL (M4), and two as erythroleukemia (M6). Twenty-five patients had chromosome abnormalities initially. In the accompanying cytogenetics report, Rowley and Potter, using Q-banding techniques, stressed that the most frequent structural rearrangement was the t(8;21), but that it may be associated with the loss of a sex chromosome [5]. In addition, nonrandom chromosome changes such as the addition of No. 8, the loss of No. 7, and a gain or loss of one No. 21 were seen. They further noted that chromosomal abnormalities decreased or disappeared during remission; however, the same abnormality recurred in relapse. Evolution of the karyotype occurred in eight patients, in five of whom an additional No. 8 was observed.

Mitelman *et al.*, in 1976 [6] reported G-banding results on 30 patients with acute myeloid leukemia (FAB classification not utilized). Seventeen patients (57%) had distinct chromosomal abnormalities at the time of diagnosis. All except two of the patients displayed trisomy 8, 9, or 21 or monosomy 7. The authors concluded that, when chromosome aberrations occurred, they were clearly nonrandom.

Alimena *et al.* [7] reported in 1977 on consistent cytogenetic abnormalities in 16 of 30 patients with a diagnosis of ANLL (FAB classification not utilized). They concluded that chromosome imbalances were apparently nonrandom.

In 1978, Golomb *et al.* reported on 40 additional ANLL patients [8]; slightly more than one-half (53%) had an abnormal karyotype. Of the total of 90 patients studied in eight years, 46 had a chromosomal abnormality at the time of admission. The most common rearrangements were a 15;17 translocation in five cases; an 8;21 translocation with associated loss of a sex chromosome in three cases and a complex variant in two others, a 6;9 translocation in two cases, and a 3;3 insertion in two cases.

Also in 1978, Philip *et al.* [9] described abnormal karyotypes in 37 (42%) of 88 consecutive cases of ANLL (FAB classification not utilized). They concluded that extra chromosome Nos. 6, 8 and 21; missing chromosome 7 and Y; and structural rearrangements t(8;21) and 5q- occurred so frequently that they were likely to be nonrandom.

In 1979, Hossfield *et al.* [10] reported on 48 patients with ANLL (FAB classification not utilized); 26 of these patients (54%) had an abnormal karyotype initially. Specific types of abnormalities were not given. Most recently, Hagemeijer *et al.* [11] reported on 86 patients with ANLL classified according to the FAB system. Forty-seven (55%) of the patients had an abnormal karyotype initially. Nonrandom aberrations were frequent, including trisomy 8 in 15 patients, monosomy 7 in seven patients, t(8;21) in seven patients, and t(15;17) in two patients. They also noted, as did Rowley and Potter in 1976 [5], that the complete remission achieved in ten cases was characterized by a normal karyotype in bone marrow metaphases. Also, when relapse occurred in four patients after a period of complete remission, the bone marrow metaphases showed the original abnormal karyotype with additional changes superimposed.

Thus, more than 400 patients with ANLL have been reported on from seven centers during the past five years; 50% of the patients had an abnormal karyotype initially (Table 2). This is similar to the figure reported by the First International Workshop on Chromosomes in Leukaemia in 1978 [12], which included some of the cases from the centers listed in Table 1. At the First Workshop 279 patients were reported on; 139 of these had chromosome abnormalities initially (50%). Twenty-two patients had a +8, 20 had a −7, 11 had a t(8;21), nine had a t(15;17), and five had a 22q-.

More recently, Yunis et al. [13] have utilized high resolution chromosome analysis to study marrow from 26 patients with ANLL. In 24, including 18 of 20 consecutive untreated patients, adequate mitoses were obtained. All demonstrated clonal chromosomal abnormalities involving a balanced translocation in 11 cases, a complete or partial monosomy in ten, and a trisomy in six. Thus preliminary results suggest that all cases of ANLL have chromosomal changes; subgroups may depend on the exact abnormality rather than the presence or absence of an abnormality.

## 5. RELATIONSHIP OF CHROMOSOME ABNORMALITIES TO PROGNOSIS AND SURVIVAL

Most reports have shown that there is a correlation between the initial karyotype and subsequent survival (Table 3). Sakurai and Sandberg, in 1973 [14], showed that the median survival was one-third as long for patients whose marrow cells had only abnormal metaphases (AA) as that of patients who had only normal metaphases (NN). They found patients with both normal and abnormal metaphases (AN) to have an intermediate survival time. Golomb et al. showed in 1976 [4] that NN patients had a median survival of ten months and AA patients a median survival of two months. When patients were separated into the two main FAB groupings, Acute Myeloblastic Leukemia (AML; M1 and M2) and Acute Myelomonocytic Leukemia (AMMoL; M4), similar complete remission rates (50% and 38%, respectively) and similar median survival times (7.5 months and 10 months) were found. However, when the AML patients were separated into those with and those without a chromosome abnormality, the median sur-

*Table 3.* Median survival of ANLL patients classified according to normal and abnormal karyotypes.

| Authors | Year | Median survival (months) | | |
|---|---|---|---|---|
| | | NN | AN | AA |
| Sakurai and Sandberg [13] | 1973 | 9.1 | 7.2 | 1.2 |
| Golomb *et al.* [4] | 1976 | 10,0 | 6.5 | 2.0 |
| Nilsson *et al.* [14] | 1977 | 8.0 | 2.5 | 1.0 |
| Alimena *et al.* [7] | 1977 | 7.0 | 2.0 | |
| Golomb *et al.* [†] [8] | 1978 | 8.0 | 6.5 | 2.0 |
| Hossfield *et al.* [10] | 1979 | 12.5 | 8.5 | 4.0 |

* Includes three cases of ALL.
† Includes 50 patients from 1976 study.
NN — Normal metaphases only.
AN — Normal and abnormal metaphases.
AA — Abnormal metaphases only.

vival times were markedly different (2 months and 18 months, respectively). Patients with AMMoL did not differ in median survival times when subgrouped according to the presence or absence of chromosome abnormalities. In addition, in a comparison of all treated AA patients with all treated AN patients, the complete remission rate was less in AA patients (10% and 42%, respectively), as was the median survival (2 months and 9 months, respectively).

In 1977, Nilsson *et al.* [15] reported a correlation between survival time and the presence of a chromosomal abnormality in the bone marrow at the time of diagnosis. Survival times averaged 8 months for 11 NN patients, 2.5 months for 10 AN patients, and 1 month for 9 AA patients. The authors suggested that, in patients with abnormal bone marrow cells, the disease has reached a more advanced stage than in those with exclusively normal diploid cells. Alimena *et al.* [7] reported a difference in survival between patients with normal and abnormal karyotypes, as shown in Table 3. Only four of 16 ANLL patients with an abnormal karyotype obtained a complete remission, whereas at least five of the 14 patients with a normal karyotype were alive and in remission at between 13 to 19 months from their first diagnosis.

In their 1978 study, Golomb *et al.* [8] confirmed the differences which they had reported in 1976 in a total of 90 ANLL patients (40 new patients since the 1976 report). The difference in survival between 37 treated patients with an initially normal karyotype (NN) and 43 treated patients with an initially abnormal karyotype (AA and AN) (10 months and 4 months) was significant (p<0.01). The survival times of these 80 patients are

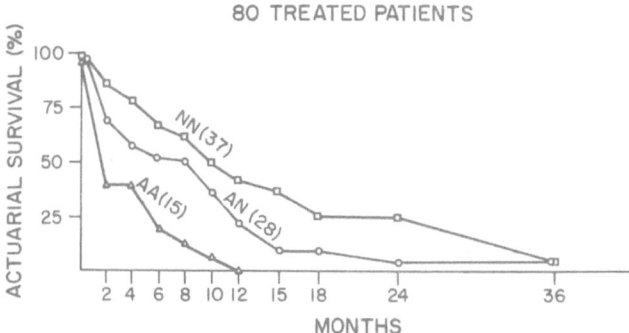

*Figure 1.* Actuarial survival of 80 treated ANLL patients (M1 through M6) according to initial chromosome findings. (Originally published as Figure 3 in Golomb *et al.*, N Engl J Med 299:613–619, 1978 [8]).

shown in Figure 1. When patients were classified as having AML or AMMoL, this difference in survival was even more pronounced (Figure 2). Of 16 treated patients with AML and a normal karyotype, 11 (69%) had a CR and the median survival was 13 months. Of eight patients with AML in whom only abnormal metaphases were observed, none had a CR, and the median survival was only two months (p~0.05). The remission rate and median survival were not significantly different in patients with AMMoL who were grouped according to initial karyotypes (Figure 2).

Hossfield *et al.* in 1979 [10] reported on 48 patients with ANLL, all of whom had been treated according to a single protocol. The remission rate of NN patients was 73%, that of the AN patients, 60%, and that of the AA

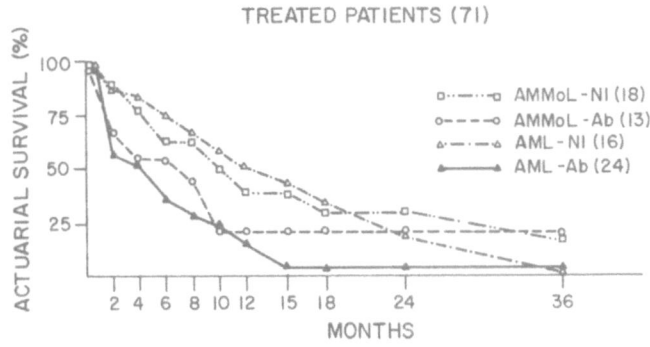

*Figure 2.* Actuarial survival of treated patients according to cytologic diagnosis (AML-acute myelogenous leukemia, or AMMol-acute myelomonocytic leukemia) and karyotype (N1-normal or Ab-abnormal). (Originally published as Figure 2 in Golomb *et al.*, N Engl J Med 299:613–619, 1978 [8]).

patients, 36%. The respective median survival times paralleled the remission rates (Table 3). The difference in remission rates and survival times between patients with normal (NN) and without normal (AA) metaphases was significant.

The data from the First International Workshop on Chromosomes in Leukaemia [12] support the results of the individual studies cited in Table 3. Of 102 patients with a normal karyotype on whom complete clinical data were available, the median survival time was six months. Of the 139 patients with an abnormal karyotype, 80 were AN with a median survival of five months and 59 were AA with a median survival of four months. The percentages of patients alive after one year in the three groups were NN — 21%, AN — 21%, and AA — 5%. When the patients were grouped as AML and AMMoL, the initial differences reported by Golomb et al. [8] were confirmed. There were 137 AML (M1 and M2) patients; median survivals were NN — 9 months, AN — 5 months, AA — 3.5 months. For the 67 AMMoL and AMoL patients, there were no observable differences, with NN — 6 months, AN — 5 months, and AA — 7 months.

The only study in the last decade which has not supported the general trend was that by Hagemeijer et al. [11]. They found a 33% CR rate for 39 NN patients, with a median survival of three months, and a 40% CR rate for 47 AA and AN patients, with a median survival of five months. Possibly, the lack of uniform treatment at the three referring hospitals could have contributed to obscuring the differences noted previously by others.

## 6. THE (8;21) TRANSLOCATION — A POSSIBLE PROTOTYPIC ABNORMALITY IN AML

In 1973, Rowley first reported on a patient with AML who had a translocation between chromosomes 8 and 21 [16]. In 1974, Sakurai et al. [17] confirmed this observation and called the t(8;21) the 'prototypic' karyotype, because he found this abnormality in 11 of 51 patients (22%). The identification of a t(8;21) with banding techniques supported the earlier observation of a unique 'complex' profile seen in AML by Hart et al. [18] and referred to as −C, +D, +E, −G. Trujillo et al. possibly had 12 of 69 patients (17%) with this profile [19]. In 1978, the First International Workshop on Chromosomes in Leukaemia reviewed the occurrence of the t(8; 21) [12]. The t(8;21) was found in 11 of 139 patients (8%) with a chromosome abnormality. Ten of the eleven patients were found to have AML (M1 and M2), and one patient was said to have AMMoL. The complete remission rate was 50%, and the median survival for these 11 patients was 6 months. For 102 patients with a normal karyotype, the CR rate was 37%

and the median survival was six months. Loss of one X chromosome in females or the Y chromosome in males occurred in more than half of the cases with t(8;21). On the other hand, no instance of a structural aberration involving a sex chromosome was found.

In 1979 Trujillo *et al.* published an updated report on the t(8;21) in AML at M.D. Anderson Hospital and Tumor Institute [20]. They reported on 546 patients with acute leukemia who had cytogenetic studies between 1968 and 1975. They found that 32 patients had similar chromosomal alterations that appeared to involve chromosomes 8 and 21. Banding studies could be done on only 15 of the patients, but a t(8;21) was confirmed in all 15. Although the patients were not classified according to the FAB system, the authors stated that each individual had typical AML with Auer rod-positive and peroxidase-positive cells. Complete remission was achieved in 27 cases (84%). The median survival time for all 32 patients was 81 weeks. Thus, Trujillo *et al.* concluded that these patients seemed to respond better to therapy than other adult patients with AML. They also supported the suggestion by Sakurai *et al.* that acute leukemia with the 8/21 translocation represents a definite subgroup of AML, but with an incidence of only 7.3%; this figure is similar to the 8% reported by the First International Workshop.

More recently, the Second International Workshop on Chromosomes in Leukemia reviewed 48 ANLL patients with t(8q−; 21q+) [21]. Bone marrow smears which were available from 44 of the 48 patients were reviewed by four hematologists and classified according to the FAB criteria. In 43 cases, the leukemic cells were classified as M2; the material was inadequate for diagnosis on one patient. In all cases, the break point was in band q22 of chromosome No. 8 and in q22 of chromosome No. 21. In 18 patients (38%), t(8;21) was the only chromosome abnormality (Group I). Loss of one sex chromosome in addition to the t(8;21) was found in 16 patients (33%) (Group II). In 14 cases (29%), other chromosome abnormalities in addition to the t(8;21) were observed (Group III). The incidence of complete remission in all patients was 74% (34 of 46 patients for whom adequate data were available). The CR rate was 72% in Group I, 63% in Group II, and 79% in Group III. The median survival times were 14, 5.5, and 15.5 months, respectively. The median survival was 9 months for all patients with AA and 14.5 months for those with AN. In Group II, AA patients had a median survival of 2 months. The improved response of AN patients was reflected in the number of such patients who were alive one year after diagnosis. Of 23 such patients, 19 had an AN pattern; 11 patients were alive at 2 years, and all had an AN pattern.

It was also found that geographic differences in the occurrence of the t(8;21) exist. The frequency was 30.4% in Saitama (Japan), 24% in Chicago,

2.8% in London, and 4% in Paris. The reason for this variation remains to be determined.

Several conclusions can be drawn regarding the t(8;21):

1. The typical bone marrow morphology in ANLL with t(8;21) is that of M2, i.e., myeloblastic with some maturation.
2. The t(8;21) in ANLL is associated with loss of one sex chromosome in a significant number of patients (33%),
3. Overall, the t(8;21) is associated with a good prognosis, particularly for patients who have some normal metaphase cells.
4. However, the acute leukemia is an especially aggressive type in patients with both a t(8;21) and a missing sex chromosome.
5. The findings to date suggest a geographic difference in the incidence of the t(8;21).

## 7. ACUTE PROMYELOCYTIC LEUKEMIA (APL) AND THE 15;17 TRANSLOCATION

Engel *et al.* [22] reported, in a pre-banding study in 1967, on a 6-year-old girl with acute promyelocytic leukemia (APL) who had a deletion of a portion of the long arm of a chromosome 17–18. It was not until 1976, however, that Golomb *et al.* [23] suggested a specific association between a chromosome 17 abnormality and APL. In a Q-banding study, two patients with acute promyelocytic leukemia and disseminated intravascular coagulation (DIC) were found to have a deletion of almost one-half of the proximal portion of the long arm of chromosome 17. The authors suggested that this might be an abnormality specific to APL. The only two patients with APL in a consecutive series of 50 ANLL patients had the same abnormality involving chromosome 17 [4]. In 1977, the University of Chicago group reported a third case of APL in which what initially appeared to be a deletion of No. 17 was found in reality to be a reciprocal translocation between No. 15 and No. 17 [24, 25]. Support for their observations came quickly from two groups in Japan, each of which reported a 15;17 translocation in a patient with APL [26, 27].

At the First International Workshop on Chromosomes in Leukemia held in Helsinki in August 1977, abnormalities associated with APL were a topic of major interest. The report published in 1978 [12] showed that there were nine patients with a t(15q+;17q−) among 139 patients who had an abnormal karyotype; all nine of these had APL. Six of the total of 17 patients with APL had a normal karyotype. Thus, the Workshop confirmed the observation that a significant number of patients with APL had a t(15q+;17q−), and that this aberration was not found in other types of ANLL.

In 1979, Van Den Berghe *et al.* [28] published a report on 16 patients with APL; 14 of these had an abnormal karyotype. Eleven patients had a consistent t(15;17) structural anomaly; one patient had a rearrangement of chromosomes 15 and 17, apparently different from that in other patients, one a No. 17 deletion without a demonstrable translocation, and one a 47,+8 karyotype. Only two of the 16 patients [both with the t(15;17) chromosomal abnormality] did not have disseminated intravascular coagulation (DIC).

According to the 1976 criteria of the FAB cooperative group [1], the diagnosis of acute promyelocytic leukemia should be made only when the 'great majority' of cells are abnormal promyelocytes whose cytoplasm is packed with coarse granules and contains prominent Auer-like bodies. It may be that these criteria are too limiting, and that the APL syndrome encompasses a broader spectrum of patients. One patient at the University of Chicago who had the t(15;17) abnormality (Figure 3), DIC, and only a small percen-

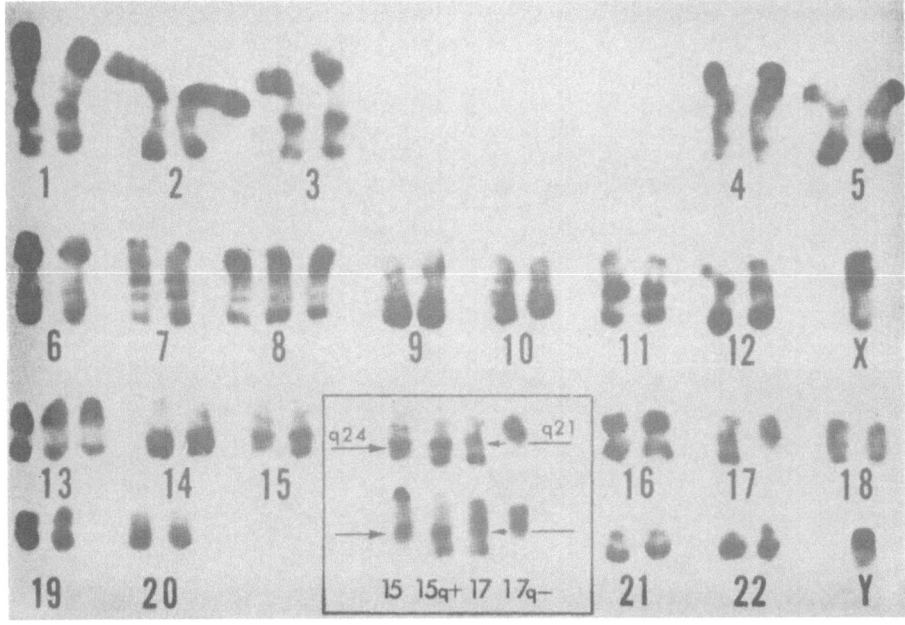

*Figure 3.* Karyotype of an R-banded metaphase cell obtained from unstimulated peripheral blood during relapse in the initial patient with atypical APL [29]. Cell has t(15;17) and extra chromosomes No. 8 and No. 13 [48, XY, +8, +13, t(15;17)]. Inset, partial karyotypes of pairs 15 and 17 from this cell (top row) and another cell. Densely stained band q24 is present both in the normal 15 and in the 15q+, suggesting a translocation breakpoint distal to q24. Two narrow bands in 17q21 are present both in the normal 17 and in the 17q-, suggesting a breakpoint at or near the junction of q21 and q22. Probable breakpoints are identified with arrows, and the number above each arrow indicates the band proximal to the breakpoint [t(15;17) (q25?; q22)]. (Originally published as Figure 3 in Testa *et al.*, Blood 52:272–280, 1978 [29]).

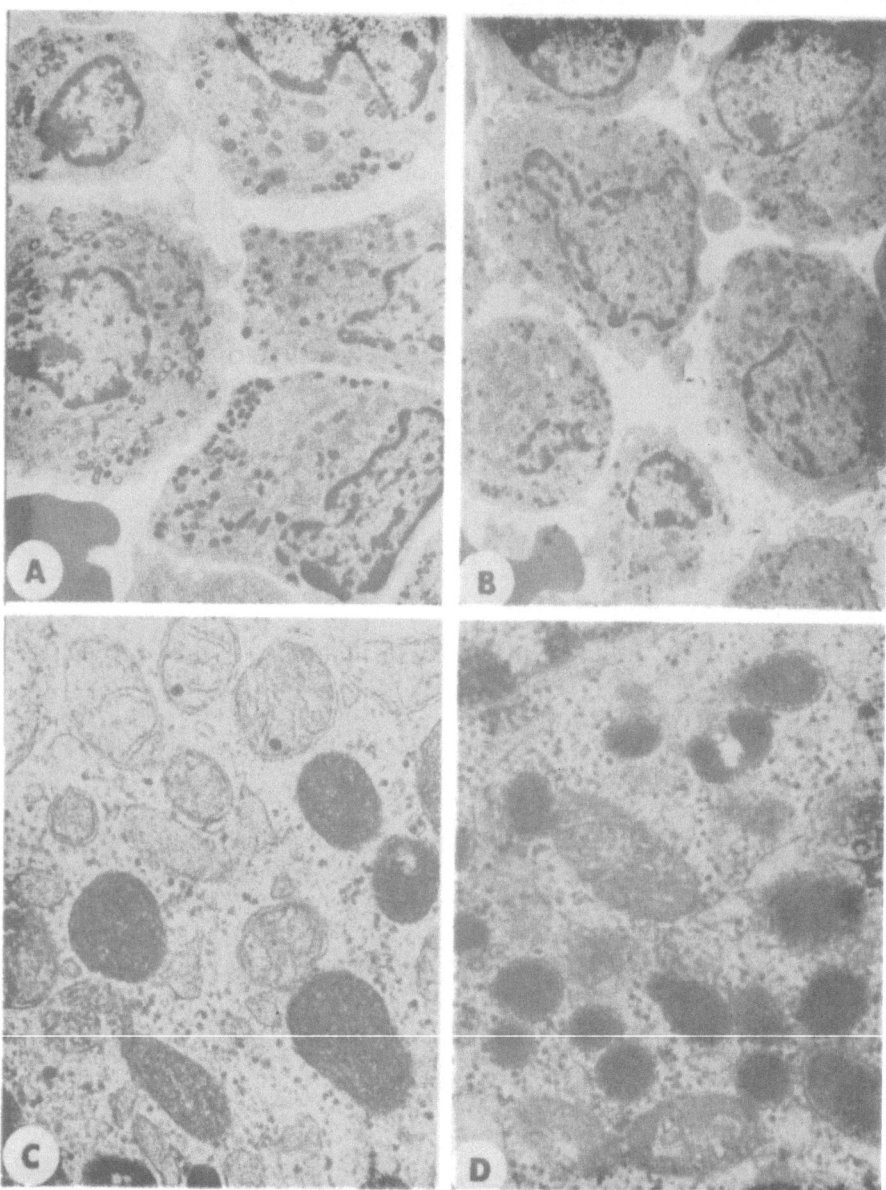

*Figure 4.* (A) Low-magnification transmission electron micrograph (TEM) of a bone marrow spicule from a previously reported case of typical APL [23], as determined by light microscopy. Note the large reniform nuclei as well as the distribution of dark primary granules throughout the cytoplasm. × 4400. (B) Low-magnification TEM of a bone marrow spicule from an atypical case [29] at the time of first admission. Large reniform nuclei are readily seen. Although the dark granules are smaller than those in Figure 4A, their distribution is similar in both cases. × 4400. (C) High-magnification view of a portion of the cytoplasm from a cell of the patient in Figure 4A. Granules are usually larger than mitochondria. × 40 300. (D) High-magnification view of a portion of cytoplasm from a cell of an atypical case. Dark granules are numerous but usually much smaller than mitochondria. × 39 700. (Originally published as Figure 2 in Testa *et al.*, Blood 52:272–280, 1978 [29]).

tage of heavily granulated cells was found by electron microscopy to have numerous, very small granules in most cells [29] (Figure 4). Since daunorubicin can induce remission in about 50% of patients, with a median duration of 26 months [30], and since heparin given prophylactically may allow a better chance of inducing remission [31], it is clearly important to make an accurate diagnosis. Since the original report of a single case of atypical APL at the University of Chicago [29], Berger et al. [32] have reported on three patients with a t(15;17) who had a type of ANLL similar to that of the patient reported by Testa et al. [29]. All three patients had DIC, and light microscopy showed the presence of reniform folded nuclei. In 1980, the FAB group recognized a variant form of hypergranular promyelocytic leukemia (M3) in which the cells are characterized by bilobed, multilobed, or reniform nuclei, and by cytoplasm with minimal or no granulation [33]. They realized that a few cells with the features typical of M3 will be present in such instances.

An explanation for these variant cases was given by Golomb et al. who described three patients with 'microgranular' APL in 1980 [34]. These patients with acute leukemia, DIC, and the t(15;17) were found by transmission electron microscopy to have the typical distribution of granules seen in promyelocytes. However, the average granule sizes were 120, 170, and 180 nm for the three patients, significantly below the 250 nm resolution of light microscopy (Figure 5).

With this information as a background, the Second International Workshop on Chromosomes in Leukemia met in Belgium in the fall of 1979 to review APL and chromosome specificity [35]. Eighty cases of APL were submitted with complete cytogenetic profiles; 73 had typical APL, and seven had the M3 variant. The 80 patients were divided into four groups: (1) normal karyotype, (2) t(15q+;17q−) only, (3) t(15q+;17q−) plus another abnormality, and (4) an abnormal karyotype without a t(15q+;17q−). There were 40 patients with a normal karyotype; their median survival was 4 months. There were 23 patients with a t(15q+;17q−) only, and their median survival was 1.0 month. Ten patients with a t(15q+;17q−) plus other abnormalities had a median survival of 1.5 months. Seven patients with other abnormalities only had a median survival of 5.0 months. Thus, patients with the t(15q+;17q−) seemed to have a poorer prognosis than other APL patients. Of the 40 APL patients who had only normal metaphases (NN), 28% were alive at one year; however, of the 19 APL patients who had only abnormal metaphases (AA), only 16% were alive at one year. Of the seven patients with the M3 variant, six had the t(15;17) only, and one had the t(15;17) plus additional material on the short arm of No. 17 in the majority of metaphases. No normal karyotypes were seen at the University of Chicago in six APL patients, and no abnormal karyotypes were

142

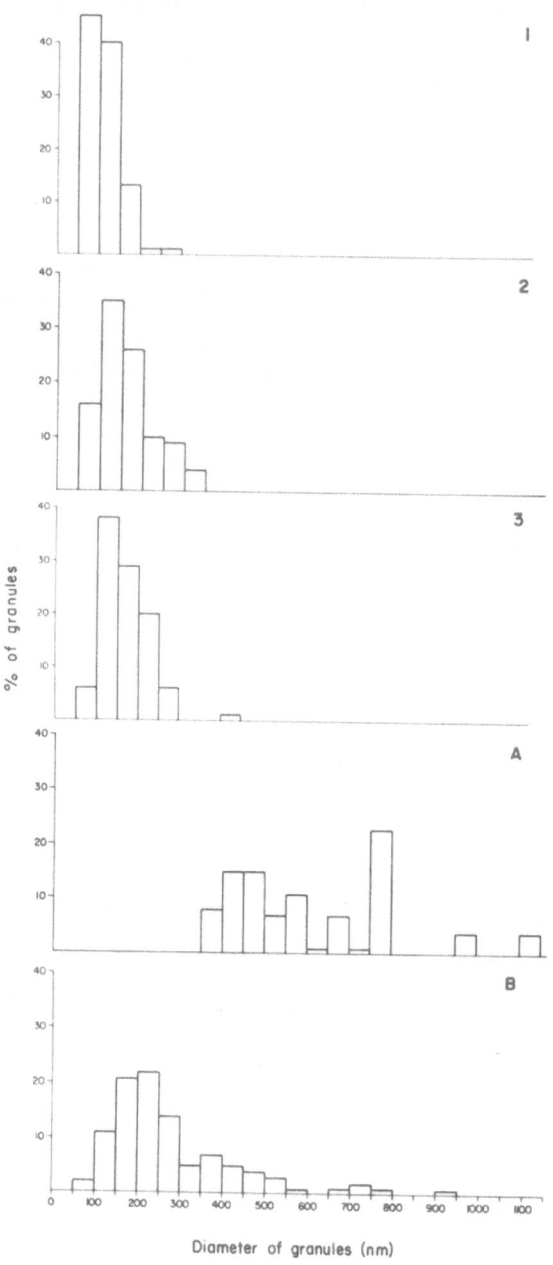

Diameter of granules (nm)

*Figure 5.* Histograms 1, 2, and 3 illustrate the distribution of primary granules in the cells of three patients with microgranular acute promyelocytic leukemia (APL). The majority of granules have a diameter less than 250 nm, the limit of resolution of light microscopy. Histograms A and B show the distribution of primary granule sizes in the cells of two previously reported patients with typical APL, diagnosed by light microscopy. (Originally published as Figure 3 in Golomb *et al.*, Blood 55:253–259, 1980 [34]).

seen in Finland in seven APL patients. At Roswell Park Memorial Institute in Buffalo, only one of 18 patients had the t(15;17), whereas 16 of 18 APL cases in Belgium had the t(15;17). The cause of this uneven geographic distribution remains to be determined. No Workshop member had observed a patient with the t(15;17) who had a disease other than APL.

Thus, several conclusions can be drawn regarding the t(15;17):

1. The t(15;17) is a specific acquired abnormality in ANLL associated with either hypergranular promyelocytic leukemia (M3) or microgranular promyelocytic leukemia (M3 variant).
2. The t(15;17) is present in approximately one-half of the patients with the M3 or M3 variant promyelocytic leukemia.
3. Patients with M3 or the M3 variant who have the t(15;17) appear to have a worse prognosis than those with a normal karyotype or with another type of karyotypic abnormality.
4. The findings to date suggest a geographic difference in the occurrence of the t(15;17).

## 8. EVOLUTION OF KARYOTYPES

Rowley and Potter reported in 1976 that eight of their 50 patients (16%) showed evolution of their karyotype in several samples. In 1979, Testa *et al.* [36] published an updated report on the evolution in the 90 patients described by Golomb *et al.* in 1978. Serial samples of leukemic cells were obtained from 60 of the 90 patients. Evolution of the karyotype was observed in 17 of the patients, seven of whom had normal chromosomes initially and ten of whom had abnormal chromosomes. All ten patients with abnormal chromosomes had structural rearrangements in the initial sample; eight of the ten also had loss of one or more chromosomes initially. The most frequent evolutionary change was a gain of one or more chromosomes (in 12 of the 17 patients). Ten of the 12 patients who acquired one or more additional chromosomes had an extra chromosome 8, and six had an extra chromosome 18. Other evolutionary changes included structural rearrangements (eight patients), loss of a chromosome (four patients), and loss of a marker (two patients). These various changes sometimes occurred in combination. The incidence of karyotypic evolution and the type and frequency of particular evolutionary changes were similar in the patients who were initially normal and in those who were initially abnormal. In all but one of the initially abnormal patients, karyotypic evolution involved the original cytogenetically abnormal clone. In no instance was a clone of chromosomally abnormal cells detected when the bone marrow was morphologically normal; single abnormal cells of clonal origin, however, were observed on a few occasions when the bone marrow morphology was normal.

The 17 patients in whom a karyotype change evolved tended to have relatively long survival times. The median survival of patients who had normal karyotypes in the first sample was longer than that of patients who were abnormal initially. Our series of 90 ANLL patients (80 of whom were treated) included 37 treated patients whose chromosomes were initially normal; the median survival of this group was ten months, compared to 17 months in the seven normal, treated patients among them who evolved. The median survival of 43 treated patients who were abnormal initially was only four months, compared to ten months for the ten treated patients among them who evolved. Thus, evolution might be observed in a larger number of ANLL patients if the overall median survival time could be prolonged.

Once karyotype evolution had occurred, the median survival was relatively short (two months), and response to further treatment was poor. Evolutionary changes may indicate the emergence of a resistant cell line and, thus, can have prognostic significance which may be useful in decisions on the aggressiveness of further therapy for the patient. After the onset of evolution, only two patients who were normal initially and one patient who was abnormal initially attained a remission. It may be significant that the percentage of cells with an abnormal clone or clones was small (<36% of cells) when evolution was first noted in these three patients. Eleven of the other 14 patients had at least 67% abnormal cells at the time of evolution; in nine of these patients, the majority of cells at this time was that with evolutionary change. Thus, evolution of the karyotype in the majority of cells might be an important sign of a poor prognosis.

## 9. CHROMOSOMAL ABNORMALITIES OBSERVED WITH BANDING IN PATIENTS WITH ACUTE LYMPHOCYTIC LEUKEMIA (ALL)

Prior to 1980, there had been published only two major banding studies on unselected ALL populations in which the frequency of chromosomal aneuploidy was determined. In 1977, Oshimura et al. [37] published results of successful banding studies on 31 of 50 unselected ALL patients. The ages of their patients ranged from less than one year to 59 years. Sixteen of the 31 patients had chromosome abnormalities (52%). Four of the patients had a similar abnormality, i.e., partial deletion of the long arm of chromosome 6. The authors found evidence of karyotypic evolution in eight cases. Of their 16 aneuploid cases, only six were patients 16 years of age or older.

In 1979, Cimino *et al.* [38] reported on banding studies of 16 ALL patients studied during 4½ years; ten were adults and six were children. Eight patients (50%) had a normal karyotype initially; however, three of them developed a chromosomal abnormality during relapse. Eight patients had a chromosomal abnormality in their initial samples. Of the 11 patients with abnormalities during the course of the disease, each had a different abnormality. A patient with B-cell ALL had a 14q+ marker in addition to other abnormalities. The only previously published case of B-cell ALL at that time was a patient in the study by Oshimura *et al.* [37], who also had the 14q+ chromosome. This patient also showed a gain of No. 7, loss of No. 13, and a 6p+; all of these were also observed in the B-cell ALL patient reported by Cimino *et al.*. The 14q+ marker occurs frequently in other lymphoproliferative cancers of B-cell origin, such as poorly differentiated lymphocytic lymphoma, diffuse histiocytic lymphoma, and African Burkitt's lymphoma. Cimino *et al.* also found that all five patients who achieved remission after having an abnormal karyotype had normal karyotypes during remission. This observation had previously been made by Zuelzer *et al.* [39].

Cimino *et al.* reported that the eight patients with initially normal karyotypes had a median survival of 17+ months (range: 11–50+ months). The eight patients with initially abnormal karyotypes had a shorter median survival of eight months (range: 2–32+ months).

Because of the limited information on chromosome abnormalities detected with banding in childhood and adult ALL, the Third International Workshop on Chromosomes in Leukemia examined this problem in a meeting held in Lund, Sweden, in July 1980 [40]. There were 157 children and 173 adults with ALL in whom cells from heavily involved marrow (92%) or blood (8%) were evaluated with chromosome banding techniques at diagnosis. Ninety-six children and 120 adults (66% of all) had clonal chromosomal abnormalities. Specific abnormalities included Ph[1] in 12%, t(4;11) in 6%, t(8;14) in 5%, other 14q+ in 5% and 6q− in 4%. Other abnormalities were grouped by the predominent chromosome number in the cells studied (modal no.): >50 (9%), 47–50 (9%), 46 (12%), <46 (5%). Ninety-one percent of children and 65% of adults achieved a complete remission. Among adults, the complete remission rate varied by karyotype; 95% of patients with normal karyotypes, but only 45% with t(8;14) or Ph[1] achieved complete remission. Among children, complete remission duration, but not rate, varied significantly by karyotype. The longest remissions were in children with modal numbers >50; the shortest remissions in those with t(4;11) or t(8;14). Significant differences in survival were seen even when other major risk factors were considered. Thus, it appears that the presence of a chromosome abnormality has prognostic significance in ALL.

## 10. ACUTE LEUKEMIA AS A SECOND MALIGNANCY

A clinically important complication of the treatment of certain hemato-logic malignancies such as Hodgkin's disease (HD), non-Hodgkin's lympho-ma (NHL), and multiple myeloma (MM) is the late development of acute leukemias, almost always of the non-lymphocytic types (see chapter by Colt-man). Although the association has been reported by several groups during the past decade [41–44], it was not until 1975 that a case was reported [45] in which the chromosomes were studied with banding.

Both the group at the University of Chicago [46] and the group at the University of Minnesota [43] recognized that secondary leukemia was a rather distinct entity. Vardiman et al. [46] reported on ten patients who had developed ANLL 29 to 132 months after a diagnosis of malignant lympho-ma was made; six of these patients had HD and four had NHL. Two of the patients had received radiotherapy, two had had chemotherapy, and six patients had received both forms. A preleukemic period with peripheral blood and bone marrow changes was noted in six patients. Nucleated red cells, macrocytosis and marked anisopoikilocytosis of red cells, and occa-sional myelocytes and promyelocytes were early changes in the peripheral blood of these patients. Erythroid hyperplasia with megaloblastoid features, a mild to moderate shift toward granulocytic immaturity, increased num-bers of megakaryocytes with cytologic abnormalities, and increased amounts of reticulin were found in the bone marrow. As overt myelogenous leukemia evolved, serial marrow studies in five of the six preleukemic patients showed a gradual increase in the numbers of blasts and in the amount of reticulin, a decrease in numbers of megakaryocytes, and a decrease in num-bers of erythroid precursors. The sixth patient developed erythroleukemia. Two of the ten patients had no apparent preleukemic phase, and informa-tion on two others was insufficient for a determination of preleukemia. Cytochemical studies in all cases confirmed the nonlymphocytic nature of the leukemia.

In 1977, Rowley et al. [47] reported on a banding study of ten patients (nine of these were included in the morphologic study of Vardiman et al.) who had ANLL following treatment for malignant lymphoma. The median time between the diagnosis of lymphoma and subsequent leukemia was 58 months. Four patients had the blast phase of a myeloproliferative syn-drome, four had acute myelogenous leukemia, one had acute promyelocytic leukemia, and one had erythroleukemia. Of four leukemic patients who received intensive chemotherapy none responded. Every patient had an abnormal karyotype. Seven of the patients had hypodiploid cell lines, two a pseudodiploid, and one a hyperdiploid cell line. Cells from every patient except one were lacking a B chromosome; in eight, this could be identified

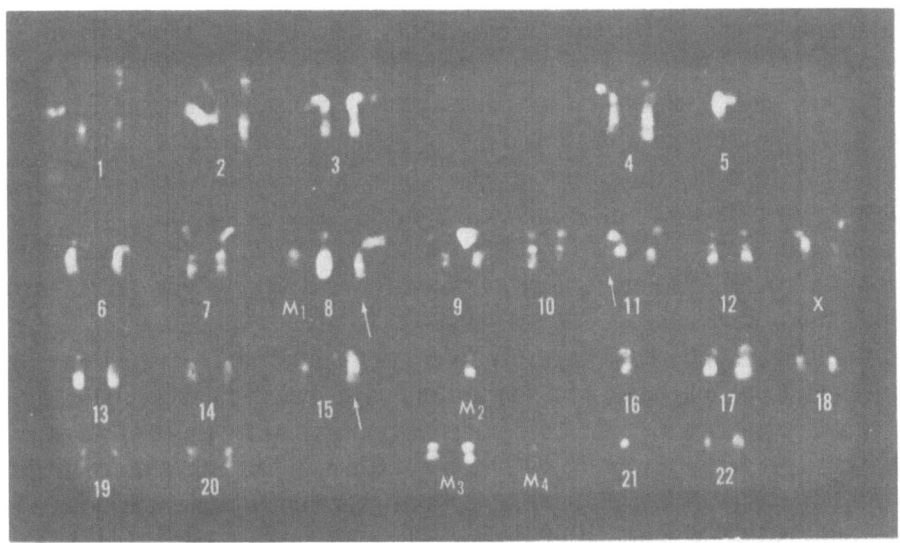

*Figure 6.* Karyotype of metaphase cell obtained from 24-hour cultures bone marrow from a patient with a secondary acute leukemia. Cell contains 48 chromosomes and is lacking one No. 5, possibly one No. 16, and one No. 21. The 8q+, 11q−, and 15p+ chromosomes are identified with arrows. M2 may be a No. 16, a 5q− chromosome, or a marker (M). Origin of M1, M3, and M4 is unknown. Karyotype: 48, XX, −5, t(8;?) (p23?;?), del(11) (q23), t(15;?) (p11;?), −16?, −21, +mar1, +mar2, +mar3, +mar3, +mar4. Quinacrine mustard. (Originally published as Figure 3 in Rowley *et al.*, Blood 50:759–770, 1977 [47]).

as a No. 5 (Figure 6). Five of nine patients lacking a B chromosome were lacking a No. 7. Loss of rearrangement of No. 17 was found in four and of No. 6 or 8 in three patients. Many of the karyotypes were bizarre, with marker chromosomes and minute chromosomes. The karyotypic pattern seen in these patients showed no correlation with the nature of the original lymphoma, the type of leukemia, or the therapy used. In this study, 70% of the patients had fewer than 46 and 40% had fewer than 45 chromosomes. In comparison, in ANLL *de novo,* less than half of the patients had fewer than 46 chromosomes, and less than 10% had fewer than 45 chromosomes.

Recently, the University of Chicago group updated its findings [48]. We now have studied 26 patients with ANLL as a second malignancy and one patient with a renal transplant who developed ANLL. Fifteen of these patients had previously received both radiotherapy and chemotherapy, eight had only chemotherapy, and four had only radiotherapy. The median times from diagnosis of the initial disease to the development of ANLL for these treatment groups were 61, 59, and 59 months, respectively. Twenty-six of the 27 patients had an abnormal karyotype; one or both of two consistent chromosome changes were noted in 23 of these patients. Eleven patients had loss of No. 5, and marrow cells from three others were lacking part of the long arm of No. 5 (5q−), whereas No. 7 was missing from cells of 18 patients and one other had loss of part of the long arm of No. 7 (7q−). Although these changes are distinctly different from those seen in lymphomas, they are similar to those seen in 25% of aneuploid patients with ANLL *de novo.* The presence of these specific abnormalities might help to identify a group of patients who have ANLL associated with exposure to environmental mutagens. Support for this proposal is provided by findings in children with ANLL *de novo,* none of whom have −5, 5q−, or −7 in their leukemic cells.

Additional support for exposure to environmental mutagens and carcinogens as a possible cause of a portion of ANLL lies in the karyotypic similarities between the 'exposed' group of patients with ANLL *de novo* of Mitelman *et al.* [49], and the University of Chicago patients with secondary ANLL. Rowley [50] recently pointed out that the highest percentage of patients with a hypodiploid modal number is seen in secondary ANLL, and that the lowest is observed in the 'nonexposed' group; the reverse is true for patients with a normal karyotype (Table 4). The exposed group of patients with ANLL *de novo* had an intermediate frequency of hypodiploid and normal karyotypes. Again, when certain specific chromosome abnormalities are examined, the highest frequency of abnormalities of nos. 5 and 7 occurs in secondary ANLL, an intermediate frequency is seen in the exposed, and the lowest frequency is seen in the nonexposed group of patients with ANLL *de novo.* All of these comparisons are based on relatively little data, and must be expanded in prospective studies. But it appears from these data that there is a gradation in the frequency and type of karyotypic abnormality which is related to a history of exposure to mutagenic agents. If one averages the frequency of various abnormalities in the exposed and nonexposed groups of patients who have ANLL *de novo,* one obtains the approximate incidence and types of chromosome changes seen in the total population with ANLL *de novo.* Thus, there might be two types of ANLL *de novo* based on the presence or absence of carcinogenic and mutagenic exposure.

Chemotherapy for treatment-related leukemias has resulted in very poor responses (see chapter by Coltman). Of the 11 treated patients in the University of Chicago series, only two had a partial remission, and each lived only four months after initiation of therapy. Casciato and Scott [51] reported that more than 90% of second malignancy patients died within six months and 68% died within two months of the development of leukemia; only two patients in their review survived for more than one year after the development of acute leukemia. Recently, Beltran and Stuckey [52] reported complete remissions in four of five patients with ANLL after malignant lymphomas which had been treated with chemotherapy. According to

*Table 4.* Modal chromosome number and specific chromosome abnormalities in patients with ANLL related to exposure to mutagenic agents.

| | ANLL *de novo* | ANLL—Sweden | | ANLL secondary |
| | | Non-exposed | Exposed | |
|---|---|---|---|---|
| No. of patients | 382 | 33 | 23 | 21 |
| Modal chromosome number | % patients | | | |
| <46 | 14 | 3 | 35 | 66 |
| 46 normal | 50 | 76 | 18 | 0 |
| 46 abnormal | 17 | 12 | 17 | 19 |
| >46 | 19 | 30 | 21 | |
| No. of aneuploid patients * | 190 | 8 | 19 | 21 |
| Frequency of specific abnormalities | % patients with aneuploidy | | | |
| −5 or 5q− | 8 | 0 | 25 | 54 |
| −7 or 7q− | 14 | 12 | 25 | 65 |
| +8 | 25 | 0 | 25 | 10 |
| +21 | 7 | 12 | 21 | 4 |

\* This is a subset of the total number of patients listed above.
(Table from Rowley, *et al.*, Br J Haematol 44:339–346, 1980 [50].

Zarrabi and Rosner [53], two of 15 patients treated for ANLL following treatment for solid tumors had complete remissions. Although additional data on the response to combination chemotherapy are needed, it can be stated that abnormal karyotypes discovered in cytogenetic studies can help to identify patients with the pre-leukemic phase of a second malignancy. In addition, the pattern of the abnormality in these patients might lead to a better understanding of a sub-type of ANLL *de novo* which could be associated with exposure to carcinogens.

## 11. SUMMARY

Chromosome abnormalities of a clonal nature can be found in approximately 50% of patients with ANLL and ALL. Among patients with ANLL, the presence of a chromosomal abnormality is associated with a worse prognosis in all cases, except if a t(8;21) is present without an associated loss of a sex chromosome. Patients with AML (M1 and M2) with only abnormal metaphases (AA) have the worst prognosis among ANLL patients, whereas AML (M1 and M2) patients with only normal metaphases (NN) have the best prognosis among ANLL patients.

The t(8;21), found in approximately 8% of patients with ANLL, has been shown to be associated exclusively with AML of the M2 type. The acute leukemia associated with a t(8;21) and a missing sex chromosome is an especially aggressive type. A t(15;17) is present in approximately 50% of patients with either hypergranular (M3) or microgranular (M3 variant) promyelocytic leukemia and in no other types of ANLL. Patients with this abnormality seem to have a worse prognosis than patients with M3 or the M3 variant who have a normal karyotype or another karyotype abnormality. Geographic differences have been found in the frequency of both translocations; the significance of these differences remains to be deterimed.

Evolution of the karyotype was seen in approximately 28% of patients with ANLL whose clinical course has been followed. Once evolution of the karyotype occurs, the median survival is approximately two months, and the response to further therapy is poor. Possibly, the evolutionary changes indicate the emergence of a resistant cell line and should suggest a change in the therapeutic plan.

Banding studies in a consecutive series of ALL patients are few; aneuploidy is seen in more than half of these patients. It now appears that aneuploidy or the presence of a specific abnormality has prognostic importance in ALL.

In patients who develop acute leukemia after previous cytotoxic or radiation therapy for a primary malignancy (usually malignant lymphoma or multiple myeloma), clonal chromosome abnormalities are almost always present. The finding of a chromosomal abnormality in a previously treated cancer patient with an isolated cytopenia or pancytopenia is diagnostic of a preleukemic phase. The specific abnormalities found in the majority of patients with second malignancies, such as loss of a No. 5 or a No. 7, as well as the hypodiploid state are found in approximately 25% of all aneuploid patients with ANLL *de novo*. These abnormalities are very similar to those in patients with ANLL *de novo* who have had documented exposure to environmental mutagens and carcinogens. These observations suggest that patients with ANLL *de novo* belong in different groups, depending on the etiology of their leukemia. Such a separation could also be of therapeutic importance if it turns out that the exposed ANLL *de novo* patients respond as poorly to chemotherapy as do patients with a second malignancy.

The study of chromosomal abnormalities by means of banding methods during the past ten years has resulted in significant discoveries and clinical associations. Further advances will require continued careful analyses of large populations of patients will acute leukemia who are carefully classified according to a unified system such as the FAB classification and sub-classified on the basis of new ultrastructural, cytochemical, and immunological methods. Careful prospective epidemiologic studies are necessary for the identification of subclasses according to etiology.

REFERENCES

1. Bennet JM, Catovsky D, Daniel M, Flandrin G, Galton DAG, Gralnick HR, Sultan C: Proposals for the classification of the acute leukaemias. Br J Haematol 33:451–458, 1976.
2. Mitelman F, Brandt L: Chromosome banding pattern in acute myeloid leukemia. Scand J Haematol 13:321–326, 1974.
3. Oshimura M, Hayata I, Kakati S, Sandberg AA: Chromosomes and causation of human cancer and leukemia. XVIII. Banding studies in acute myeloblastic leukemia (AML). Cancer 38:748–761, 1976.
4. Golomb HM, Vardiman J, Rowley JD: Acute non-lymphocytic leukemia in adults: correlations with Q-banded chromosomes. Blood 48:9–21, 1976.
5. Rowley J, Potter D: Chromosome banding patterns in acute non-lymphocytic leukemia. Blood 47:705–721, 1976.
6. Mitelman F, Nilsson PG, Levan G, Brandt L: Non-random chromosome changes in acute myeloid leukemia: chromosome banding examination of 30 cases at diagnosis. Int J Cancer 18:31–38, 1976.
7. Alimena G, Annimol L, Balestrazzi P, Montuoro A, Dallapiccola B: Cytogenetic studies in acute leukaemias: prognostic implications of chromosome imbalances. Acta Haematol 58:234–239, 1977.
8. Golomb HM, Vardiman JW, Rowley JD, Testa JR, Mintz U: Correlation of clinical findings with quinacrine-banded chromosomes in 90 adults with acute nonlymphocytic leukemia. N Engl J Med 299:613–619, 1978.
9. Philip P, KroghJensen M, Killman SA, Drivsholm A, Hansen NE: Chromosomal banding patterns in 88 cases of acute nonlymphocytic leukemia. Leukemia Res 2:201–212, 1978.
10. Hossfield DK, Faltermeier M, Wendehorst E: Relations between chromosomal findings and prognosis in acute nonlymphoblastic leukemia. Blut 38:377–382, 1979.
11. Hagemeijer A, Hählen K, Abels J: Cytogenetic follow-up of patients with non-lymphocytic leukemia. Cancer Genet Cytogenet 3:109–124, 1981.
12. First International Workshop on Chromosomes in Leukaemia: chromosomes in acute non-lymphocytic leukaemia. Br J Haematol 39:311–316, 1978.
13. Yunis JJ, Bloomfield CD, Ensrud K: All cases of acute non-lymphocytic leukemia may have a chromosomal defect. N Engl J Med 305:135–139, 1981.
14. Sakurai M, Sandberg AA: Prognosis of acute myeloblastic leukemia: chromosomal correlation. Blood 41:93–104, 1973.
15. Nilsson PG, Brandt L, Mitelman F: Prognostic implications of chromosome analysis in acute non-lymphocytic leukemia. Leukemia Res 1:31–34, 1977.
16. Rowley JD: Identification of a translocation with quinacrine fluorescence in a patient with acute leukemia. Ann Genet (Paris) 16:109–112, 1973.
17. Sakurai M, Oshimura M, Kakati S, Sandberg AA: 8–21 translocation and missing sex chromosomes in acute leukemia. Lancet ii:227–228, 1974.
18. Hart JS, Trujillo JM, Freireich EJ, George SL, Frei III E: Cytogenetic studies and their clinical correlation in adults with acute leukemia. Ann Intern Med 75:353–360, 1971.

19. Trujillo JM, Cork A, Hart JS, George SI, Freireich EJ: Clinical implications of aneuploid cytogenetic profiles in adult leukemia. Cancer 33:824–834, 1974.

20. Trujillo JM, Cork A, Ahearn MJ, Youness EL, McCredie KB: Hematologic and cytologic characterization of 8/21 translocation of acute granulocytic leukemia. Blood 53:695–706, 1979.

21. Second International Workshop on Chromosomes in Leukemia: Cytogenetic, morphologic, and clinical correlations in acute nonlymphocytic leukemia with t(8q− ; 21q+). Cancer Genet Cytogenet 2:99–102, 1980.

22. Engel E, McKee LC, Bunting KW: Chromosomes 17–18 in leukaemias. Lancet i:42-43, 1967.

23. Golomb HM, Rowley J, Vardiman J, Baron J, Locker G, Krasnow S: Partial delection of long arm of chromosome 17; a specific abnormality in acute promyelocytic leukemia? Arch Intern Med 136:825–826, 1976.

24. Rowley JD, Golomb HM, Dougherty C: 15/17 translocation, a consistent chromosomal change in acute promyelocytic leukaemia. Lancet i:549–550, 1977.

25. Rowley JD, Golomb HM, Vardiman J, Fukuhara S, Dougherty S, Potter D: Further evidence for a consistent chromosomal abnormality in acute promyelocytic leukemia. Int J Cancer 20:869–872, 1977.

26. Kaneko Y, Sakurai M: 15/17 translocation in acute promyelocytic leukaemia. Lancet i:961, 1977.

27. Okada M, Miyazaki T, Kumota K: 15/17 translocation in acute promyelocytic leukaemia. Lancet i:961, 1978.

28. Van den Berghe H, Louwagie A, Broeckaret-Van Orshoven A, David G, Verwilghen R, Michaux JL, Ferrant A, Sokal G: Chromosome abnormalities in acute promyelocytic leukemia (APL). Cancer 43:558–562, 1979.

29. Testa JR, Golomb HM, Rowley JD, Vardiman JW, Sweet DL: Hypergranular promyelocytic leukemia (APL): Cytogenetic and ultrastructural specificity. Blood 52:272–280, 1978.

30. Bernard S, Weil M, Boiron M: Acute promyelocytic leukemia: results of treatment by daunorubicin. Blood 41:489–496, 1973.

31. Drapkin RL, Gee TS, Dowling MD: Prophylactic heparin therapy in acute promyelocytic leukemia. Cancer 41:2484–2490, 1978.

32. Berger R, Bernheim A, Daniel MT, Valensi F, Flandrin G, Bernard J: Translocation t(15;17), leucemie aiguë promyelocytaire et non promyelocytaire. Nouv Rev Fr Hématol 21:117–131, 1979.

33. Bennet JM, Catovsky D, Daniel MT, Flandrin G, Galton DAG, Gralnick HR, Sultan C, (FAB 1980): A variant form of hypergranular promyelocytic leukemia (M3). Ann Intern Med (Ltr) 92 1:261, 1980.

34. Golomb HM, Rowley JD, Vardiman JW, Testa JR, Butler A: 'Microgranular' acute promyelocytic leukemia: a distinct clinical, ultrastructural, and cytogenetic entity. Blood 55:253–259, 1980.

35. Second International Workshop on Chromosomes in Leukemia: Chromosomes in acute promyelocytic leukemia. Cancer Genet Cytogenet 2:103–107, 1980.

36. Testa JR, Mintz U, Rowley JD, Vardiman JW, Golomb HM: Evolution of karyotypes in acute non-lymphocytic leukemia. Cancer Res 39:3619–3627, 1979.

37. Oshimura M, Freeman AI, Sandberg AA: Chromosomes and causation of human cancer and leukemia. Cancer 40:1161–1172, 1977.

38. Cimino MC, Rowley JD, Kinnealey A, Variakojis D, Golomb HM: Banding studies of chromosomal abnormalities in patients with acute lymphocytic leukemia. Cancer Res 39:227–238, 1979.

39. Zuelzer WW, Susumu I, Thompson RI, Ottenbreit MJ: Long-term cytogenetic studies in acute leukemia of children; the nature of relapse. Am J Hematol 1:143–190, 1976.

40. Bloomfield CD: Clinical significance of chromosomal abnormalities in acute lymphoblastic leukemia. A preliminary report of the Third International Workshop on Chromosomes in Leukemia. Proc Am Soc Clin Oncol 22:477, 1981.

41. Rosner F, Grünwald H: Hodgkin's disease and acute leukemia. Report of eight cases and review of the literature. Am J Med 58:339–353, 1975.

42. Coleman CN, Williams CJ, Flint A, Glatstein EJ, Rosenberg SA, Kaplan HS: Hematologic neoplasia in patients treated for Hodgkin's disease. N Engl J Med 297:1249–1252, 1977.

43. Foucar K, McKenna R, Bloomfield CD, Bowers TK, Brunning RD: Therapy-related leukemia. A panmyelosis. Cancer 43:1285–1296, 1979.

44. Bergsagel DE, Bailey AJ, Langley GR, MacDonald RN, White DF, Miller AB: The chemotherapy of plasma-cell myeloma and the incidence of acute leukemia. N Engl J Med 301:743–748, 1979.

45. Lundh B, Mitelman F, Nilson PG, Stenstam M, Söderström N: Chromosome abnormalities identified by banding technique in a patient with acute myeloid leukaemia complicating Hodgkin's disease. Scand J Haematol 14:303–307, 1975.

46. Vardiman JW, Golomb HM, Rowley JD, Variakojis D: Acute non-lymphocytic leukemia in malignant lymphoma. Cancer 42:229–242, 1978.

47. Rowley JD, Golomb HM, Vardiman J: Non-random chromosomal abnormalities in acute nonlymphocytic leukemia in patients treated for Hodgkin's disease and non-Hodgkin's lymphomas. Blood 50:759–770, 1977.

48. Rowley JD, Golomb HM, Vardiman JW: Nonrandom chromosome abnormalities in acute leukemia and dysmyelopoietic syndromes in patients with previously treated malignant disease. Blood 58:759–767, 1981.

49. Mitelman F, Brandt L, Nilsson PG: Relation among occupational exposure to potential mutagenic/carcinogenic agents; clinical findings, and bone marrow chromosomes in acute nonlymphocytic leukemia. Blood 52:1229–1237, 1978.

50. Rowley JD: Chromosome changes in acute leukemia. Br J Haem 44:339–346, 1980.

51. Casciato DA, Scott JL: Acute leukemia following prolonged cytotoxic agent therapy. Medicine 58 1:32–47, 1979.

52. Beltran G, Stuckey WJ: Successful therapy of acute myelogenous leukemia (AML) in patients with malignant lymphomas. Blood 52:239a, 1978.

53. Zarrabi MH, Rosner F: Acute nonlymphocytic leukemia following treatment for solid tumors: report of 18 cases. Blood 52:281a, 1978.

# 6. An Integrated Approach to the Study and Treatment of Acute Myelocytic Leukemia

HARVEY D. PREISLER

CONTENTS

## 1. INTRODUCTION

Acute myelocytic leukemia results from the proliferation of immature myeloid cells whose ability to differentiate is markedly impaired. Failure to

*C. D. Bloomfield (ed.), Adult leukemias 1, 155–197. All rights reserved.*
*Copyright © 1982 Martinus Nijhoff Publishers, The Hague/Boston/London.*

differentiate confers an extended reproductive life time on the leukemic cells so that their numbers progressively increase. These cells not only fail to differentiate but their very presence inhibits normal hematopoiesis resulting in anemia, granulocytopenia, and thrombocytopenia. Recent studies have suggested that the conventional view of the kinetics of leukemia cell proliferation should be revised. The low $^3$HTdR labeling indices reported in the past have been interpreted as indicating that leukemic cells proliferate more slowly than normal immature myeloid elements [1, 2]. Tritiated thymidine suicide studies of leukemic progenitors which clone *in vitro* have demonstrated that the proportion of clonogenic cells which are synthesizing DNA is comparable to that of normal progenitor cells at a comparable level of maturation and is in fact 3–5 times that which would be projected from conventional labeling index studies [3, 4]. Furthermore, labeling index studies of leukemic cells obtained from bone marrow biopsies as opposed to marrow aspirates have also demonstrated a greater proportion of cells in S phase than had been formerly estimated [5]. Hence, the concept of acute leukemia being a disease of slowly proliferating cells is probably incorrect. It is of interest that in an early report Gavosto attempted to determine the compartment size and turnover time of leukemic cells and concluded that the myeloblast population per se was not self-maintaining and that there had to be a precursor compartment which fed cells into the blast compartment [6]. Perhaps the cloning studies are providing a window for viewing this precursor pool.

At the time that leukemia is usually diagnosed, the majority of cells in the bone marrow are leukemic. It has been estimated that at this stage of the disease the body contains $1\text{-}4 \times 10^{12}$ leukemic cells [7]. The strategy of remission induction therapy is to reduce the number of leukemic cells by at least 2–3 logs producing marrow hypocellularity thereby releasing the residual normal hematopoietic elements from leukemia-induced suppression. Cytogenetic studies have demonstrated that this is in fact the most likely mechanism of remission induction. The leukemic cells of many patients possess a chromosomal abnormality which is unique to the individual patient [8, 9]. When remission is induced this abnormality usually disappears [10]. It reappears upon relapse of the leukemia.

## 2. REMISSION INDUCTION THERAPY

The general strategy of remission induction therapy is to administer two or more cytotoxic agents for short courses in relatively high doses so as to induce bone marrow aplasia as quickly as possible. This is in contrast to the early attempts at remission induction therapy when cytotoxic agents were usually administered on a daily basis until toxicity occurred. The administration of cytotoxic therapy in short courses resulted from the dual recognition that the shorter the time to aplasia the faster the marrow can begin to regenerate and that maximal marrow toxicity was often manifested 7-10 days after the cessation of chemotherapy.

The 7+3 regimen of cytosine arabinoside (ara C) and daunorubicin (DNR) is probably the most commonly used regimen [11]. Successful remission induction rates are generally 70-75% at institutions which care for a large number of patients [12, 13] and 50-60% in cooperative group studies [14, 15]. Recently 6-thioguanine has been added to regimens containing cytosine arabinoside and an anthracycline antibiotic in an attempt to increase the therapeutic efficacy of the regimen [16-18]. Table 1 compares the drug schedule and the therapeutic efficacy of several TAD regimens and it is apparent that the range of complete remission rates is quite variable. A recently initiated CALGB study (Figure 1), designed to determine whether or not 6TG increases the therapeutic efficacy of the standard '7+3' regimen, is in its early stages but with 25 patients entered/arm the remission induction rates of arms I and III are both 63% [19]. It is possible, and perhaps likely, that the fact that some institutions obtain 80-85% CR rate with TAD while others using similar regimens with or without TG achieve remission rates of 70% is more a reflection of inter-institutional differences in patient referral patterns rather than the result of significant differences in the induction regimens themselves. For example, it is extremely uncommon for patients being treated at Addlesbruck Hospital in Cambridge to die of infection during the first three weeks of remission induction therapy [20]. This is a unique situation which is not understood but clearly plays a significant role in the 85% CR rate reported from this institution [18].

Further improvement in remission induction therapy requires either the development of more effective and less toxic agents or a more rational approach to treatment through the individualization of therapy.

*Table 1.* Comparison of drug doses in TAD regimens.

| | Vogler et al. [11] | Wiernik et al. [25] | Gale et al. [16] | Rees et al. [18] | Arlin et al. [17] |
|---|---|---|---|---|---|
| DNR * | $10 \times 5$ | $75 \times 1$ | 60 d 5, 6, 7 | $50 \times 1$ | $60 \times 3$ |
| ara C * | $200 \times 5$ | $150 \times 5$ | $200 \times 7$ | $200 \times 5$ | $200 \times 5$ |
| TG * | $200 \times 5$ | $150 \times 5$ | $200 \times 7$ | $100 \times 5$ | $200 \times 5$ |
| CR rate | 48% | 50% | 79% | 85% | 78% |

* Dosages in $mg/m^2$ per day. Note that route and timing of administration vary among regimens.

Schema for CALGB Protocol 7921

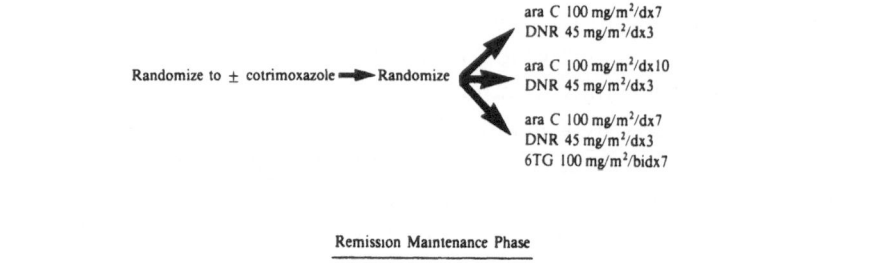

Remission Induction Phase

Randomize to ± cotrimoxazole ➡ Randomize

ara C 100 mg/m²/dx7
DNR 45 mg/m²/dx3

ara C 100 mg/m²/dx10
DNR 45 mg/m²/dx3

ara C 100 mg/m²/dx7
DNR 45 mg/m²/dx3
6TG 100 mg/m²/bidx7

Remission Maintenance Phase

if CR ➡ ara C 100 mg/m²bidx5d
6TG 100 mg/m²bidx5d ➡ ara C 100 mg/m²/bidx5d
vincristine 2 mg/m²xl
prednisone 40 mg/m²/dx5 ➡ ara C 100 mg/m²bidx5d
DNR 45 mg/m²x2d ➡ are C 100 mg/m²bidx5d
vincristine 2 mg/m²xl
prednisone 40 mg/m²/dx5 ➡ ....

*Figure 1.* Schema for the current Cancer and Leukemia Group B protocol for the treatment of acute myelocytic leukemia or one of its variants. The protocol is designed to determine if antimicrobial prophylaxis with cotrimoxazole will decrease the incidence of infection during remission induction therapy causing a reduction in deaths due to intercurrent disease and hence a higher remission rate. With respect to remission induction therapy two modes of increasing the intensity of 7 + 3 therapy are being tested: an increase in the duration of administration of cytosine arabinoside to 10 days and the addition of 6-thioguanine. Once patients enter remission and receive 8 courses of maintenance therapy they are randomized to stop all therapy or to continue to relapse, thus determining if prolonged maintenance therapy is necessary.

## 3. THERAPY ONCE COMPLETE REMISSION IS INDUCED

It has been somewhat fashionable to argue that maintenance therapy has not been demonstrated to prolong either the duration of remission or patient survival. Close examination of available data however clearly demonstrates that some therapy administered after a patient enters remission does in fact increase the duration of remission. Table 2 provides remission duration data for several representative studies. [A more exhaustive review of the literature can be found in reference 21.] The shortest median duration of remission is reported for those studies which provided little or no post-remission therapy [22–24] or alternatively for regimens that utilized relatively ineffective agents during maintenance therapy [25, 26]. The more intensive regimens which include cytosine arabinoside and an anthracycline antibiotic have produced the longest remission durations [27, 28].

Remissions which exceed three years are currently seen in 10–25% of patients who enter complete remission [29–31]. While a small proportion of

*Table 2.* Effect of consolidation and maintenance therapy on remission duration.

| Study # | Experimental design | MDR (mo.) |
|---------|---------------------|-----------|
| 1 [22] | ara C induction then (R) → no maint. | 1.25 |
|  | ⤷ ara C maint. | 7.5 |
| 2 [113] | POMP or DNR induction. no maint. | 2.25 |
| 3 [24] | TAD induction → 2 consol. (R) → no maint. | 6.7 |
|  | ⤷ monthly maint. | 10.3 |
| 4 [112] | ara C + DNR → 3 consol. → no rx. | 6.3 |
| 5 [114] | pred-VCR-ara C-adr → 3 consol. → main. to relapse | 18.0 |
| 6 [27] | ara C-anthra → courses of rx. to relapse | 15.0 |
| 7 [115] | ara C-DNR → courses of rx. to relapse | 12.0 |
| 8 [32] | ara C-adr-pred-VCR → courses of rx. × 14 months | 20+ |

(R) = randomize
MDR = median duration of complete remission
rx. = therapy

patients may experience prolonged remissions without receiving post-remission induction therapy, it is clear that the majority of patients will benefit from therapy with appropriate drugs. The optimal length of maintenance therapy will probably vary from regimen to regimen with the most intensive regimens requiring the shortest durations of therapy. This question is under intensive investigation at the present time.

Recent interest has been focused on administering much more intensive maintenance therapy than had hitherto been administered in an attempt to produce still longer remissions. Studies at the Sidney Farber Cancer Center where courses of intensive therapy are administered each month for 14 months have produced a median duration of remission of approximately 24 months [32]. A similar study in progress at Roswell Park Memorial Institute appears to be producing similar results [33].

Other investigators have attempted to prolong the duration of remission by administering 'immunotherapy.' These studies have employed both 'specific' and 'nonspecific' immunotherapy with occasional studies appearing to demonstrate a clinical advantage [34, 35]. However, to the present time these studies have not been reproducible and the role of such therapy is currently unknown [36, 37]. This is not surprising in view of the absence of evidence for the existence of a tumor specific antigen in man. On the other hand, the presence of an abnormal combination of normal differentiation antigens might render a tumor cell susceptible to immunologic attack so that the field of immunotherapy may become relevant at some time in the future when more knowledge of the immune system is acquired.

Recently attention has been focused on the use of allogeneic bone marrow transplantation in patients who are in their first remission [38–40]. Previous experience with marrow transplantation in patients in relapse demonstrated a small but significant cure rate in these patients [41]. These observations have been interpreted as indicating that bone marrow transplantation was clearly a potentially curative therapeutic modality but that in this latter setting its therapeutic effects were limited by the clinical problems of advanced disease and the larger tumor load present in such patients. Hence the focus turned to marrow transplantation for patients in complete remission. The initial results have been quite encouraging with the major problem being those of the transplantation procedure itself and graft versus host disease. Leukemic relapse has been an uncommon problem in the early reports. Nevertheless the high early mortality among transplanted patients has resulted in an overall patient survival which at the present time is not significantly better than that seen with potent chemotherapeutic regimens.

A major difficulty with this therapeutic modality is the fact that at the present time it is limited to individuals under 45 years of age who have a histocompatible sibling. Transplantation across HLA barriers has recently been initiated and perhaps the introduction of cyclosporin A as an immunosuppressive agent will make such transplantations feasible [42]. In any event, it is too early to come to any conclusions regarding the role of marrow transplantation in patients in remission. It is not known if the very low incidence of leukemic relapse will continue as the studies become extended in time. If it does, ultimate patient survival may very well exceed that for patients treated with current chemotherapeutic regimens. On the other hand, the long-term effects of total body irradiation and high dose cyclophosphamide therapy are not known and it is possible that there may be a high rate of secondary neoplasms or accelerated aging of vital organs.

Despite the advances in the treatment of AML it is clear that therapy is far from satisfactory for the majority of patients. Even under the best of circumstances 20–30% of patients do not enter remission and by the third year 80% of the patients who entered remission have relapsed. Long term survival is limited at the present time to approximately 10–15% of patients with this disease.

### 3.1. Analysis of Remission Induction Failures

Recognition of the fact that 20–30% of patients do not enter complete remission identifies a problem without suggesting a potential solution. Without knowing the proportion of patients who do not enter complete remission because of drug resistant leukemia, the proportion who die because of excessive marrow toxicity or because of intercurrent disease one cannot decide as to how the current therapeutic regimens should be modified to increase the complete remission rate. To deal with this problem we introduced a system for classifying remission induction failures [43]. That this was not done in the past was most likely due to the psychology of the physicians.*

A modification of the original classification system is presented in Table 3. The utility of this system is illustrated in Table 4 where one of our recent treatment protocols has been analyzed. Using this approach it is clear that approximately 10–15% of patients expired while hypoplastic or shortly after therapy was initiated while a comparable percent of patients had disease which was clearly resistant to therapy with ara C and an anthracycline antibiotic.

Figure 2 illustrates the possible effects of remission induction therapy on leukemic cells. The leukemic cells of patients who enter complete remission

*Table 3.*

| Failure types | |
|---|---|
| I | 'Significant' drug resistance—administration of a course of remission induction therapy fails to produce significant marrow hypoplasia in a patient who survives for seven or more days after the completion of drug administration. |
| II | 'Relative' drug resistance: |
| | a) a course of chemotherapy produces severe marrow hypoplasia but leukemic cells repopulate the marrow within 40 days of completion of the course of therapy |
| | b) severe marrow hypoplasia is produced by a course of chemotherapy and leukemic cells repopulate the marrow. Normal elements also reappear and the patient enters partial remission status (return of peripheral blood white blood cell count to >2500/µl with >50% mature granulocytes, and platelet count returns to >50 000/µl. |
| III | Regeneration failure—chemotherapy renders the marrow severely hypoplastic and it remains so for >40 days after the end of the course of chemotherapy. |
| IV | Hypoplastic death—patient expires during a period of severe marrow hypoplasia. If this death occurs >40 days after the end of a course of therapy the patient is considered to be a type III failure. |
| V | Inadequate trial—patient expires <7 days after the end of a course of chemotherapy with a cellular bone marrow. |
| VI | Patient achieves complete hematologic remission status but leukemic cells persist in extramedullary sites (i.e., CSF, liver, spleen, etc.). |

* Physicians, like others, prefer to deal with their successes and to forget their failures. Hence in common parlance a patient who does not enter complete remission is referred to as having 'failed' therapy when in fact it is the physician who has failed to deliver effective therapy. This attitude accounts for the fact that the very significant differences between patients in the group in which remission is not induced have been ignored.

*Table 4.* Response to remission induction therapy and causes of failure in patients treated on Protocol 950501.

Response to Course #1

Complete remission—19 patients
Death during induction—12 patients
   Type II failure—1
   Type IV failure—4
   Type V failure—7

| Survived and received Course #2 | Response to Course #2 |
|---|---|
| Type I failure—5  ⟶ | CR—1, type I failure—1, type IV failure—3 |
| Type II failure—5  ⟶ | CR—4, type II failure—1 |
| Type VI failure—1  ⟶ | CR |
| Unknown  ⟶ | CR—2, type IV failure—1 |

after a single course of therapy are sufficiently drug sensitive that the single course of therapy reduced the leukemic cell number to $10^8$ cells (see text accompanying Figure 2) permitting normal hematopoietic elements to reappear. Patients who do not enter remission because of relative drug resistance (type II failures) are usually retreated before their leukemic cells increase in number to pretherapy levels so that the second course of therapy further reduces leukemic cells numbers to that required for complete remission to occur. Hence, four out of the five patients described in Table 4 who were type II failures after the first course of therapy entered complete remission after a second course was administered.

It appears that the leukemic cells of patients who do not enter remission because of significant drug resistance (type I failures) are reduced by a second course of therapy to that level to which the leukemic cells of patients who manifested relative drug resistance were reduced after the first course of therapy. This level of leukemic cell reduction is not sufficient to permit the regrowth of normal marrow elements. Hence these patients tend to expire since they have been profoundly pancytopenic for a long period of time. One would assume that had they lived longer leukemic cells would have repopulated the marrow of these patients and that the administration of a third course of therapy would have resulted in a complete remission since it would have reduced the leukemic cell load to a level which permits the regrowth of normal hematopoietic elements. Hence, the patients who enter complete remission together with the patients who manifest relative

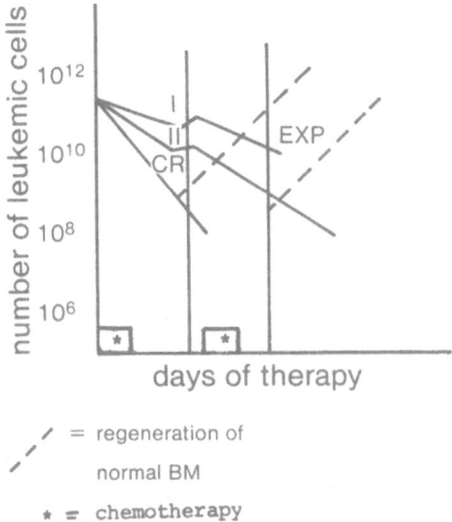

*Figure 2.* Effect of remission induction therapy on the number of leukemic cells present in a patient. The first course of chemotherapy only slightly reduces the number of leukemic cells present in patients who are type I treatment failures after the first course of therapy. A second course of therapy renders these patients hypoplastic and then they generally expire. Therapy produces a greater reduction in leukemic cell numbers in patients who are type II failures, and a second course of therapy reduces leukemic cells numbers to the point that normal marrow cells can regenerate. This occurs after a single course of therapy for patients who enter remission with one course of chemotherapy.

drug resistance and those who manifest significant drug resistance actually represent a continuous spectrum of drug sensitivity-resistance with the leukemic cells of patients who manifest relative drug resistance bridging the gap between the drug sensitive cells of patients who enter complete remission and the drug resistant cells of patients who are felt on clinical grounds to manifest significant drug resistance.

This interpretation of the data also suggests that the drug sensitivity of the majority of leukemic cells in any individual patient is relatively uniform. This hypothesis is reinforced by the fact that we have not as yet observed a single patient who manifested relative drug resistance to a first course of therapy who manifested a significant drug resistance to a second course of the same therapy. This would be expected if the leukemic cells of patients who were type II failures (relative drug resistance) consisted of a majority of drug sensitive cells with a minority of drug resistant cells and that marrow hypoplasia was the result of a drug effect on the drug sensitive cells and that the drug resistant minority population was unaffected by the treatment and was responsible for repopulation of the marrow. In this case such a progression from relative drug resistance to significant drug resistance would have been expected if repopulating leukemic cells were resistant to the therapy being administered. As noted above we have not as yet observed such a progression. Similarly in several patients whose leukemic cells were studied before and after an unsuccessful course of remission induction therapy we have found an increase in *in vitro* drug sensitivity rather than a decrease; the latter would have been expected if the course of therapy killed a drug sensitive cell population leaving a drug resistant cell to repopulate the marrow. As discussed below, a resistant cell subpopulation may in fact be present at the time the disease is diagnosed but those cells would constitute a very small portion of the leukemic cells at this time. Ultimately, however, they may increase in number causing relapse.

The analysis of treatment failures permits several conclusions. For some patients current regimens need to be augmented with respect to anti-leukemic potency, while for other patients an increase in drug dosages or in the duration of therapy will not be beneficial and may in fact be harmful. Barring the appearance of less toxic but more potent agents, future advances in remission induction therapy will have to be based upon recognizing differences between patients so that treatment regimens can be designed to suit the needs of the individual. Hence, some patients might benefit more from a regimen which produces less than maximal antileukemic effects but one which also produces fewer severe side effects. Other patients who are able to tolerate severe side effects would be candidates to receive even more aggressive therapy. As might be expected, the outcome of remission induction therapy is determined by the interaction of many factors including the biological status of the patient and the drug sensitivity of his leukemic cells.

## 4. FACTORS AFFECTING THE OUTCOME OF REMISSION INDUCTION THERAPY

### 4.1. Clinical Aspects

Table 5 lists the factors which are known to significantly affect the outcome of remission induction therapy. The most obvious are those which are related to a patient's general condition, which in essence determines whether or not a patient will survive long enough to enter remission. For patients who enter complete remission after a single course of therapy, the minimum time to remission is 18 days, with most patients in this group entering remission between 24 and 35 days of the initiating of therapy. Needless to say the clinical conditions of patients may range from those who enter the hospital in shock or after a subarachnoid hemorrhage and who have essentially no chance of entering remission to those young patients whose disease was found during a routine physical examination. Between these two ex-

*Table 5.* Factors which affect the outcome of remission induction therapy.

| General physical status | Clinical condition | Property of leukemic cells |
|---|---|---|
| 1. Age | 1. Fever | 1. Drug sensitivity of leukemic cells |
| 2. Past medical history | 2. Documented infection | 2. Regenerative capacity of leukemic cells. |
|    a) prior radiation therapy<br>   b) prior therapy with alkylating agents<br>   c) preleukemic condition |    a) severity | |
| 3. Number of residual normal hematopoietic elements | 3. Major medical problems<br>   a) shock<br>   b) subarachnoid hemorrhage<br>   c) cardiac, renal, pulmonary insufficiency | |
| 4. Ability of patient to metabolize and excrete antileukemic drugs | | |

tremes are the patients who are infected when they enter the hospital. Superimposed upon these clinical conditions is the general physical status of the patient as determined by the patient's biological age. While the influence of age has long been recognized, only recently has its effects been quantified [44].

A history of having received chemotherapy or radiation therapy prior to the development of AML indicates a reduction in the probability of entering complete remission to the order of 10% with median patient survivals of one month from the initiation of intensive remission induction therapy (see chapter by Coltman).

While these patients clearly are usually 'resistant' to therapy, clinical resistance is not necessarily synonymous with leukemic cell resistance to the agents employed in therapy. Analysis of the causes of treatment failure in these patients suggests that in many cases it was due to inadequate regenerative potential of the normal marrow perhaps because of residual damage from prior exposure to DNA damaging agents [45, 46]. In other cases drug resistant leukemic cells were clearly present. The exact proportion of treatment failures due to inadequate regeneration of normal elements or to leukemic cell resistance awaits study of larger numbers of patients.

The fact that patients who develop leukemia after experiencing a preleukemic syndrome (hyperplastic refractory anemia, aplastic anemia, etc.) seem to have a worse prognosis than patients who have not had a prodromal syndrome may be explained in one or more ways. The preexisting hematologic syndrome may be indicative of a reduced number and/or of limited proliferative potential of normal hematopoietic stem cells and hence of impaired regenerative potential after chemotherapy for leukemia. On the other hand, these leukemias may involve more primitive cells than the usual leukemias and these more primitive cells may be relatively resistant to the chemotherapeutic agents employed to treat the more common kinds of acute myelocytic leukemia.

If the latter explanations were correct they might tie together several other superficially unrelated observations. The syndrome of acute erythroleukemia clearly involves a primitive multipotential cell since while it often begins with the isolated involvement of the erythroid series and in essentially all cases it evolves to include the myeloid series as well. This variant of acute myelocytic may be more resistant to therapy than other subtypes of leukemia [47, 48]. The leukemias associated with prior therapy with alkylating agents or radiation therapy appear to bridge the gap between the leukemias which follow a prodromal hematologic syndrome and acute erythroleukemia in that the leukemias associated with prior therapy are usually preceded by a prodromal period similar to the classical preleukemic states and often evolve into acute erythroleukemia [45]. Hence, these three syndromes (leukemias preceded by a prodromal period, erythroleukemia, and leukemia associated with prior therapy) which are often thought of as three distinct entities may represent a similar biological problem in that all may be associated with impaired marrow regenerative potential and/or the involvement of a primitive hematopoietic stem cell whose drug sensitivities may differ significantly from that of cells involved in the more common variants of AML.

## 4.2. Prognostic Significance of General Biological Characteristics of Leukemic Cells

Several measurable biological properties of leukemic cells are of substantial prognostic significance. For example, the chromosomal constitution of the bone marrow cells of leukemic patients is a strong predictor of a patient's survival time [49, 58] and in fact is an indicator of the likelihood that a patient will enter remission [52]. Patients in whom only normal metaphases are seen (NN) have a much greater likelihood of entering remission than do patients in whom only aneuploid metaphases are seen (AA). Patients in whom both normal and abnormal metaphases are detected (NA) have a prognosis which is intermediate between patients with NN or AA

*Table 6.* Outcome of therapy vs cytogenetic characteristics of the bone marrow chromosomal type.

|  | NN | NA | AA |
|---|---|---|---|
| CR | 34/47 (72%) | 12/22 (55%) | 5/15 (33%) |
| | Failure types | | |
| Failure type | Individuals who received only one course of therapy | | |

|  | NN | NA | AA |
|---|---|---|---|
| I | 1 | 3 | – |
| II | – | 2 | 1 |
| III | – | – | 1 |
| IV | 3 | 1 | 4 |
| V | 5 | 3 | 1 |
| unknown | – | 1 | 1 |

Four NN patients received two courses of chemotherapy. One entered CR and three were type IV failures. All were initially type I failures. Two AA individuals received two courses of therapy and both were type IV failures. Both were type I failures after their first course of therapy.

karyotypes. The respective remission rates for NN, NA and AA patients at Roswell Park who were treated with cytosine arabinoside and an anthracycline antibiotic are 75%, 59%, and 30%, respectively [50]. Preliminary analysis of the distribution of remission failure types in these patients is also given in Table 6. While five of the eight AA patients who did not enter remission expired with hypoplastic marrow, only three of the 14 treatment failures classified as NN or NA expired with hypocellular marrows. These data suggest that the absence of normal metaphases reflects an absence of or a severe reduction in the number of residual normal hematopoietic stem cells with consequent impairment of the regenerative potential of the residual normal hematopoietic cells. By similar reasoning, the good prognosis of NN patients could result from the persistence of substantial numbers of normal cells in these patients, the metaphases of which would be indistinguishable from the leukemic metaphases when conventional techniques are used. Clearly many more patients need to be studied to confirm or refute this hypothesis.

On the other hand, several other explanations are also possible. Perhaps aneuploid leukemic cells are more biologically adaptable than euploid leukemic cells in that the former cells are the product of a more extensive clonal evolution than the euploid leukemic cells with a consequent greater biological adaptability for survival. Such adaptability might be reflected in the ability to suppress competing normal cells and in a more flexible cellular constitution conferring the ability to adapt to adverse environmental conditions including the presence of chemotherapeutic agents. Both of these properties would have an adverse effect on response to chemotherapy. Studies reported by Broxmeyer *et al.* have in fact demonstrated that leukemic cells as a group produce substances which inhibit the proliferation of normal progenitor cells [51]. Nevertheless the exact nature of the normal metaphases present in these patients is unknown. Are they (at least in part) residual normal cells or are they in fact leukemic cells which are at an early stage of clonal evolution?

The cloning characteristics of the leukemic cells *in vitro* have also been reported to be of prognostic significance. In general, patients whose leukemic cells produce large-sized clusters or colonies when cloned in agar *in vitro* have a lower remission rate than patients whose leukemic cells either fail to clone or produce small clusters *in vitro* [52–54]. One report has noted that the leukemic cells of these patients seemed to be more resistant to therapeutic attack *in vivo* [55]. The prognostic significance of leukemic cell growth *in vitro* has also been studied from a different vantage point. Leukemic cells were cloned in methylcellulose *in vitro*, recovered seven days later, and then replated [56]. The cloning efficiency of the second plating was then compared with that of the initial plating. The idea behind this approach was to measure the self-renewal capability of the clonogenic leukemic cells, i.e., their ability to produce other clonogenic cells. There is, in fact, a weak but statistically significant direct correlation between secondary cloning efficiency and failure of the patient to enter complete remission [56]. The conventional interpretation of this observation is that the ability of the clonogenic cells to produce other clonogenic cells (i.e., the stem cell or self-renewal potential of the leukemic cells) is a reflection of the capacity of the leukemic cell population to increase its numbers after chemotherapeutic attack.

In our own studies we have not found a correlation between colony or cluster size and either $^3$HTdR labeling index of the leukemic population as a whole or the suicide index of the clonogenic cells. Therefore, the differences in the size of the clusters or colonies produced in agar by marrow specimens obtained from different patients are not due to differences in proliferative rate. It appears then that differences between patients' leukemic cell growth *in vitro* under the conditions employed may be related to differences in the adaptability of patients' leukemic cells to adverse conditions since *in vitro* growth conditions are undoubtedly less than optimal. If this hypothesis were correct then the reported correlations between the size of leukemic cell clusters *in vitro* and between self-renewal capacities and the outcome of remission induction therapy would be readily understandable since *in vitro* studies would be a reflection of the leukemic cells' general ability to survive under adverse conditions, conditions including *in vivo* chemotherapy. It is especially unfortunate that the papers reporting a relationship between *in vitro* growth characteristics and response to chemotherapy *in vivo* did not classify the failure type of the patients studied since the use of such a classification system would perhaps have provided answers to this hypothesis. If the hypothesis was correct the failure types should have been predominantly types I and II.

Other factors which have been reported in the past to be of adverse prognostic significance include the percent of leukemic cells in S phase at the time of diagnosis [57, 58], the presence of acute promyelocytic leukemia [59], and an extremely high white blood cell count [60]. The first factor is no longer by itself of prognostic significance with respect to remission induction probably because of the introduction of more potent chemotherapeutic regimens while the latter two are also no longer significant because of recognition of the unique problems that they present and the use of supportive care directed at these problems.

## 4.3. Biology of Remission Induction

The goal of remission induction therapy is to significantly reduce the numbers of or to ablate the leukemic cell population while preserving enough residual normal hematopoietic cells to permit restoration of normal hematopoietic function. The reduction of leukemic cell numbers is in itself a complex phenomenon since it represents the net effects of several factors: the proportion of leukemic cells destroyed by chemotherapy, the number of residual leukemic stem cells and their rate of proliferation, and the rate of proliferation of the leukemic cell population as a whole. The exact same factors determine the restoration of normal hematopoiesis. The relationship between the killing of leukemic cells, the regenerative potential of normal hematopoietic cells, and the outcome of remission induction therapy is illustrated in Figure 2.

Clearly little is known about these various phenomena. For patients who enter complete remission the antileukemic chemotherapy must have had a substantially greater effect upon the leukemic cells than on normal cells, otherwise remission could never occur. In these patients the normal stem cells may be less sensitive than the leukemic cells to the drugs employed. We have observed, for example, that the proportion of normal CFUs killed by cytosine arabinoside does not exceed the percent of CFUc which are in S phase during exposure to the drug [61]. By contrast, the percent of leukemic CFUc killed by cytosine arabinoside may greatly exceed the percent of cells in S phase [84]. Hence some leukemic CFUc may be more intrinsically metabolically sensitive to chemotherapeutic agents than are normal hematopoietic elements. Another possible mechanism may be related to the fact that essentially all of the chemotherapeutic agents employed in remission induction regimens are cell cycle specific. Hence if leukemic-produced inhibitory factors have put the normal progenitors out of cycle then a further differential sensitivity would result. Finally it should not be assumed that the drug sensitivity of the CFUc of normal patients or of remission patients are reflective of the drug sensitivities of the residual hematopoietic elements present at the time of florid disease because essentially nothing is known about these cells.

The relative differential sensitivity of normal and leukemic cells may also be related to the regenerating abilities and rate of proliferation of the normal and leukemic stem cells which survive chemotherapy. One additional factor which must be considered is the endogenous death rate of the cells in question. If the spontaneous death rate of leukemic cells under post chemotherapy conditions were substantially higher than that of the surviving normal stem cells then a significant growth advantage would accrue for the regenerating normal cells.

### 4.4. Assessment of the Properties of Leukemic Cells In Vitro

As described above it may be possible to derive an estimate of the biological adaptability of leukemic cells by studying their growth characteristics *in vitro* and/or the ability of the leukemic cells to produce clonogenic cells *in vitro* since these properties may in fact be a reflection of the leukemic cell's general ability to survive under adverse conditions. These general measurements do not, however, provide information regarding the leukemic cell's sensitivity to specific chemotherapeutic agents.

*4.4.1. General Approach.* Three questions must be answered before effective and reliable tests for measuring the drug sensitivity of leukemic cells become available: which cells should be studied, what studies should be carried out, and how should the efficacy of the *in vitro* assays be determined.

*Which Cells Should Be Studied.* Tumor cell populations are believed to be organized into a pattern which is similar to the pattern of organization of normal hematopoietic cells: there is a stem cell pool which replicates itself and also gives rise to cells of limited replicative ability and an additional cell population which in essence is in the process of dying. While the latter two cell populations may be important with respect to the effects they produce in the patient, therapeutic attack need only be directed against the stem cell population since they sustain the disease. At the present time there is no information as to the relative sizes of these leukemic cell subpopulations nor can they be distinguished from each other with any degree of certainty. The existence of these different cell subpopulations greatly complicates the development of *in vitro* predictive assays since the properties of the population as a whole or of some of the subpopulations may not be reflective of the properties of the clonogenic cells. In fact, we have demonstrated that the proportion of leukemic cells in the bone marrow population as a whole which are synthesizing DNA is much less than the proportion of clonogenic leukemic cells synthesizing DNA [3]. We have also demonstrated that the effects of cytosine arabinoside on the population of murine myeloid leukemic cells as a whole are not reflective of its effects on the clonogenic leukemic cells [62]. Hence drug sensitivity studies must be directed at the relevant target cells and since the properties of the population as a whole are not necessarily reflective of the properties of the leukemic stem cells one must not overinterpret *in vitro* studies.

The situation is further complicated by the fact that the leukemic cell population consists of two kinetically distinct subpopulations: kinetically active and kinetically quiescent cells [63–65]. These populations differ in cell size as well as in kinetic activity and may also differ in their ability to take up and metabolize drugs [66]. For example, we have recently found that small quiescent leukemic cells as a whole phosphorylate less cytosine arabinoside than do kinetically active cells. The enzyme system which breaks down cytosine arabinoside triphosphate may be similar, however, since the retention of cytosine arabinoside triphosphate by kinetically active and kinetically quiescent leukemic cells was indistinguishable. In general leukemic cells in the peripheral blood tend to be kinetically quiescent while those in the bone marrow are much more kinetically active. At least a portion of the quiescent cells can become kinetically active [67]. Recent flow cytometric studies suggest that leukemic cells are not in a 'deeply quiescent' $G_0$ state as are normal lymphocytes or tissue culture cells grown to and maintained in a confluent state [68]. Such deeply quiescent cells have a distinct acridine orange staining pattern since their RNA content is extremely low. Human leukemic cells do not manifest this pattern of staining [68]. This recent observation is compatible with earlier studies in which $^3$HTdR was administered by continuous infusion and which demonstrated that 98% of leukemic cells synthesized DNA at some time during a 2-week period [69]. Hence, it appears that the majority of human leukemic cells do not enter a deeply quiescent $G_0$ state.

While under the usual culture conditions *in vitro* only the kinetically active subpopulation will clone [70]; by changing the *in vitro* conditions we have now been able to clone a portion of the kinetically quiescent cells as well [71]. Taken together, then, at least five leukemic cell populations can be recognized: a clonogenic population and a nonclonogenic population, each of which contains cells which are kinetically active and kinetically quiescent and an end stage population of dying cells. The situation is further complicated by the fact that we do not know if the cells which clone *in vitro* are in fact leukemic stem cells. (The implications of this problem will be discussed below.) In any event, leukemic cell populations are quite complex and at the present time methods are being developed to separate and/or recognize these subpopulations.

Since the only clinically relevant measurements are those which are reflective of the properties of leukemic stem cells and since the properties of the population as a whole are not necessarily reflective of the properties of the stem cells, the relevance of drug studied on the former cells must be validated by parallel studies of leukemic stem cells or by rigorous parallel evaluation of the outcome of therapy *in vivo*.

A final question relates to whether or not peripheral blood leukemic cells are suitable for study. It is clear that at least the cell cycle characteristics of peripheral blood leukemic cells are different from those of the leukemic cells present in the bone marrow. This was believed in the past to result from the fact that the circulating cells were smaller in size thus representing a greater proportion of kinetically quiescent cells. However, we have recently compared comparably sized blood and marrow leukemic cells and found that while the small sized cells of the blood and marrow were similar in RNA content and proliferative activity, the large marrow cells were more kinetically active and contained more RNA than identically sized peripheral blood cells [68]. On the other hand the Toronto Group has reported that by using 'special' *in vitro* conditions they could clone leukemic stem cells from the peripheral blood of patients and that these cells could be used to estimate the drug sensitivity of leukemic cells [72]. We have directly compared the properties of the cells grown in our standard *in vitro* assay with those of the cells which proliferate under the conditions used by the Toronto Group and have not found any differences [73].

*Potential Measures of Drug Sensitivity.* A variety of *in vitro* methods were tested in an attempt to develop an accurate means for estimating the drug sensitivity of leukemic cells. The two most common approaches have been pharmacologic studies of drug uptake and metabolism [74, 75] and determination of the effects of drugs on macromolecular synthesis [76, 77]. These assays have several disadvantages. In the first place they measure the properties of the leukemic cell population as a whole and perhaps not of the relevant cells. While failure to take up a drug or to activate it (when necessary) probably indicates drug resistance, the converse is not necessarily true in that drug uptake and activation do not guarantee antileukemic effect. Similarly, inhibition of macromolecular synthesis is not necessarily indicative of a lethal effect upon a cell since the inhibition may be reversible and the metabolic pathway being studied may in fact not even be a relevant

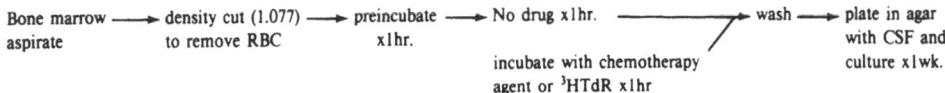

*Figure 3.* Method for measuring the drug sensitivity and <sup>H</sup>TdR suicide index of donogenic lenkemic cells.

metabolic pathway. Studies of the effects of cytosine arabinoside on leukemic cells provide an excellent illustration of these points. Cytosine arabinoside must be taken up and phosphorylated to the triphosphate form for it to be active [78]. As the triphosphate it can inhibit DNA synthesis [79]. The DNA inhibitory effect may be reversible [80] and in fact it has not been demonstrated to the present time that inhibition of DNA synthesis is relevant since the mechanism by which the drug kills cells is unknown. Lethal effects may be the result of chromosomal breakage [81] perhaps secondary to errors in DNA replication [82, 83] or to the incorporation of cytosine arabinoside triphosphate into DNA. Hence, even for this extensively studied drug, the actual mechanism by which it kills sensitive cells is unknown. It remains possible, however, that the failure of cytosine arabinoside to inhibit DNA synthesis, as is failure of the cell to phosphorylate the drug, may be useful as an indication of drug resistance.

Given the above it would seem logical to assume that an assay which directly measures cell killing would avoid the above problems. We have been studying the possibility of estimating leukemic cell drug sensitivity by measuring the killing of the clonogenic leukemic cells by chemotherapeutic agents [84]. The method is illustrated in Figure 3. While our studies have demonstrated that the ability of cytosine arabinoside to inhibit DNA synthesis by the leukemic cell population as a whole does not necessarily indicate that the drug will kill or even inhibit DNA synthesis by the clonogenic leukemic cells [62], the studies illustrated in Table 7 demonstrate that there

*Table 7.* Relationship between outcome of remission induction therapy and the killing of clonogenic cells *in vitro*.

|  | *in vitro* sens to DNR | | *in vitro* sens. to DNR + ara C | |
|---|---|---|---|---|
|  | # pts. | % LCFUC* killed | # pts. | % LCFUC killed |
| Complete remission[†] | 8 | 45±8 | 9 | 50±7 |
| Drug resistant[†] | 6 | 23±5 | 5 | 10±2 |

* LCFUC = leukemic CFUC.
[†] All patients treated with daunorubicin-cytarabine combinations.

is a good correlation between the ability of drugs to kill the clonogenic cells and the outcome of remission induction therapy [84].

The development of *in vitro* clonogenicity techniques as tools to study leukemic cells have also led to an integration of cell cycle measurements with measures of drug effects. During the development of these methods it became clear that when the sensitivity of leukemic CFUc to an S phase specific agent such as cytosine arabinoside was being measured a parallel determination had to be made of the percent of leukemic CFUc which were in S phase during the time that the cells were exposed to cytosine arabinoside [61]. This was accomplished by carrying out a $^3$HTdR suicide index study [3]. In this way an accurate measurement of sensitivity of the leukemic CFUc to cytosine arabinoside can be derived by determining the percent of CFUc which were in S phase and which were killed by the drug. The utility of this approach is illustrated in Table 8 where what appears to be a discordance between *in vitro* sensitivity to cytosine arabinoside and *in vivo* response to chemotherapy is demonstrated to be an artifact. This general approach undoubtedly applies to other S phase specific drugs whose intracellular retention time is low.

The assessment of drug sensitivity before and after a course of chemotherapy in patients whose leukemic cells manifest drug resistance *in vivo* (type I and II therapeutic failures) is beginning to shed some light on the biology of remission induction. In one patient we have found evidence that his initial failure to respond to therapy appeared to be due to the fact that too few of his clonogenic leukemic cells were actively cycling to permit cytosine arabinoside to kill a substantial number of these cells [84]. An initial course of combination chemotherapy resulted in the apparent recruitment of cells into cycle due to the killing of leukemic cells by daunorubicin, thus rendering them sensitive to cytosine arabinoside (Table 8). In two other initial treatment failures we have found that drug sensitivity increased after a course of therapy for reasons not due to changes in the cell cycle characteristics of the leukemic cells. Intuitively one would have expected the

*Table 8.*

| Pt. # | % CFUC killed by ara C | $^3$HTdR Si | % killed by ara C Si | Outcome of therapy |
|---|---|---|---|---|
| 1 (a) | 0 | 0 | – | Type I failure |
| (b) | 64 | 74 | 0.86 | CR |
| 2 | 23 | 29 | 0.79 | CR |
| 3 | 21 | 62 | 0.34 | Type I failure |
| 4 | 2 | 70 | 0.03 | Type I failure |

opposite in that the administration of cytosine arabinoside-daunorubicin should have killed the sensitive cells leaving drug resistant cells. That this did not occur might be due to the production of sublethal damage by the initial course of therapy with the additional damage produced by the second course of therapy resulting in a lethal intracellular event. The ability of damaged cells to survive for a time and to replicate with the persistence of either sublethal or lethal damage is well known in both the carcinogenesis and radiation therapy literature.

The apparent utility of this measure of drug sensitivity as compared to previous studies in this area raises the question as to why the clonogenicity studies appear to be far more reliable than the latter. The clonogenicity studies represent two methodological departures. The first and most obvious difference is that clonogenicity assays utilize cell killing as the end point. If the sole advantage of this method is related to the detection of cell killing, then there may be other and simpler ways to measure killing. The ability to exclude Trypan blue is one such measurement which is employed in many laboratories as an estimate of cell viability. Some studies with tissue culture cells have suggested that the Trypan blue dye exclusion test does not provide an accurate means for measuring a loss of clonogenicity [85]. On the other hand, there has been at least one report claiming that the killing of acute lymphocytic leukemic cells *in vitro* by drugs as measured by Trypan blue dye exclusion correlates quite well with the outcome of remission induction therapy utilizing these agents *in vivo* [86].

A second difference between the clonogenicity drug sensitivity systems and the usual pharmacologic approaches relates to the fact that in the former only the drug sensitivity of the cells which clone *in vitro* are being studied. The cells which clone differ from the population as a whole in being both clonogenic *in vitro* and in being more kinetically active than the population as a whole [71]. Whether the killing of these clonogenic cells can occur in the absence of the killing of the population as a whole and whether the population as a whole can be killed while the clonogenic cells are spared is unknown. Direct studies of this problem are under way and are of great importance because of the studies described above, which demonstrated that in some circumstances there is a dissociation of the properties between the clonogenic cells and the populations as a whole.

Given that it is likely that the cells which clone *in vitro* are a special subset whose drug sensitivity can be used to estimate the response of leukemic cells to chemotherapy *in vivo*, are these cells necessarily the most appropriate targets, i.e., the leukemic stem cells? It is possible that the clonogenic cells are in fact more primitive than the population as a whole and that these cells are close to the leukemic stem cell. In the studies under discussion all clusters *in vitro* which consist of four or more cells are

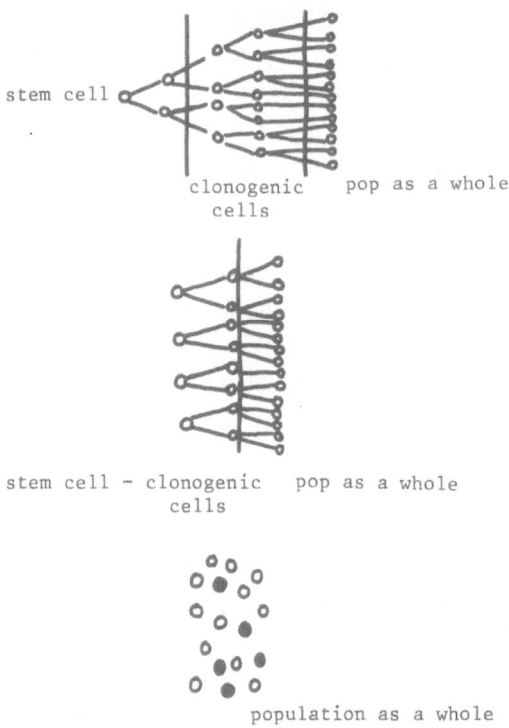

stem cell

clonogenic    pop as a whole
cells

stem cell - clonogenic    pop as a whole
cells

population as a whole

*Figure 4.* The schema in the top third of the figure represents the situation where the leukemic stem cell is a unique cell different from the cells which clone *in vitro* and from the population as a whole. Since this cell could be very rare it could be resistant to the drugs administered to a patient and yet the patient could still enter remission if the cells which clone *in vitro* and/or the leukemic cell population as a whole were sensitive to these agents. In this situation the *in vitro* drug sensitivity test would predict for remission induction success but not for cure.

The middle third of the figure illustrates the situation which could exist if the cells which clone *in vitro* were identical to the leukemic stem cell and had properties which were different from those of the population as a whole. In this situation only the drug sensitivity of the clonogenic cells would be therapeutically relevant and could theoretically predict for cure as well as the outcome of remission induction therapy.

The lower portion of the figure represents the situation that would exist if all leukemic cells were equivalent in properties with only 'chance' determining whether or not a cell clones *in vitro*. In this situation, the properties of the leukemic cells as a whole would be representative of the properties of the clonogenic cells and would predict for the outcome of remission induction therapy and also for cure.

counted, with the clusters generally consisting of 8–12 cells. This represents a range of cell replications of from two to four, a number which would be much less than that expected of a stem cell. However, these cells may have a much greater replicative potential *in vivo* and their limited replication *in vitro* may be a reflection of inadequate *in vitro* conditions. Alternatively, true leukemic stem cells may not proliferate at all *in vitro* under the conditions which are currently employed. It must be recognized that the true clonogenic potential of leukemic cells can never be estimated by *in vitro* studies unless 100% of the cells clone since a cloning efficiency which is less than 100% can always be attributed to inadequate culture conditions *in vitro*. Figure 4 illustrates these three possibilities, each of which is compatible with a good correlation between the drug sensitivity of the leukemic cells which clone *in vitro* and *in vivo* response. If the middle or bottom panels are correct then there should be a correlation between drug effects *in vitro* and both the remission induction rate as well as remission duration and curability. If the first possibility is correct then there would not necesarily be a correlation with curability and such a correlation would occur only when methods are developed which permit the direct measurement of the drug sensitivity of the true leukemic stem cells.

*Evaluation of In Vitro Assays.* A major difference between the studies described here and previous attempts to develop *in vitro* assays predictive of drug sensitivity *in vivo* also relates to the approach used to analyze clinical response to therapy. In the previous studies patients were divided into two groups: those that entered remission and those that did not. As already discussed above, patients who do not enter remission are a diverse group including some individuals whose disease is drug sensitive. Hence, by failing to classify the remission induction failures into drug resistant and indeterminant groups, patients who did not enter remission and who may have had drug sensitive disease were included in the drug resistant group. This is illogical since one cannot expect an *in vitro* test of drug sensitivity to predict death due to intercurrent disease of a patient with drug sensitive leukemia. In our studies, patients who entered complete remission were classified as having drug sensitive disease but the drug resistant group included only those patients in whom drug resistance was documented—i.e., the type I and II treatment failures [84, 87]. These are patients in whom the failure to enter remission could be ascribed to the presence of leukemic cells with significant or limited drug resistance. All other patients were excluded since a determination of their *in vivo* drug sensitivity could not be made.

Theoretically there should be differences in the drug sensitivity of the leukemic cells of patients whose cells manifest significant or relative drug resistance. These differences may become apparent when a larger number of patients are studied. Hence, the evaluations of drug sensitivity studies carried out in the past may have been confounded by the failure of the investigators to classify the remission induction failures.

### 4.5. Delivery of Drugs to the Leukemic Cells

Regardless of the degree of leukemic cell sensitivity to chemotherapeutic agents, patients will not enter remission unless adequate serum drug levels

178

are attained for an adequate length of time. The critical role of serum levels is illustrated by a case we have recently studied. Fifty percent of this patient's clonogenic leukemic cells were killed by *in vitro* exposure to cytosine arabinoside-daunorubicin, a cell kill so high that one would have expected that complete remission would occur. The patient was, however, a type I treatment failure. The serum daunorubicin levels achieved during therapy were much lower than that usually achieved, suggesting that inadequate serum levels were the cause for the failure of this course of therapy (see Figure 5, patient in question indicated by arrow). The variability of serum levels achieved between patients further complicates the prediction of response since very high serum drug levels may convert a case of borderline *in vitro* drug sensitivity to a case with very clinically responsive disease. Clearly the converse could be true as well. The serum drug levels attained in patients appears to be a function of endogenous patient factors as well as prior exposure to the drug. For example, in a study of adriamycin levels attained during chemotherapy patients who had been treated with adriamycin within the previous 2 years had upon treatment significantly lower

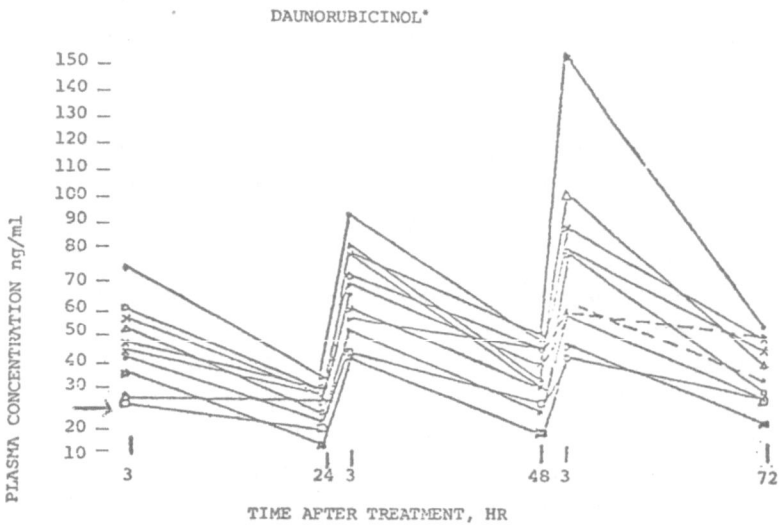

DAUNORUBICINOL*

*Figure 5.* Serum daunorubicinol levels attained in 8 patients treated with daunorubicin 45 mg/m²/day on days 1, 2, and 3 of therapy. The patient whose serum levels are indicated by the lower ■ — ■ was referred to in the text as being a relapsed patient whose leukemic cells were very sensitive to cytosine arabinoside and daunorubicin but who was a type I failure when treated with these agents.

* *Studies carried out in collaboration with Dr. Teresa Gessner, Roswell Park Memorial Institute.*

serum levels of adriamycin than patients who had never been treated with the drug [88].

Extremes of serum drug levels attained during therapy could have profound effects on the outcome of treatment since very high levels might produce intolerable toxicity while high levels may increase the likelihood that a patient whose leukemic cells are only moderately drug sensitive will enter remission while very low serum levels would not induce remission in any patient regardless of the drug sensitivity of his leukemic cells.

An even more difficult problem is represented by leukemic cells located in a sanctuary where adequate drug levels cannot be attained. Clearly the central nervous system represents one such potential site and is probably of greatest significance for patients with acute myelomonocytic and acute monocytic leukemia [89]. Whether other privileged sites exist (comparable to the testis in children with acute lymphocytic leukemia) is not known at the present time.

### 4.6. Clinical Implications of In Vitro Studies

On the basis of our clinical experience approximately 10–15% of previously untreated patients have leukemia which is resistant to cytosine arabinoside-anthracycline antibiotic chemotherapy and 10–15% fail to enter remission because of early death or inadequate marrow regeneration. For relapsed patients the percent of patients with drug resistant disease is much higher with 80% of patients who fail to enter complete remission with the first course of chemotherapy having clinically documented drug resistant disease (Table 9).

It is clear, however, that recognition of those patients in whom clinical drug resistance is due to leukemia cell resistance will permit a change in

Table 9. Outcome of courses of remission induction therapy.

|  | Previously untreated patients | Patients with relapsed disease |
|---|---|---|
| # patients | 90 | 44 |
| # courses of therapy | 112 | 69 |
| # complete remissions | 59 | 20 |
| # with drug resistant disease | 10 | 40 |
| Hypoplastic deaths | 11 | 2 |
| Inadequate trial | 12 | 3 |
| Unknown failure type | 8 | 4 |
|  | ∴ 10% w/ resistant disease | ∴ 29% w/ resistant disease |

180

therapeutic approach. If low serum levels are a problem then the dosage of drug could be increased since low serum levels would also be accompanied by reduced toxic side effects as well thus permitting dosage escalation without the production of lethal side effects. That the latter is the case is suggested by our observations that patients in whom chemotherapy fails to produce an adequate antileukemic effect frequently do not suffer from the nausea usually associated with chemotherapy.

If, on the other hand, the leukemic cells of a patient were found to be resistant to one or more of the usually employed chemotherapy agents then these agents could be avoided and other agents substituted. For patients whose leukemic cells were drug resistant because few of the leukemic cells were actively cycling, perhaps the administration of a noncycle specific agent would reduce cell numbers to the point that enough cells would begin active cycling to permit the use of more conventional remission induction therapy. In any event coordination of *in vivo* and *in vitro* studies will permit the individualization of chemotherapy and thus the avoidance of toxicity produced by clinically ineffective drugs as well as permitting the selection of clinically useful agents.

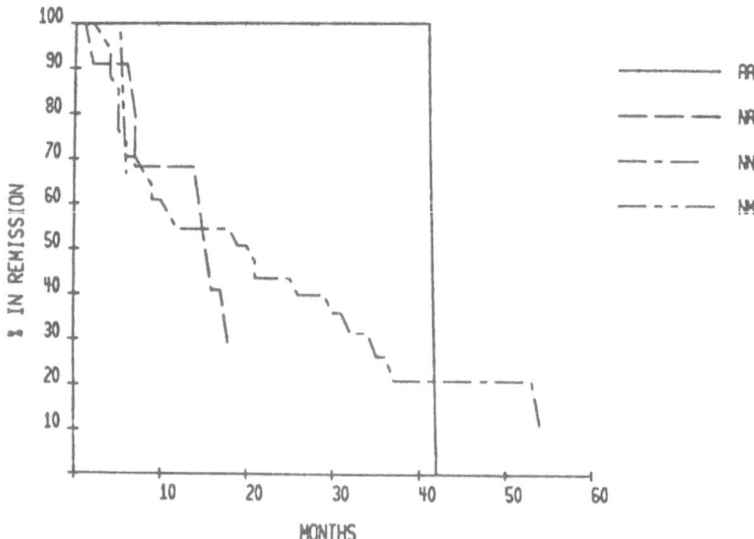

*Figure 6.* Remission durations of patients with NN, NA, or AA karyotypes. NM indicates those patients in whom metaphases were not detected *in vitro*. There is no significant difference between the median durations of remission.

5. THE PROBLEM OF REMISSION DURATION AND RELAPSE

### 5.1. Prognostic Factors

The clinical factors which are of prognostic significance with respect to remission induction outcome are not of prognostic significance for remission duration since they basically are related to a patient's ability to survive remission induction therapy. This is illustrated in Figure 6 where it is demonstrated that the pretherapy cytogenetic studies which are so highly predictive of outcome of remission induction therapy are not predictive of remission duration [50]. Much less is known about factors which may be useful in predicting remission duration. At the present time serum LDH and fibrinogen levels [90] and the $^3$HTdR labeling index appear to be of prognostic significance possibly as nonspecific measures of leukemic cell load and 'aggressiveness' of the disease. The prognostic significance of the number of courses required to induce a complete remission is not universally accepted but intuitively it seems logical in that the number of courses that are required to produce a remission would be related to the drug sensitivity of the leukemic cells and to the serum drug levels achieved and hence to the number of leukemic cells killed during remission induction therapy as well as of the probable effect of maintenance therapy on residual leukemic cells. On the other hand if remission consolidation-maintenance therapy were effective, a correlation between courses to remission and remission duration might not be detectable. The ability of pretherapy leukemic cells to phosphorylate cytosine arabinoside and retain cytosine arabinoside triphosphate has been found to be related to remission duration [91]. Recent studies have confirmed our initial observations [92].

The significance of these potential prognostic factors lies in the fact that their measurement at the time of diagnosis may permit separation of AML patients into high and low risk categories and thus permit recognition of those patients who need and those who do not need continued intensive chemotherapy after complete remission is attained. At the present time, however, the measurement of the known prognostic parameters does not appear to distinguish between patients who will relapse late and those who will not relapse. Perhaps the simultaneous determination of several of these factors will permit a more precise prognostication to be made.

### 5.2. Causes of Relapse

It is generally assumed that relapse occurs because of the development of leukemic cell resistance to chemotherapy. Indeed most clinical observations are in accord with this assumption in that relapse usually occurs despite the administration of courses of maintenance therapy which produce pancytopenia (with the production of pancytopenia during maintenance therapy being taken as an indication of an 'adequate' therapeutic effect). In addition, the presence of clinical evidence of increased leukemic cell resistance to chemotherapy at the time of relapse (see Table 9) appears to confirm this hypothesis. Other observations, however, suggest that a significant number of exceptions may exist. As we study increasing numbers of relapsed patients we have found that the leukemic cells of some relapsed patients are still quite sensitive to the drugs which were used in maintenance therapy.

If the leukemic cells were still sensitive, why did the relapse occur? In some cases relapse undoubtedly occurred because of the administration of inadequate drug dosages during maintenance therapy, dose levels which had been lowered from that originally administered because of increasing pancytopenia during maintenance therapy. The production of pancytopenia during maintenance therapy cannot be used as an indication that the dose-time levels of drugs being administered were adequate with respect to anti-leukemic effects since profound pancytopenia may have been produced because a progressive reduction in normal marrow stem cell reserve occurred during maintenance therapy despite relatively low serum drug levels. These low levels may have been adequate to suppress normal hematopoiesis but may have produced few if any effects on the residual leukemic cells.

Several months before leukemic relapse is documented some patients manifest marked intolerance to chemotherapy, an intolerance which necessitates a significant reduction in maintenance therapy. It is not clear whether impending relapse caused the marked decrease in tolerance to chemotherapy or if the reduction in chemotherapy resulted in relapse. The former possibility is raised by the studies of rat myeloid leukemia where when as little as 2 % of marrow cells are replaced by leukemic cells suppression of normal hematopoiesis occurred [93]. Hence, it is possible that in some patients when dosages are reduced because of hematopoietic toxicity an increase in the intensity of chemotherapy or a change to other agents would have been more appropriate.

Finally, it is possible that the occurrence of relapse in patients whose leukemic cells are still drug sensitive (as determined by the *in vitro* clonogenicity assay) is merely a reflection of an inadequacy in the sensitivity assay itself. If, as discussed earlier, the properties of the leukemic cells which clone *in vitro* are not identical with or at least reflective of the drug sensitivity of the true leukemic stem cells then relapse with 'drug sensitive' cells could occur if the majority of relapsed cells were leukemic stem cells which did not clone *in vitro* and hence, whose drug sensitivity were not being measured by the drug sensitivity assay. Opposed to this possibility is the observation that the administration of cytosine arabinoside-daunorubicin therapy to patients with relapsed disease where leukemic cells still manifest sensitivity *in vitro* to these agents results in the production of severe marrow hypoplasia and often in the induction of a complete remission. Of significant concern, however, is the possibility that the correlation of *in vitro* and *in vivo* responsiveness may be less for relapsed patients than for previously untreated patients and also that the duration of remission in these patients appears to be quite short, in some cases despite marked *in vitro* sensitivity of the leukemic cells to the drugs being administered. These observations are confounded, however, by a lack of measurement of serum drug levels produced during chemotherapy with the possibility that low serum drug levels during therapy resulted in a lesser reduction in leukemic cell levels than is usually produced in patients who have not received chemotherapy in the past, despite similarity in the drug sensitivity of the two different sets of patients leukemic cells.

## 5.3. Prediction of Relapse

The ability to recognize regrowth of leukemic cells prior to the clinical reappearance of the disease would be of great clinical utility. It would permit intensification of maintenance chemotherapy and/or a change to other chemotherapeutic agents. It would also permit recognition of those patients in whom the appearance of drug intolerance during maintenance therapy was due to the regrowth of leukemic cells. Table 10 lists four methods which are purported to be of use in diagnosing impending relapse. The first three methods make use of an alteration in the cell cycle characteristics of remission bone marrow cells in that two are based upon a reduction of the percentage of cells in S phase [94, 95] and the third utilizes recognition of an increase in the proportion of cells in late $G_1$ phase [96]. These phenomena are presumably due to the effects of leukemic cells upon normal marrow

*Table 10.* Prediction of relapse in patients with acute leukemia.

| Investigator | Measurement | Successful pred. of relapse | Med. time to relapse * | (Month–range) |
|---|---|---|---|---|
| Hillen et al. [95] | ↓ % S phase cells on DNA histogram | 10/14 | ? | (1–5 months) |
| Stryckmans et al. [96] | ↓ ³HTdR Li marrow myeloblasts | 8/17 | 8 | (5–12 months) |
| Hittelman et al. [97] | ↑ Proliferative potential index | 11/14 | 3.5 | (1¼–11 months) |
| Baker et al. [98] | ↑ Reactivity to antileukemia antisera | 21/26 | 3.7 | (1–6 months) |

* Months from when abnormal measurement first noted.

elements. Interestingly these three reports came from three different groups of investigators, in three different countries, using three different methodologies, and essentially provide the same lead time to clinical relapse.

The fourth method utilizes the appearance of cells which are reactive with a murine antibody directed against human AML cells [97]. The basis for this assay is not easily understood since there are as yet no well-documented reports of tumor specific antigens in man. Nevertheless this approach warrants further testing.

Given the situation described above, it would appear that a combination of these relapse predictor assays with an assessment of the number of residual normal hematopoietic stem cells by measuring CFUc [98], BFUe [99], and the mixed cell assay [100] would be of help in determining whether chemotherapy should be increased or decreased in a patient who became 'sensitive' to maintenance chemotherapy.

## 5.4. Treatment of Relapsed Disease

From the data already accumulated it would appear that relapse is a much more heterogeneous state than was previously suspected with great variation in the drug sensitivity of leukemic cells and in the serum drug levels achieved during therapy. Hence, rational decisions for treatment of relapsed disease must be based upon evaluations of prognostic factors and of measurements of drug sensitivity. Such studies will be described below.

## 6. ESTIMATION OF MARROW REGENERATIVE CAPACITY

Implicit in the discussion regarding the selection of potent antileukemic drugs is the fact that it is not very difficult to design a regimen which will destroy most of the leukemic cells in a patient's bone marrow. This can be done with essentially any of the regimens used for marrow transplantation (the appearance of recurrent disease in the majority of patients who are transplanted while in leukemic relapse attests to the difficulty in destroying every leukemic cell when a large number are present). The obvious limitation of this approach is the necessity of sparing enough normal hematopoietic stem cells so that normal marrow regeneration can occur once leukemic cell reduction is effected. As already mentioned there are several clues that can be sought in a patient's past history which can provide a rough estimate as to whether or not a patient is likely to have adequate reserves of normal marrow. Needless to say this clinical-historical approach presents the problem of not providing adequate information about the regenerative potential of the marrow of a specific individual patient, which clearly ranges from high to low even among patients who have never received chemotherapy or radiation therapy in the past, who have a normal chromosomal constitution, and who did not have a prodromal preleukemic syndrome.

The information which would be most desired is: 1) an estimate of the number of residual normal hematopoietic elements, 2) an estimate of the ability of marrow stroma to support regrowth of these elements, and 3) an estimate of the drug sensitivity of residual normal hematopoietic elements and or normal marrow stroma. In the ideal situation, one would like to be able to distinguish between normal and leukemic clusters during growth in agar and hence derive an estimate not only of the relative proportion of each but also of the drug sensitivity of each. Unfortunately, this would require cytogenetic characterization of each cluster or colony since other available markers could not make the necessary distinctions. The impossibility of such a task is self-evident. In fact, it is assumed that all of the *in vitro* growth of leukemic marrow and peripheral blood under CFUc conditions reflects only leukemic cell growth. This fact has never been proven but appears likely at least for newly diagnosed patients because of the nature of the cluster-colony distribution, the bizarreness of the cells which are growing and the good correlation of *in vitro* and *in vivo* drug sensitivity.

An alternate approach could be to look at the ability of bone marrow and peripheral blood to produce BFUe *in vitro*. It is possible that with the possible exception of the erythroleukemias, in the majority of patients the erythroid cell line is not directly involved in the leukemic process but rather is suppressed by the disease. A review of papers purporting to demonstrate that the erythroid cell line is involved in AML shows that for the most part the morphology of the leukemic cells is not adequately described so that some of the patients may have had erythroleukemia [101, 102]. Given that there do appear to be differences in the number of clonable erythroid elements among leukemic patients [103], it may be that such differences correlate with the number of residual primitive hematopoietic elements. Hence, quantitation of the number of residual hematopoietic elements and perhaps their drug sensitivity may provide a measure of the residual normal hematopoietic stem cell pool as well as their drug sensitivity.

Several observations have suggested that there are differences in the ability of the hematopoietic microenvironments of different patients to support normal cell growth. Recent studies have suggested that the ability of the bone marrow and/or peripheral blood of patients to produce colony stimulating factor (CSF) *in vitro* prior to the initiation of remission induction therapy is correlated with the outcome of therapy [104, 105]. A possible explanation for this observation is that what is being measured may be an estimate of the likelihood of normal cell regeneration after chemotherapy. Unfortunately, the investigators did not classify the remission induction failures in their studies and had they done so one would expect that if the above explanation were correct, the patients with low CSF production would have expired due to a failure of regeneration of normal marrow after remission induction chemotherapy. Hence, it is possible that the measurement of CSF production by bone marrow and peripheral blood cells before and after remission induction therapy may be useful in deriving an estimate of the capacity of a patient's marrow to support endogenous repopulation. A further sophostication would be to determine the effects of chemotherapeutic agents upon CSF production.

Clearly the development of a reliable means of predicting marrow repopulation capacity would significantly complement the studies of drug sensitivity and resistance.

## 7. *IN VIVO* ESTIMATES OF RESPONSE TO REMISSION INDUCTION THERAPY

While under ideal circumstances it would be preferable to have an *in vitro* test available which could be used to determine the optimal therapeutic regimen prior to initiating therapy, studies carried out during the administration of chemotherapy appear to provide the possibility of altering the initial chemotherapeutic regimen so that its effectiveness can be increased. Since 1975 bone marrow aspirates and biopsies have been performed after six days of remission induction therapy. The data illustrated in Figure 7 demonstrate that by determining the marrow cellularity one can distinguish between the majority of patients who will not enter remission because of persistance of leukemia (significant and relative drug resistance) and those who will either enter remission or not enter remission for reasons other than drug resistance [27]. Hence, in our current study the end of the first course of remission induction therapy will be intensified in those cases where the marrow monitoring studies predict remission induction failure due to inadequate leukemic cell kill.

The ability to monitor serum levels of cytosine arabinoside and the anthracycline antibiotics may also permit modification of a therapeutic regimen while it is being administered. As described earlier, there appears to be an occasional patient whose leukemic cells are quite sensitive to the agents administered but who fails to enter remission because inadequate serum levels of drugs were produced during therapy. Figure 5 illustrates the range of serum daunorubicinol levels achieved during remission induction therapy. Once a larger number of patients are studied and the lower limits of serum levels which produce effective antileukemic action *in vivo* are recognize it will be possible to insure that therapeutic serum drug levels are attained.

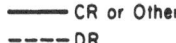

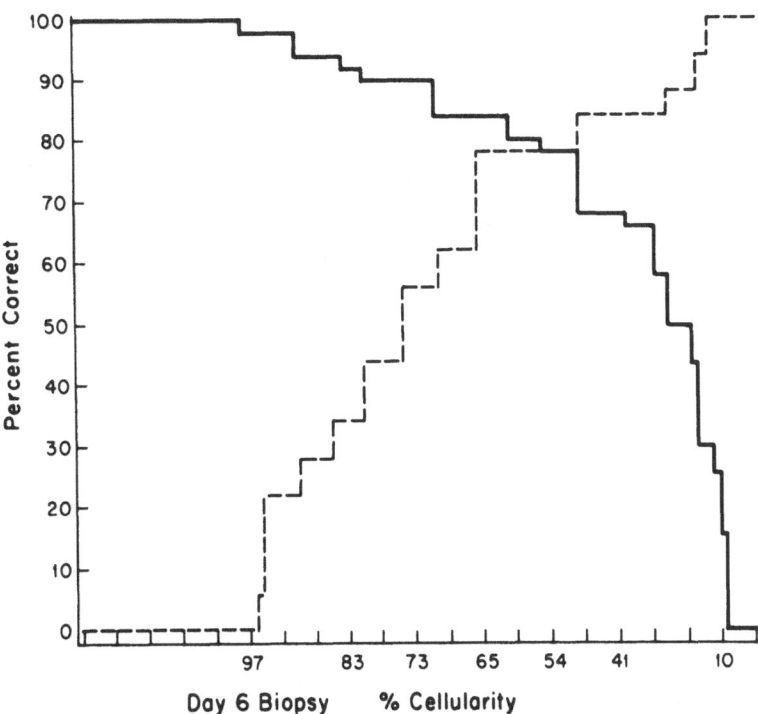

*Figure 7.* The probability of correctly predicting the outcome of remission induction therapy based on estimating the percent of marrow cellularity on the 6th day of remission induction therapy. By taking the 65% cellularity line one can correctly predict 85% of the patients who will enter remission or die of intercurrent disease and 70% of the patients who will fail to enter remission because of drug resistant (DR) disease.

Finally, the advent of flow cytometry offers the possibility of precisely monitoring the *in vivo* effects of drugs on leukemic cells at a level of sophistication which has not been possible in the past. While attempts to correlate the outcome of therapy with changes in the DNA histograms of leukemic cells have not been helpful, the advent of multiparameter measurements may make this approach more fruitful. For example, one could simultaneously measure DNA-protein or DNA-RNA content in individual cells looking not only for the arrest of cells in a particular phase of the cell cycle, but also for evidence of unbalanced cell growth which may be an indication of a loss of clonogenic potential and hence a marker for the production of lethal damage in cells [106]. Recent flow cytometric studies have demonstrated the feasibility of detecting intracellular adriamycin on the basis of the native fluorescent properties of this anthracycline antibiotic [107]. This approach raises the possibility of sampling a patient's bone marrow and/or peripheral blood during chemotherapy so that the ability of the leukemic cells to take up the chemotherapeutic agent under the conditions of *in vivo* chemotherapy can be assessed. This approach would permit an assessment of the final result of the interaction of the serum drug levels and the ability of the individual cells to take up the drug. Perhaps an increase in anthracycline dosages or a change in schedule would result in an increase in adriamycin uptake by cells which fail to do so with conventional chemotherapy schedules.

Hence, it seems possible to directly modify a course of chemotherapy on the basis of studies carried out while the course is in progress. This will permit an increase in drug dosage for those patients with relatively resistant disease as well as perhaps a reduction in the intensity of remission induction therapy for those patients in whom moderate therapy will suffice.

## 8. INDIVIDUALIZATION OF CHEMOTHERAPY FOR ACUTE MYELOCYTIC LEUKEMIA

The major clinical prognostic parameters have in all likelihood been defined. The reasons for their influence on the outcome of therapy are well understood for the most part, and their adverse effects would be reduced if better means of supportive care were developed to prevent and/or treat such complications. The adverse effects of some factors [such as karyotypic constitution (see chapter by Golomb), history of prior chemotherapy (see chapter by Coltman)) have to be better defined in order for the problems that they are associated with to be corrected.

With respect to utilizing *in vitro* tests to assess drug sensitivity certain principles appear to be emerging. While the usual pharmacologic techniques of studying the leukemic cell population as a whole with regard to the metabolism of drugs by cells and the effects of drugs upon cellular metabolism may provide some useful information, to date the measurement of the killing of cells which clone *in vitro* appears to provide the most clinically meaningful information. The cloning systems however present several problems: they are tedious to carry out, they require 7-10 days to provide information, cells from 25-30% of patients cannot be cloned *in vitro* at the present time, and finally, it is extremely unlikely that cloning assays will be sensitive enough to detect one drug resistant cell in 1 000 or 10 000, a cell which may ultimately cause a patient's death.

Studies attempting to deal with these problems are in progress. For example, while no one study of the leukemic cell population as a whole appears to be able to replace the clonogenicity assays, it is possible that measurement of two or more parameters of drug metabolism together with quantitating the effects of chemotherapeutic agents on macromolecular synthesis may be able to do so if there were some dissociation of the properties of the cell population as a whole and those of the clonogenic cells. The studies listed in Table 11 are presently being carried out with this being one of the goals. As already discussed, the advantage of the cloning systems over the other measurements may be related to the fact that cell killing is the end point of the former. With this possibility in mind we are attempting to develop flow cytometric techniques to detect irreversible cell damage as well as to directly detect the death of cells. Clearly the ability of flow systems to rapidly analyze large numbers of cells would provide several advantages: the assays would be rapid and reliably free of human counting errors; they could be carried out on cells obtained from any patient and not be limited to those patients whose cells clone *in vitro*; they would provide information on very large numbers of individual cells, thus perhaps permitting the recognition of drug resistant cells which may be very rare at the time of diagnosis.

Needless to say, the integration of such a large number of clinical and laboratory measurements is quite complex and could not even be attempted without some form of computer assistance for both data collection and analysis. The development of multivariate analytic techniques such as log-

*Table 11.* Pretherapy *in vitro* studies of leukemic cells.

---

*General Properties*
ability to form clusters/colonies
repopulating potential

*Cell Cycle Characteristics*
[3]HTdR labeling index
acridine orange DNA-RNA measurement (DNA histogram + RNA content)
[3]HTdR suicide index

*Drug Sensitivity*

  *Cytosine Arabinoside*
  ability of cells to take up and phosphorylate ara C and to retain ara CTP
  effects of ara C on DNA synthesis
  ability of ara C to kill the clonogenic leukemia cells

  *Adriamycin*
  ability of cells to take up and retain adriamycin
  effects of adriamycin on DNA integrity
  ability of adriamycin to kill clonogenic leukemia cells

  *Adriamycin—ara C*
  ability to kill clonogenic leukemia cells

---

istics regression [108] and Cox Modeling [109] have revolutionized our ability to interpret large amounts of data. Such studies require very large numbers of patients, at least ten per variable under study. Since no one institution has access to such a large number of patients, an interinstitutional study of clinical variables together with the laboratory measurement of drug sensitivity listed in Table 11 has recently been initiated.

## 9. CURRENT APPROACHES TO THERAPY

With respect to remission induction therapy for previously untreated patients, there are several intensive regimens which produce a high rate of remission after a single course of therapy. For the majority of patients less than 70 years of age any one of these regimens would seem to be suitable. For older patients and for those individuals in whom compromised marrow function is suspected, probably a reduction in the intensity of therapy is indicated. From the data already described the augmentation of therapy in those patients in whom an adequate antileukemic effect is not obtained after six days of therapy appears to be indicated. Given the present high remission induction rates in previously untreated patients the effectiveness of such treatment modification would probably best be studied in patients with relapsed disease. The specific tailoring of remission induction regimens on the basis of patient characteristics will probably be ready for testing within the next two years.

The high relapse rates in patients who receive no therapy after entering complete remission emphasizes the fact that substantial numbers of leukemic cells remain in patients who enter remission. Accordingly some form of post remission induction therapy is indicated. The very elegant work by Skipper and his colleagues provides the basis for Figure 8. It can be seen that for the majority of patients repeated courses of therapy are indicated once a patient enters remission. When patients are being treated with curative intent these courses of 'consolidation' theapy should be intensive enough so that the reduction in leukemic cell numbers is so great that leukemic cell proliferation between these courses cannot return leukemic cell numbers to what they were or to a higher level than they were prior to the course of chemotherapy.

It appears that there are two basic causes of leukemic relapse: inadequate reduction of drug sensitive cells and the appearance of leukemic cells which are resistant to the drugs being used to treat the patient. Thus it seems logical that more courses of very intensive chemotherapy be administered than are usually given and that these courses should include drugs for which cross-resistance do not occur. The optimal duration of such intensive con-

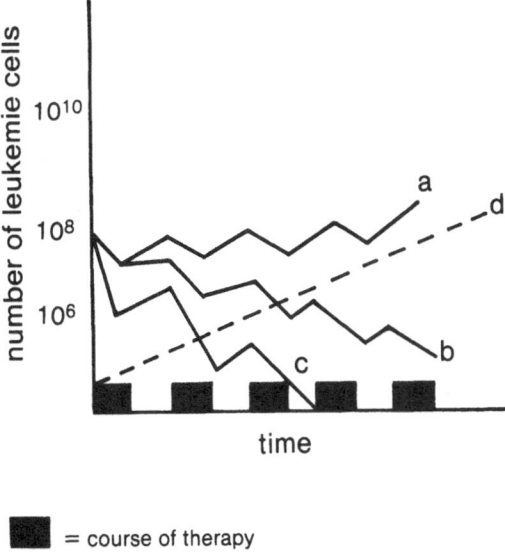

= course of therapy

*Figure 8.* The effect of post-remission chemotherapy on leukemic cell numbers in patients who have entered remission. As discussed in the text it appears that the majority of leukemic cells are similar in their drug sensitivity. The possible effects of therapy on these cells are indicated by the solid lines. The effect of courses of chemotherapy on these cells is illustrated by curves a, b, and c. While the cells whose numbers are described by curve a are somewhat drug sensitive, the courses of chemotherapy are not intense enough or close enough together to effect a steady reduction in cell numbers, since the rate of growth of the leukemic cells exceeds the rate at which they are being killed. Curves b and c represent the effect of therapy on moderately and on highly sensitive cells. Long-term remissions and cure are possible. More intensive therapy (higher doses or more closely spaced courses) would result in greater cell kill, thus altering the slopes of the curves. Less intensive therapy would have the opposite effect. Hence, even for patients with only 'drug sensitive' leukemic cells, relapse could occur despite chemotherapy if the latter was not sufficiently intense.

The broken line indicates another mechanism of leukemic 'relapse.' In this situation, at the time remission is induced, a few drug resistant leukemic cells are present. These cells increase in number despite the administration of chemotherapeutic agents which continue to produce reduction in the drug sensitive cell populations. Eventually, the drug resistant cells replace the drug sensitive cells and relapse occurs with drug resistant disease.

solidation therapy is unknown but this will vary from patient to patient. The tailoring of such high risk intensive therapy to individual patients awaits the outcome of many of the studies which have already been described. The use of prophylactic platelet transfusions and the administration of cotrimoxazole reduce the incidence of the hemorrhagic and infectious complications associated with intensive chemotherapy administered during remission to the point that the outpatient administration of such therapies is practical for individuals being treated at institutions which have extensive experience in the treatment of AML [110].

While several factors are known which can be used to prognosticate for remission duration (see chapter by Keating), at the present time we cannot distinguish between patients who will have long remissions and those who will be cured. Hence, it seems logical that the therapeutic aproach described above should be made available to all patients who are to be treated with curative intent. On the other hand, when the treatment intent is not to obtain a cure but rather to obtain a long remission because the patient is not likely to survive intensive therapy, it may already be possible to distinguish between those patients who will have long remissions when treated with currently employed regimens. Once the ability to distinguish between these two groups of patients is sufficiently reliable it will be possible to administer less intensive therapy to those patients in whom the goal of treatment is palliation.

REFERENCES

1. Mauer AM, Fisher, V: In vivo study of cell kinetics in acute leukemia. Nature 197:574–577, 1963.
2. Killmann SA: Acute leukemia. The kinetics of leukemia blast cells in man. An analytical review. Ser Haematol 1:38–102, 1968.
3. Preisler H, Shoham D: Comparison of triatiated thymidine labeling and suicide indices in acute myelocytic leukemia. Cancer Res 38:3681–3684, 1978.
4. Minden MN, Till JE, McCulloch EA: Proliferative state of blast cell progenitors in acute myeloblastic leukemia (AML). Blood 52:592–600, 1978.
5. Hiddemann W, Buechner T, Andreef M, et al. Bone marrow biopsy – a new approach for cell kinetics in acute leukemia. Amer Assoc Cancer Res Abst. 742, p 185, 1980.
6. Gavasto F, Pileri A, Gabutto V, Masera P: Non-self maintaining kinetics of proliferating blasts in human acute leukemia. Nature 216:188–189, 1967.
7. Frei Ill, E, Fraireich EJ: Progress and perspectives in the chemotherapy of acute leukemia. Adv Chemotherapy 2:269–295, 1965.
8. Golomb HM, Vardiman J, Rowley JD: Acute nonlymphocytic leukemia in adults: correlations with Q-banded chromosomes. Blood 48:9–21, 1976.
9. Lawler SD, Secker Walker LM, Summersgill BM et al. Chromosome banding studies in acute leukemia at diagnosis. Scand J Haematol 15:312–320, 1975.
10. Fitzgerald PH, Crossen PE, Hamer JW: Abnormal karyotypic clones in human acute leukemia. Their nature and clinical significance. Cancer 31:1069–1077, 1973.
11. Yates JP, Wallace HJ, Ellison RR, Holland JF: Cytosine arabinoside and daunorubicin therapy in acute nonlymphocytic leukemia. Cancer Chemotherapy Rep 57:485–488, 1973.
12. Preisler HD, Bjornsson S, Henderson ES, Hryniak W, Higby D: Remission induction in acute nonlymphocytic leukemia: comparison of a 7–day and 10–day infusion of cytosine arabinoside in combination with adriamycin. Med Pediatr Oncol 7:269–275, 1979.
13. Glucksberg H, Buckner DC, Fefer A, Kjobech C, Hill AS, Dittman W, Nieman PE, DeMarsh Q, Coleman D, Dobrow RB, Huff J, Cheever MA, Einstein AB, Thomas D: Chemotherapy for acute nonlymphoblastic leukemia in adults. Cancer Chemotherapy Rep 59:1131–1137, 1975.

14. Coltman C: For the Southwest Oncology Group, personal communication, 1980.

15. Rai K, McIntyre R, Holland JF: Subcutaneous cytosine arabinoside is superior to intravenous route maintenance therapy of acute myelocytic leukemia. Proc Amer Assoc Cancer Res. 20:407, 1979.

16. Gale RP, Cline MJ: High remission induction rate in acute myeloid leukemia. Lancet i:497–499, 1977.

17. Arlin Z, Gee T, Fried J, et al.: Rapid induction of remission in acute nonlymphocytic leukemia. Proc Amer Assoc Cancer Res 20:112, 1979. Abstract # 452.

18. Rees JKH, Sandler RM, Challener J, Hayhoe FGJ: Treatment of acute myeloid leukemia with a triple cytotoxic regime: DAT. Br J Cancer 36:770–776, 1977.

19. Preisler HD: Unpublished observations.

20. Rees JKH: Personal communication.

21. Preisler HD: Acute myelocytic leukemia. In: Leukemia. Henderson, ES, Gunz F (eds). New York: Grune and Stratton, 1981 (in press).

22. Ellison RR, Holland JF, Weil M: Arabinosyl cytosine: a useful agent in the treatment of acute leukemia in adults. Blood 32:507–523, 1968.

23. Thompson I, Hall TC, Moloney WC: Combination therapy of adult acute myelogenous leukemia. Experience with the simultaneous use of vincristine, amethopterin, 6-mercaptopurine, and prednisone. N Engl J Med 273:1302–1307, 1965.

24. Embury SH, Elias L, Heller RH et al.: Remission maintenance therapy in acute myelogenous leukemia. West J Med 267–272, 1977.

25. Wiernik PH, Schimpf SC, Schiffner CA, Lichtenfeld L. Aisner J, O'Connell MJ, Fortner C: Comparison of daunorubicin alone with a combination of daunorubicin, cytosine arabinoside, 6 thioguanine, and pyrimethamine for the treatment of acute nonlymphocytic leukemia. Cancer Treat Rep 60:41–53, 1976.

26. Wiernik PH, Serpick AA: A randomized clinical trial of daunorubicin and a combination of prednisone, vincristine, 6 mercaptopurine, and methotrexate in adult acute nonlymphocytic leukemia. Cancer Res 32: 2023–2026, 1972.

27. Preislen HD, Bjornsson S, Henderson ES, et al.: Treatment of acute nonlymphocytic leukemia. Use of anthracycline-cytosine arabinoside induction therapy and a comparison of two maintenance regimens. Blood 53 (3):455–464, 1979.

28. Keating MJ, Smith TL, McCredie KB: A four year experience with anthracycline, cytosine arabinoside, vincristine, and prednisone combination chemotherapy in 325 adults with acute leukemia. Submitted 1980.

29. Rai K, Brunner K, Obrecht JP, Preisler HD, et al.: Treatment of acute myelocytic leukemia: a study by Cancer & Leukemia Group B. Blood 58:1203–1212, 1981.

30. Ellison RR, Glidewell O: Improved survival in adults with acute myelocytic leukemia. Proc Amer Assoc Cancer Res 20:161, 1979. Abst. # 651.

31. Coltman CA, Savage RA, Gehan E: Long term survival of adults with acute leukemia. Proc Amer Assoc Cancer Res 20:389, 1978. Abst. # C-405.

32. Weinstein HJ, Mayer RJ, Rosenthal DS et al.: Treatment of acute myelogenous leukemia in children and adults. N Engl J Med 303:473–478, 1980.

33. Preisler HD, Browman G, Tebbi C: Acute myelocytic leukemia: remission induction and maintenance therapy in patients thirty years of age and less. Semin Oncol (in press) 1980.

34. Powles RL, Russell J, lister TA: Immunotherapy for acute myelogenous leukemia: analyses of a controlled clinical study 2½ years after the entry of the last patient. In: Progress in cancer research and therapy vol. 6. Immunotherapy of cancer: present status of trials in man. Terry WE, Windhortst D (eds). New York: Raven Press, 1978, p 315.

35. Holland JF, Bekesi JG: Comparison of chemotherapy plus VCN – treated cells in acute

myelocytic leukemia. In: Immunotherapy of cancer: present status of trials in man. Terry WD, Windhorst D. New York: Raven Press, 1978, p 347.

36. Omura GA, Vogler WR, Lynn MJ: A controlled clinical trial of chemotherapy vs BCG immunotherapy vs no further therapy in remission maintenance of acute myelogenous leukemia. Proc Amer Soc Clin Oncol Abstract C23, 1977, p 272.

37. Zittoun R. In: EORTC. Personal communication.

38. Thomas EO, Buckner CO, Clift RA *et al.*: Marrow transplantation for acute nonlymphoblastic leukemia in first remission. N Engl J Med 301:597–599, 1979.

39. Blume KG, Beutler E, Brass KJ, *et al.*: Bone marrow ablation and allogenic marrow transplantation in acute leukemia: clinical candidacy and outcome. N Engl J Med 301:1041–1046, 1979.

40. Powles RL, Clark HM, Bandini F, *et al.*: The place of bone-marrow transplantation in acute myelogenous leukemia. Lancet i:1047–1050, 1980.

41. Thomas ED, Bruckman CD, Banaji M: One hundred patients with acute leukemia treated by chemotherapy, total body irradiation, and allogenic marrow transplantation. Blood 49:511–533, 1977.

42. Powles RL, Clink HM and Spence D: Cyclosporin A to prevent graft-versus-post disease in man after allogeneic bone marrow transplantation. Lancet i:327, 1980.

43. Preisler HD: Failure of remission induction in acute myelocytic leukemia. Med Pediatr Oncol 4:275–276, 1978.

44. Gehan EA, Smith TL, Freireich AJ, Bodey G, Rodriguez V, Speer J, McCredie K: Prognostic factors in acute leukemia. Semin Oncol 3:271–282, 1976.

45. Preisler HD, Lyman GH: Acute myelogenous leukemia subsequent to therapy for a different neoplasm: clinical features and response to therapy. Am J Hematol 3:209–218, 1977.

46. Botnick LE, Hannon EC, Hellman S: Limited proliferation of stem cells of surviving alkylating agents. Nature 262:68–70, 1976.

47. Gunz FW: Erythroleukemia in hematology, Williams, WJ, Bentley E, Esten AJ, *et al.*, eds. New York: McGraw-Hill, 1972.

48. Tamura K, Preisler HD: Treatment of erytholeukemia with anthracycline antibiotics and cytosine arabinoside. Submitted 1980.

49. Sakurai M, Sandberg AA: Prognosis of acute myeloblastic leukemia: chromosomal correlation. Blood 41:93–104, 1973.

50. Rothman H, Preisler HD, Pothier L, Marinello M. Paper in preparation.

51. Broxmeyer HE, Jacobsen N, Kurland J, *et al.*: In vitro suppression of normal granulocytic stem cells by inhibitory activity derived from human leukemia cells. J Natl Cancer Inst 60:497–511, 1978.

52. Moore MAS, Spitzer G, Williams N, *et al.*: Agar culture studies in 127 cases of untreated acute leukemia. The prognostic value of reclassification of leukemia according to in vitro growth characteristics. Blood 44:1–18, 1974.

53. Vincent PC, Sutherland R, Bradley M *et al.*: Marrow culture studies in adult acute leukemia at presentation and during remission. Blood 49:903–912, 1977.

54. Goldberg J, Tice P, Nelson DA, Gottlieb AJ: Predictive value of in vitro colony and cluster formation in acute nonlymphocytic leukemia. Amer J Med Sci 277:81–84, 1979.

55. Spitzer G, Dicke KA, Gehan EA, *et al.*: A simplified in vitro classification for prognosis in adult acute leukemia: the application of in vitro results in remission-predictive models. Blood 48:795–807, 1976.

56. Buick RN, Minden MD, McCulloch EA: Self-renewal in culture of proliferative blast progenitor cells in acute myeloblastic leukemia. Blood 54:95–104, 1979.

57. Hart JA, George SL, Frei E, *et al.*: Prognostic significance of pretreatment proliferative activity in adult acute leukemia. Cancer 39:1603–1617, 1977.

58. Crowther D, Beard MEJ, Bateman CJT, *et al.*: Factors influencing the prognosis in adults with acute myelogenous leukemia. Br J Cancer 32:456–464, 1975.

59. Valdivieso M, Rodriguez V, Drewinko B, *et al.*: Clinical and morphological correlations in acute promyelocytic leukemia. Med Pediatr Oncol 1:37–50, 1975.

60. Gunz FW, Burns EW: Prognosis in acute leukemia in adults. N Z Med J 64:555–560, 1965.

61. Preisler HD, Epstein J: A comparison of methods for determining the sensitivity of myeloid clonogenic cells to cytosine arabinoside. Br J Haematol (in press), 1980.

62. Epstein J, Preisler HD: Effects of cytosine arabinoside on DNA synthesis and the olonogenicity of RF/UN murine myeloid leukemia cells. Exp Hematol (in press), 1980.

63. Mauer AM: Cell proliferation in acute leukemia. Blood 24:833–834, 1964.

64. Lin MS, Bouroncle BA: The size and transit time of nondividing subpool of precuser cells in acute leukemia. Blood 29:63–76, 1967.

65. Gavasto F, Pileri A, Gabutti V, Masera P: Cell population kinetics in human acute leukemia. Eur J Cancer 3:301–307, 1967.

66. Ayulo M, Preisler HD: Prednimustine in acute non-lymphocytic leukemia. Submitted 1980.

67. Saunders EF, Mauer AM: Reentry of nondividing leukemic cells into a proliferative phase in acute childhood leukemia. J Clin Invest 48:1299–1305, 1969.

68. Preisler HD, Darynkiewicz Z: Characterization of proliferative and quiescent leukemic cells by flow cytometry. Submitted 1980.

69. Clarkson BD: Review of recent studies of cellular proliferation in acute leukemia. In: National Cancer Inst Monogr vol 30:81–119, 1969.

70. Preisler HD: Clonogenic potential in vitro of proliferative and quiescent leukemic cells. Leukemia Res 4(2):245–248, 1980.

71. Preisler HD, Epstein J: Clonal growth of leukemic cells in vitro. Cell and Tiss Kin (in press), 1980.

72. Lau L, McCulloch EA, Till JE, Price GB: The production of hemopoietic growth factors by PHA-stimulated leukocytes. Exp Hematol 6:114–121, 1978.

73. Kubota K, Preisler HD, Sagawa K, Minowanda J: A comparison between agar and the myelcellolose cultures of human leukemic cells. Submitted 1980.

74. Smythe JF, Robins, AO, Leese CL: The metabolism of cytosine arabinoside as a predictive test for clinical response to cytosine arabinoside in acute myeloid leukemia. Eur J Cancer 12:567–573, 1976.

75. Greene W, Huffman D., Wiernik PH *et al.*: High dose daunorubicin therapy for acute nonlymphocytic leukemia: correlation of response and toxicity with pharmacokinetics and intracellular daunorubicin reductive activity. Cancer 30:1419–1427, 1972.

76. Zittoun r, Bouchard M, Facquet-Danis J, Prediction of the response to chemotherapy in acute leukemia. Cancer 35:507–513, 1975.

77. Raich PC: Prediction of therapeutic response in acute leukemia. Lancet i:74–76, 1978.

78. Kessel D, Hall TC, Wodinsky I: Transport and phosphorylation as factors in the antitumor action of cytosine arabinoside. Science 156:1240–1241, 1967.

79. Kessel D, Hall TC, Rosenthal D: Uptake and phosphorylation of cytosine arabinoside by normal and leukemic human blood cells in vitro. Cancer Res 29:459–463, 1969.

80. Epstein J, Preisler HD: Effects of cytosine arabinoside on DNA synthesis as a predictor for AML patient's response to chemotherapy (in press), 1981.

81. Karon M, Benedict WF: Chromatid breakage: differential effect of inhibutors of DNA synthesis during $G_2$ phase. Science 178:62, 1972.

82. Woodcock DM, Cooper IA: Aberrant double replications of chromosomal DNA following DNA synthesis inhibition by cytosine arabinoside. Exp Cell Res 123:157–166, 1979.

83. Woodcock DM, Fox RM, Cooper IA: Evidence for a new mechanism of cytotoxicity of I-B-D-arabinofuranosyl cytosine. Cancer Res 39:1418–1424, 1979.

84. Preisler HD: Prediction of response to chemotherapy in acute myelocytic leukemia. Blood 56:361–367, 1980.

85. Roper PR, Drewrinko B: Comparison of in vitro methods to determine drug-induced cell lethality. Cancer Res 36:2181–2188, 1976.

86. Laurie HC, Willoughby MLN: In vitro prediction of clinical response to chemotherapy in childhood acute leukemia. Combination of daunorubicin, vincristine, and prednisone. Br J Haematol 17:251–256, 1969.

87. Preisler HD: Evaluation of in vitro predictive assays in acute myelocytic leukemia. Blut 41:393–396, 1980.

88. Gessner T, Robert J, Bolanowska W, Preisler HD, Rustum Y: Effects of previous treatment with anthracycline on subsequent therapy with adriamycin. Submitted 1980.

89. Meyer RJ, Ferreire PPC, Cuttner J, Greenberg ML, Goldberg J, Holland JF: Central nervous system involvement at presentation in acute granulocytic leukemia. Am J Med 68:691–694, 1980.

90. Freireich EJ, Keating MJ, Gehan EA et al.: Therapy of acute myelogenous leukemia. Cancer 42: 874–882, 1978.

91. Rustum YM, Preisler HD: Correlation between leukemic cell retention of 1-B-D-arabinosylcytosine-5'-triphosphate and response to therapy. Cancer Res 39:42–49, 1979.

92. Preisler HD, Rustum YM: In preparation.

93. Hoelzer D, Harris EBb: The failure of normal haemopoieses in rats during the development of acute leukemia. Acta Haematol 49:36–47, 1973.

94. Hillen HFP, Burghouts j, Haanen C: The application of pulse cytophotrometry for the early detection of the relapse in acute leukemia. In: 3rd International Symposium Pulse Cytophotometry 3/31-4/1, 1977. Vienna.

95. Stryckmans P, Debrusscher L, Ronge-Collard E, et al.: The labelling index of marrow myeloblasts: a predictive test for relapse of acute nonlymphoblastic leukemia. Leukemia Res 4:79–87, 1980.

96. Hittelman WN, Broussard LC, Dosik G, McCredie K: Predicting relapse of human leukemia by means of premature chromosome condensation. N Eng J Med 303:479–484, 1980.

97. Baker MA, Falk JA, Carter WH, et al.: Early diagnosis of relapse in acute myeloblastic leukemia. N Engl J Med 301:1353–1357, 1979.

98. Pike BL, Robinson WA: Human bone marrow colony growth in agar gels. J Cell Physiol 76:77–84, 1970.

99. Iscove NN, Sieber F: Erythroid progenitors in mouse bone marrow detected by macroscopic colony formation in culture. Exp Hematol 3:32–43, 1975.

100. Fauser AA, Messner HA: Granulo-erythropoietic colonies in human bone marrow, peripheral blood, and cord blood. Blood 52:1243–1248, 1978.

101. Jensen MK, Killmann SA: Chromosome studies in acute leukemia. Evidence for chromosomal abnormalities common to erythroblasts and leukemic white cells. Acta Med Scand 181, Sosc 1:47–53, 1967.

102. Blackstock AM, Garson DM: Direct evidence in involvement of erythroid cells in acute myeloblastic leukemia. Lancet: 1178–1179, 1974.

103. Urabe A, Murphy mJ, Haghlin M, Gee TSb: Erythroid progenitors CBFUe and CFUC in acute leukemia. J Clin Pathol 32:666–669, 1979.

104. Greenberg, PL, Mara B, Heller P: Marrow adherent cell colony-stimulating production in acute myeloid leukemia. Blood 52:362–378, 1978.

105. Hornsten P, Granstrom M, Waliren B, Galiston G: Prognostic value of colony-stimulating

and colony-forming cells in peripheral blood in acute nonlymphoblastic leukemia. Acta Med Scand 201:405–410, 1977.

106. Ross DW: Volume growth after cell cycle block with chemotherapeutic agents. Cell Tissue Kinet 9:379–387,1976.

107. Krishan A, Ganapathi R: Laser flow cytometric studies on the intracellular fluoresence of anthracycline. Cancer Res 40:3895–3900, 1980.

108. Cox DR: In: The analysis of binary data. London: Methuen and Co., 1970.

109. Cox DR: Regression models and life tables. Stat Soc B 34:187–220, 1972.

110. Preisler HD, Early AP, Hytniuk W: Prevention of infection in leukemic patients receiving intensive remission maintenance therapy. Submitted 1980.

111. Vogler R: For the Southeastern Oncology Group, personal communication, 1980.

112. Wiernik PH, Serpick AA: A randomized clinical trial of daunorubicin and a combination of prednisone, vincristine, 6-mercaptoperine, and methrotrexate in adult acute nonlymphocytic leukemia. Cancer Res 32:2023–2036, 1972.

113. Coltman CE: For the Southwest Oncology Group, personal communication, 1980.

114. Cassileth PA, Katz ME: Chemotherapy for adult acute nonlymphocytic leukemia with daunorubicin and cytosine arabinoside. Cancer Chemotherapy Rep 61:1441–1445, 1977.

# 7. Acute Nonlymphocytic Leukemia in the Elderly: Biology and Treatment

CONTENTS

1. Introduction
2. Characteristics of Leukemia in the Elderly
3. Tolerance of the Elderly to Leukemia and Chemotherapy
4. Chemotherapy of Acute Nonlymphocytic Leukemia in the Elderly

## 1. INTRODUCTION

Since the introduction of chemotherapy for adults with acute nonlymphocytic leukemia, the adverse impact of advancing age on prognosis has been repeatedly demonstrated [1–22]. Age has consistently been one of the most important clinical factors that can predict the outcome of treatment and, consequently, the length of survival [23–30]. The degree to which the age of the patient affects the results of treatment has not remained uniform over time, but perception of it as a major prognostic factor continues to influence the philosophy of treatment. Although it is no longer considered fitting to routinely withhold potentially beneficial treatment from the elderly, there is a residual sentiment to employ only conservative therapy and, thus, not cause the older patient any harm. However, since the identification of an adverse prognostic factor such as advanced age, regardless of importance, does not simultaneously establish the optimal choice among therapeutic options for patients characterized by that specific factor, it becomes relevant to evaluate the reasons elderly patients are perceived to do poorly following treatment and the methods by which therapeutic success for them might be increased.

In the early trials with single chemotherapeutic agents that did relatively little to alter the clinical course of acute nonlymphocytic leukemia, only

C. D. Bloomfield (ed.), Adult leukemias 1, 199–235. All rights reserved.
Copyright © 1982 Martinus Nijhoff Publishers, The Hague/Boston/London.

small differences were noted in the length of survival of cohorts of patients analyzed according to age. As the results of treatment began to improve, the rate of response in older patients did not keep pace with that observed in younger patients. Now, with present intensive chemotherapy and the comprehensive supportive care programs that are available to contend with the complications arising during the induction period, the variation in prognosis of individuals with acute nonlymphocytic leukemia that can be attributed to age is declining. However, despite the reduction of differences in the outcome of treatment, they have not yet been eliminated.

Another reason for exploring the impact of age on prognosis in acute nonlymphocytic leukemia is the frequency of this group of diseases in the elderly population. In clinical trials containing large numbers, the median age of the patients is most often around 50 years and, frequently, 35–40% of all of the adults encountered are over 60 years of age [6, 15, 30–34]. The elderly constitute a prominent segment of patients afflicted by acute leukemia and are characterized by at least one major adverse prognostic variable, age. The importance of this observation is further enhanced by data suggesting that the incidence of acute leukemia is rising, particularly in elderly patients [35–38]. In the locales where an increasing incidence has been documented, it has been accelerating mostly since the mid-1960s.

The group of patients for whom the incidence of acute nonlymphocytic leukemia appears to be increasing the most is the male population over 50 years of age [35, 36, 38]. While the incidence has remained relatively stable in younger individuals, it has nearly doubled in the elderly male population. In Sweden in 1970, the mean incidence of acute myelocytic leukemia in males who were under 50 years of age was reported at approximately 2–3 cases per 100 000 population [35]. In males over 50 years of age, the incidence was more than twice that and had risen considerably from the previous decade. In Olmsted County in Minnesota, the incidence of acute leukemia in men over 50 years of age rose from approximately 10 cases in 1960 to nearly 22 cases per 100 000 population in 1970 [38]. The increase in some instances may possibly have resulted from exposure to potential leukemogens earlier in life [35, 39]. The striking increase in the incidence of leukemia observed in the elderly and the accompanying fact that the population of the United States is proportionately growing older combine to make the occurrence of acute nonlymphocytic leukemia in aged individuals a significant health problem.

The influence of age on the clinical course of patients with acute leukemia has been chiefly explained by two suppositions. First, some types of acute non-lymphocytic leukemia that occur in elderly patients are postulated to be clinically and biologically distinct from those usually seen in younger patients and are inherently less sensitive, or even refractory, to the effects of cytotoxic agents. Second, aged individuals tolerate the rigors of having leukemia and the effects of chemotherapeutic intervention, particularly the prolonged period of bone marrow aplasia, less well than do younger patients and have, consequently, a larger proportion of treatment-related deaths. Although there is evidence for both hypotheses, current experience tends to support the second explanation as the major reason for the poorer prognosis observed in the elderly.

The chronological age of a given patient provides only an imprecise estimation of the cumulative effects of both the aging process and intercurrent illness on the individual. Thus, the negative influence on the prognosis of adults with acute nonlymphocytic leukemia associated with advancing age undoubtedly represents the aggregation of many factors derived from both normal aging and pathological experiences. What the most important host characteristics are, or how they operate and interrelate to adversely affect the clinical course has not been delineated. For this reason, age remains a convenient, although inexact, measure. Since a variety of criteria have been used to define the lower age limit of elderly or poor prognosis populations in clinical studies, the specific age categories used in each referenced publication will be indicated in the following discussion.

## 2. CHARACTERISTICS OF LEUKEMIA IN THE ELDERLY

Most suggestions that important differences exist in the clinical and biologic characteristics of the acute leukemias relative to the age of the patient first appeared when chemotherapy was relatively ineffective, although still toxic, and considerable disparity existed by age in the rates of response and length of survival [1, 2, 4, 15, 17–20, 40–44]. Prominent differences do occur in the biology of leukemia concomitantly with aging. For example, acute lymphoblastic leukemia, most commonly seen in children, is relatively infrequent in the elderly, while the chronic leukemias are more often seen in an older population. However, little attention has been directed towards documenting specific biologic features associated with the age of patients with acute nonlymphocytic leukemia that might explain the differences observed in the results of treatment. Sufficient clinical and laboratory data are available to permit only a limited analysis of potential relationships between age and important disease characteristics. Most of these attributes have been previously evaluated as potential prognostic factors that reflect the likelihood of obtaining a complete remission, the major determinant of survival in acute nonlymphocytic leukemia [23–30]. Recently, other factors specifically related to the duration of complete remission have also been identified [26, 45].

Hematologic parameters, which are easily and rapidly determined at the time of diagnosis, convey prognostic information and may indirectly reflect the biologic activity of the disease. An inverse relationship between survival and either total leukocyte or absolute myeloblast count has frequently been reported [15, 23, 25–30, 46–50]. Prior to effective chemotherapy, high leukocyte counts were associated with an extremely short period of survival. The importance of this relationship for predicting successful remission induction with chemotherapy was also noted, but may be waning in the face of current therapy [6, 15, 26–28, 47, 51, 52]. Berg *et al.* found a slight tendency for patients with acute nonlymphocytic leukemia and initial leukocyte counts higher than $100 \times 10^9/l$ to be older [46], but this observation is not confirmed by data included in two larger studies [25, 31]. In one study where median leukocyte counts were compared by age, no differences were detected [31]. In another series consisting of 458 patients, no differences in the distribution of total leukocyte counts relative to the ages of the patients were apparent [25]. An overall relationship between length of survival and the total leukocyte level was noted in the younger patients, but not in those who were over 60 years of age. In the elderly, the brief survival of the entire group erased any detectable effect specific leukocyte counts might have had on life span. Anemia and thrombocytopenia also affect prognosis in some studies, but significant differences have not been reported in the medians or distributions of either hemoglobin or platelet counts relative to age [16, 31].

Severe infiltration of the bone marrow by leukemia cells, often defined as a hypercellular bone marrow containing myeloblasts in excess of 75 %, has also been associated in the past with a poor prognosis [25, 47]. In general, important age differentials in the cellularity or median percentages of leukemic blasts in bone marrows have not been substantiated [31, 52]. However, the use of statistical medians might result in overlooking true differences which occur at the extremes of a given range. Rai *et al.* reported that 38 % of 787 patients younger than 60 years of age had 90 % or more leukemic cells in their bone marrows at diagnosis compared to only 19 % of 105 patients who were over 60 years of age [16]. The frequency of a 'packed' marrow in either age group was nearly identical. At the other extreme, hypocellularity and relatively low percentages of leukemic cells occur more commonly in bone marrows of aged individuals [12, 13, 53–57]. Oligoleukemia, defined as acute leukemia in which the percentages of blasts in the marrow is less than 50 % or the marrow infiltrate, calculated from the degree of cellularity and percentages of myeloblasts and promyelocytes, is less than 50 % and there are less than $10.0–20.0 \times 10^9/l$ circulating blasts [12, 13, 56], usually presents in patients over 50 or 60 years of age.

The subtypes of acute nonlymphocytic leukemia identified by morpho-

*Table 1.* Age at diagnosis in acute nonlymphocytic leukemia classified according to the French-American-British (FAB) criteria.

| FAB Class | Foon *et al.* [61] (n = 52) | | Mertelsmann *et al.* [63] (n = 193) | | Sultan *et al.* [65] (n = 243) | |
|---|---|---|---|---|---|---|
| | Number of patients | Age–years | Number of patients | Age–years | Number of patients | Age–years |
| M1 | 15 | 55 * (21–80) ‡ | 18 | 57 * | 53 | 51 † (21–92) ‡ |
| M2 | 16 | 32 (7–67) | 57 | 49 | 80 | 48 (14–90) |
| M3 | 2 | 34 (33, 34) | 31 | 39 | 40 | 41 (16–73) |
| M4 | 14 | 55 (45–82) | 16 | 44 | 39 | 52 (17–74) |
| M5 | 5 | 43 (21–63) | 11 | a) 62 § | 31 | 52 (18–76) |
| | | | 54 | b) 38 § | | |
| M6 | 0 | — | 6 | 56 | 0 | — |

* Median.
† Mean.
‡ Range.
§ M5a—acute monocytic leukemia 'without maturation.'
  M5b—acute monocytic leukemia 'with maturation.'

logic and cytochemical features have now been standardized by the adoption of the French-American-British (FAB) classification [58, 59]. Although these criteria distinguish categories of acute leukemia with specific morphologic characteristics, the biologic differences and prognostic significance of these subtypes have not yet been completely delineated (see chapter by Bennett). In most reports utilizing FAB criteria to classify adult leukemias, significant differences in age distribution have not been observed when patients are grouped according to morphologic subtypes [60–65], with the exception of hypergranular promyelocytic leukemia (M3) [49, 63, 65] (Table 1). In a series of patients from the Medical Research Council of Great Britain where a classification scheme similar to the FAB system was utilized, the only distinct relationship between age and morphologic category was detected in hypergranular promyelocytic leukemia (M3), which occurred mainly in young patients [49]. Only three of 19 cases (16%) with M3 leukemia included in the series were over the age of 40. A tendency for patients with acute monoblastic leukemia with evidence of differentiation to be younger has also been reported [63], but M5 leukemia regardless of differentiation occurs in older patients as well [60, 64, 65]. No association has been established between specific age groups and the level of serum lysozyme [32] or the presence of Auer rods [65].

Two related factors that have emerged as prognostic variables and frequently reflect the activity of the disease are the duration of time that symptoms have been present prior to diagnosis and the documented presence of an antecedent hematologic disorder prior to the emergence of leukemia. Early clinical papers remarked that acute nonlymphocytic leukemia in elderly patients frequently had an insidious onset and the duration of symptoms prior to diagnosis tended to increase with advancing age [33, 34, 66]. The prognostic significance of these findings was not initially addressed, but it was subsequently demonstrated that longer intervals from the onset of symptoms to the time of diagnosis could be correlated with shorter survival [30]. Although not all studies supported this conclusion [11, 27], others have found that a history of an antecedent hematologic problem existing prior to the diagnosis of leukemia is also a strong indicator of a relatively poor prognosis [12, 13]. Patients with abnormalities in peripheral blood leukocytes or documented cytopenias for periods longer than one month prior to the diagnosis of acute leukemia are predominantly over 50 years of age. Approximately a third of all patients in this age group have been noted to have such a history [12]. In older patients with a pre-existing hematologic problem, the complete remission rate following treatment is lower when compared to patients without such a history, and responsiveness to chemotherapy declines progressively as the duration of the antecedent disorder increases. The relationship of these observations to what has been called smoldering acute leukemia has not been addressed.

Rheingold *et al.* in 1963 reported several patients who clearly had acute nonlymphocytic leukemia but presented with an indolent history and had a quiescent course that persisted over months or years with little or no change in either hematologic parameters or symptoms [67]. Although one of the original cases was under 50 years of age, 17 of 18 cases subsequently reported were over 50 years [68]. Unfortunately, the identification of these patients is primarily dependent on the nature of the clinical course and not the pathologic findings. Rheingold stressed the presence of a prolonged symptomatic period preceding the diagnosis of leukemia which should raise suspicion of smoldering disease. However, the bone marrows varied considerably from being markedly infiltrated with leukemic myeloblasts to containing only a slight but detectable excess, and could be hypercellular, hypocellular, or normocellular. In an individual case the bone marrow findings were not useful for predicting the subsequent clinical course, but did distinguish these patients who clearly had leukemia from those with pre-leukemic states [69, 70].

Others have tried to evaluate and characterize this group of patients more fully [53–55, 71, 72]. Speer *et al.* attempted to delay the initiation of chemotherapy in adults with acute leukemia until there was either a life-threatening complication, demonstrable progression of the leukemia, or the peripheral blasts increased to greater than $10.0 \times 10^9/l$ [72]. Four of 39 patients

(10%) were identified who remained clinically and hematologically stable for longer than three months and were then diagnosed as having smoldering leukemia. Evensen and Stavem diagnosed smoldering leukemia when the bone marrow contained less than 30% myeloblasts and promyelocytes at the time of diagnosis and there was absence of progression to a fulminant stage of leukemia during the initial six months of observation [55]. Over a ten-year period, 11 of 194 patients (6%) seen at their institution met these criteria. These patients ranged in age from 48 to 77 years (mean 66), and had a median survival of 29 months. A relatively small fraction of patients with acute nonlymphocytic leukemia exist who are usually more advanced in age and experience an atypical smoldering clinical course. However, it remains that pathologic criteria such as the cellularity of the bone marrow [53, 68], morphology [54], and percentage of blasts [55] cannot be used to identify these patients. Patients with smoldering leukemia can be recognized reliably only after being observed closely for several months following the diagnosis of acute leukemia.

Patients with either a prolonged symptomatic interval preceding diagnosis, an antecedent hematologic disorder, or smoldering leukemia apparently respond poorly to chemotherapy [13, 54, 57]. Whether or not the leukemic cells in these circumstances are actually more resistent to chemotherapy is unknown, but some data would suggest that the cells might be relatively insensitive to current therapeutic programs [13]. However, despite claims that the common acute leukemias arising in the aged generally exhibit greater primary resistance to chemotherapy, most evidence suggests that equivalent proportions of both older and younger patients have leukemias that are sensitive to the cytotoxic effects of the drugs and that these patients constitute a clear majority [12, 56, 73]. Weil *et al.* in 1976 found only 16–28% of patients regardless of age resistant to treatment with a variety of regimens [56]. More recently, even smaller numbers of patients have been regarded as resistant to chemotherapy [73] including 12% of patients over 50 years of age [12]. Many of these patients with resistant leukemia had antecedent hematologic disorders before their leukemia was diagnosed.

Clinical and pathologic data constitute the majority of information used to routinely characterize acute leukemia in the elderly. Specialized *in vitro* laboratory tests have recently also been employed, but to a more limited extent. Many of the laboratory techniques assess the proliferative activity of the leukemia or other growth characteristics by measuring the proportion of malignant cells actively synthesizing DNA. When the labelling index of leukemic cells is determined prior to therapy, the ability of the results to predict subsequent response to chemotherapy and ultimate prognosis has been inconsistent [24, 74]. However, no obvious correlation between the patient's age and *in vitro* biologic characteristics of the leukemia as measured by the labelling index has been established [74]. Similarly, age-related differences have not been detected in the size of the S-phase compartment of myeloid leukemic cell populations when analyzed by DNA flow cytometry [75]. It is not yet clear whether the lack of findings related to age reflects the absence of any biologic differences or the preliminary nature of the investigations. In general, growth patterns of leukemic cells in short-term cultures have also not varied significantly from older to young patients [76–79] with the possible exception of an increased frequency of cell cultures that demonstrate no growth in the elderly [78]. These patients may respond more poorly to chemotherapy.

Only preliminary data are available concerning the interaction of chemotherapeutic agents and leukemic cells and the importance of the results of these *in vitro* studies to subsequent response. Older patients have been reported to have lower levels of daunorubicin reductase and it has been suggested that this might have some bearing on the putative lack of response to daunorubicin in the elderly [80, 144]. Other pharmacologic investigations suggest a relationship between *in vitro* uptake and retention of 1-$\beta$-D-arabinofuranosylcytosine triphosphate by leukemic cells and the response of patients to treatment regimens that include cytosine arabinoside [81, 82]. However, these studies have not as yet uncovered any relationship between the metabolic activity of the leukemic cells and the age of the patient [82]. Similar investigations will undoubtedly extend our understanding of the interaction of leukemic cells and cytotoxic drugs, and they may identify important pharmacological characteristics occurring specifically in acute nonlymphocytic leukemia of the elderly, but sufficient data have not yet been accumulated to permit a meaningful assessment of the findings to date and any potential relationship to age.

The introduction of newer techniques for banded chromosome analysis has already yielded specific cytogenetic information that can be correlated with response to therapy and survival and may relate in some instances to the age of the patient (see chapter by Golomb). In general, patients with acute nonlymphocytic leukemia and normal karyotypes have a more favorable outlook when compared to those with abnormal karyotypes [64], and certain nonrandom cytogenetic anomalies found in leukemia also have specific biologic and prognostic implications. A translocation between chromosome No. 15 and No. 17 appears to be limited to patients with hypergranular promyelocytic leukemia (M3) [83, 84]. As indicated earlier, these patients tend to be young. Another abnormality, first recognized by Kamada *et al.* [85] and precisely defined by Rowley as a balanced translocation between chromosomes No. 8 and No. 21 [86], occurs in about 8% of all cases of acute nonlymphocytic leukemia and appears to be restricted to young patients with M2 morphology. In a series collected from the literature, no patient with this translocation, which is associated with a relatively favorable prognosis, was older than 50 years of age [39].

Rowley has combined the data from several published cytogenetic studies of patients with M1 and M2 acute nonlymphocytic leukemia [39]. Of 128 patients, the percentage with abnormal karyotypes, except for those with t(8; 21), rose with advancing age and increased particularly after 50 years of age. Most of the cytogenetic abnormalities recorded were associated with chromosomes No. 5, No. 7, and No. 8. Since abnormalities involving chromosomes No. 5 and No. 7 have been most consistently seen in those patients with acute nonlymphocytic leukemia developing after cytotoxic chemotherapy given for other diseases [39, 87], this observation may support the hypothesis that the rise in the incidence of leukemia, particularly in older men, is associated with exposure to leukemogens [39, 88], and has potential relevance for the postulated intrinsic resistance to cytotoxic drugs in some cases of acute leukemia in the elderly since current clinical results point to the unresponsiveness, or resistance, of treatment-induced leukemia [89].

## 3. TOLERANCE OF THE ELDERLY TO LEUKEMIA AND CHEMOTHERAPY

In view of the limited evidence in support of distinctive age-related characteristics in most cases of acute leukemia that can explain the poorer prognosis of the elderly, the primary reason most likely relates to their inability to tolerate the consequences of having leukemia and/or undergoing therapy. Aging, the result of both normal physiologic and pathologic changes, affects a variety of organs and tissues over time. Several systems, including the musculoskeletal, renal, cardiovascular, respiratory, and immunologic systems, undergo functional deterioration with normal aging [90–92]. Often, the impairment of these organ systems is not apparent until the particular system or the entire organism is placed under stress. Then, the exigencies of the situation are not met. Since the presence of leukemia and the rigors of treatment create both acute and chronic stress, it may become impossible for the aged individual with leukemia to meet the additional demands, and decompensation in the midst of a critical situation ensues.

The physiologic consequences of aging can result in important alterations in the pharmacologic behavior of drugs, and resultant changes in absorption, metabolism, binding, and excretion in the aged could either decrease the efficacy of a given chemotherapeutic agent or enhance its toxicity. Many drugs that are used commonly in the elderly for the management of non-malignant diseases have been investigated for age-related pharmacologic effects [93–95], but potential deviations in the pharmacology of the antineoplastic drugs associated with aging have not been extensively evaluated. Decreased activity of microsomal and non-microsomal hepatic enzyme systems could substantially alter the activation, detoxification, and hepatic clearance of certain chemotherapeutic agents. Since renal function diminishes with age, the delay in excretion of drugs or their active metabolites could also have serious clinical consequences. Important alterations in the pharmacologic behavior of supplementary drugs such as anti-emetics and antibiotics might also complicate the care of the elderly as can the number of drugs elderly patients frequently require for chronic intercurrent disease and the increased potential for adverse drug interactions.

Certain factors, clinically identifiable at diagnosis, add to the patient's burden of stress and influence the likelihood of achieving remission [23, 24, 26–30, 47]. Several of these characteristics directly reflect biologic aspects of the leukemia and have already been discussed in the preceding section. Others result from or indirectly reflect the predicament precipitated by the presence of leukemia and add stress or impair the individual's ability to tolerate it (Table 2). The presence of a fever higher than 101 °F or a proven infection influences the outcome of treatment for patients of all ages with acute nonlymphocytic leukemia [25–27, 47]. However, possible interrelationships of the frequency of fever and infection with respect to age have not been adequately delineated. In one study, fever at diagnosis appeared to be less common in patients who were over 60 years of age (58 %) than in younger patients (85 %) [31], but Rai et al. found a slightly greater incidence of fever in the elderly (50 % versus 39 %) [16]. In other studies, neither fever [96] nor infection [27] appears to be specifically related to patient age. Since a conspicuous relationship between age and the status of a patient with respect to infection or fever at diagnosis apparently does not exist, the mere presence of either of these findings could not contribute to the significant age-related differences in the rate of response to chemotherapy unless the elderly were particularly unable to tolerate the consequences of fever or infection.

Table 2. Physical findings at diagnosis in acute nonlymphocytic leukemia.

| Symptoms and signs | Bloomfield and Theologides [31] | | Rai et al. [16] | |
| | <60 years (n = 81) | >60 years (n = 53) | <60 years (n = 247) | >60 years (n = 105) |
| --- | --- | --- | --- | --- |
| Fever–infection | 76 % | 58 % | 39 % | 50 % |
| Hemorrhage | 63 % | 64 % | – | – |
| Splenomegaly | 32 % | 25 % | 18 % | 15 % |
| Hepatomegaly | 14 % | 22 % | 25 % | 25 % |
| Lymphadenopathy | 49 % | 41 % | 34 % | 14 % |

Hepatomegaly and splenomegaly at diagnosis are also unfavorable prognostic findings in patients with acute nonlymphocytic leukemia [25, 27]. In patients over 50 or 60 years of age, the presence of hepatomegaly has been specifically associated with a poorer prognosis [12, 52]. Where the frequency of splenic or hepatic enlargement can be compared between patients younger than, or older than, 60 years of age, no difference has been detected [16, 31]. It is conceivable that the adverse effect of organomegaly on hepatic or splenic function, while no more frequent, may be more severe or less well-tolerated in the aged. However, data with respect to these possibilities are not available.

The performance status of an individual, more accurately than chronological age, represents an overt summation of important host characteristics. Among the factors that interrelate to affect activity level are the status of baseline physiologic functions and the presence or absence of significant underlying or intercurrent illness. If the ability to perform normal activities is sufficiently compromised, the ability to withstand the added burdens of having leukemia and undergoing treatment, including sepsis, hemorrhage and anemia, will be impaired even further. Although the age of a patient estimates additional latent factors that are not included in the measurement of performance status but may cause unsuspected problems, performance status, when diminished, is more important for predicting how well individual patients will do [2, 25, 59, 97].

Although it seems reasonable that the elderly are more likely to possess lower performance ratings than younger patients, this has not been documented in large numbers of patients with acute nonlymphocytic leukemia. When 250 patients were evaluated for the presence of pretherapeutic morbidity that could affect performance status at diagnosis, hemorrhage and/or infection classified as severe were more common in patients who were over 40 years of age [98]. Other factors that might also influence performance were not analyzed. In another report of 54 patients, 42% of the patients over 50 years of age were determined to have a poor performance status at diagnosis compared to only 14% of patients less than 50 years of age [97]. These investigators found that performance status, more than age or any other variable, influenced response to treatment and ultimate prognosis in patients with acute nonlymphocytic leukemia.

One of the major elements in the ability to withstand or recover from treatment, in particular, is the resiliency or regenerative capacity of the aging bone marrow following intensive chemotherapy. Not only is chemotherapy myelotoxic, but the presence of leukemic cells frequently has inhibitory effects on the normal bone marrow cells. The amount of hematopoietic tissue normally present ordinarily declines with advancing age. This is reflected in the increasing degree of hypocellularity accepted as within the limits of normal for elderly patients [99]. However, the apparent amount of hematopoietic tissue present in the marrow sample may not precisely indicate the capacity to either provide adequate numbers of normal cellular elements under stress or to regenerate following a myelotoxic insult. Hematologic values in normal populations, including hemoglobin, leukocytes and platelets, do not appear to change very much with advancing age [100, 101], but some aged individuals may not be capable of mounting an appropriate leukocytosis in the face of infection. Although evidence is being developed in animal systems suggesting that marrow function declines with increasing age [102], specific data on the capacity of the normal bone marrow in elderly human beings to regenerate are limited. Observations to date of colony forming cells in short term cultures do not support the concept of decreased marrow function in the elderly [78]. However, *in vitro* tests may not accurately reflect the quantitative *in vivo* activity of an entire bone marrow.

Data regarding the regenerative capacity of bone marrow cells relative to age are also difficult to obtain from clinical observations. In the evaluation of chemotherapeutic agents, the tolerance of elderly patients to myelosuppresive and other toxic effects has at times been poorer than in younger patients. The reason for this is not obvious, and does not necessarily relate to a greater susceptibility of the aged bone marrow to myelotoxic insults. Differences in metabolism and/or elimination of the drugs associated with aging might also exist. When patients with acute nonlymphocytic leukemia enter complete remission following intensive induction chemotherapy, the time it takes for marrow regeneration and remission to occur, with rare exception [15], does not differ substantially between younger and older individuals [12, 13, 16]. Thus, it should not be concluded that the inability of an elderly patient's bone marrow to regenerate following treatment routinely plays any major role in lowering the response rates.

Despite similar intervals of bone marrow aplasia following treatment, the ability to survive that period of aplasia appears to be compromised in the elderly. This is indicated primarily by the high proportion of early, presumably treatment-related or disease-related, deaths in older populations. When acute nonlymphocytic leukemia is untreated, the elderly suffer more deaths within a brief time of diagnosis [28, 34]. When patients undergoing treatment are analyzed according to the time of death, with occasional exception [103], the elderly again experience more early deaths in the course of treatment [1, 15, 16, 22, 25]. In the past, up to a third of patients over 50 years of age who primarily received supportive care or chemotherapy of limited effectiveness died within 7–10 days of diagnosis [28, 34]. This is more than twice the frequency of early deaths observed in concurrent younger patients and suggests age-related differences in the ability of patients to withstand the consequences of having leukemia. Within two months of more intensive treatment directed at achieving complete remission, Ellison *et al.* found that 80% of patients with acute nonlymphocytic leukemia who were 20–29 years of age were still alive compared to 35–40% of those over 60 years and only 30% over 70 years [25]. These findings were accounted for by the inability of the elderly to tolerate chemotherapy and their consequent steep decline in survival time.

Another way to determine the ability of patients to withstand therapy is to measure the percentage surviving long enough to receive an 'adequate trial' of chemotherapy. An adequate trial is usually defined as the completion of two or three courses of induction treatment. The Southwest Oncology Group reported that approximately 50% of individuals 50–65 years of age and more than 70% of patients over 65 years of age did not survive long enough, approximately four weeks, to receive what the investigators considered an adequate therapeutic trial of chemotherapy with a variety of different regimens [5]. By comparison, only 30% of the patients less than 50 years of age died prior to receiving an adequate trial. In a recent study of the Cancer and Leukemia Group B, 53% of the patients over 60 years of age died within several weeks of treatment compared to 26% of the younger patients [16]. Similar data have been reported from a number of other sources [1, 13, 44]. These results indicate that the untreated elderly are more susceptible to early deaths from leukemia, but when the elderly die following intensive chemotherapy, they die as a result of the toxicity and complications of treatment rather than from persistence of the leukemia. In most cases, patients regardless of age will either successfully complete therapy and enter complete remission or die in the attempt [1, 16, 22, 44].

The common causes of death in both younger and older individuals undergoing induction treatment for acute nonlymphocytic leukemia, with minor exceptions, are similar. Certain infrequent causes, such as cardiac, cerebrovascular, and renal complications, appear mostly in the elderly. The most frequent cause of death for all patients undergoing induction chemotherapy is infection [104]. Infectious complications of treatment in one study were seen in 61% of patients over 60 years of age and 44% of the younger patients [16]. The elderly patients in this study also had a higher incidence of infections prior to the institution of therapy. Although 53% of the elderly died following chemotherapy, specific causes of death were not reported. In a series of 100 patients over 55 years of age, nearly a third of the patients died of infection early in the treatment period [51]. In another study of 96 patients over 50 years of age, 32 of the 48 patients (67%) who failed to achieve complete remission died within six weeks [12]. Infection, most commonly septicemia and pneumonia, accounted for 78% of these deaths.

Differences are apparent in the ability of the elderly to withstand serious infections when compared to younger patients. Although a loss of general immunocompetence occurs concomitantly with aging, the function of normal phagocytic cells important in eradicating bacterial and fungal infections is maintained ]90]. However, the higher mortality from infection observed in older patients, particularly those who are granulocytopenic, exists for a number of reasons [105]. Antibiotics are crucial to the management of febrile, neutropenic patients. In a cooperative trial of antibiotic therapy for infections in cancer patients who were febrile and granulocytopenic, the incidence of severe antibiotic-related renal dysfunction in patients over 60 years of age who were receiving cephalothin plus gentamicin was 27% compared to 7% for those under 60 years of age [106]. The only parameters that were found to predict antibiotic-related renal damage were age and the initial level of serum creatinine. Also, the infections in the older patients in this study responded more poorly to the antibiotics. Others have found that clinically significant deterioration of renal function happens approximately three times more often in the elderly than in young patients being treated specifically for acute leukemia [16]. Since underlying renal function decreases with age, it is not surprising that renal toxicity attributed to antibiotics and subsequently compromising the management of the patient by limiting the type or amount of further antibiotics that can be administered occurs more often in patients over 60 years of age.

Hemorrhage is an uncommon cause of death in individuals being treated for acute leukemia now that platelet transfusions are readily available. Certainly, bleeding remains a major problem in the management of patients with hypergranular promyelocytic leukemia (M3), but most of these patients are relatively young. In the other morphologic subtypes of acute nonlymphocytic leukemia, hemorrhagic complications occur in approximately equal proportions of both young and old patients [16]. Perhaps, because of underlying structural abnormalities resulting from degenerative vascular changes secondary to atherosclerosis or hypertension and associated with aging, the elderly may be more susceptible to lethal intracranial hemorrhages. However, these account for only a fraction of the overall deaths.

Of major concern in the elderly is the underlying status of the coronary circulation and the myocardium and the heart's ability to withstand the stress presented by hemorrhage, anemia, infection, and the potential cardiotoxic effects of the anthracycline antibiotics. Chang *et al.* found the heart to be one of the most frequent sites of organ failure in the elderly accounting for death in 4% of all patients [104]. The majority of these cases were associated with atherosclerotic cardiovascular disease. Others have also found the cardiac problems that occur during treatment for acute leukemia to be primarily a problem of the elderly [16, 51, 107]. These are almost certainly related to the increased frequency of underlying cardiac disease in the elderly population. The anthracyclines which can cause significant heart damage are among the most effective drugs used in the treatment of acute non-lymphocytic leukemia. Although in the early experience with daunorubicin, clinical cardiac toxicity appeared to occur most frequently in the elderly [40], it is now apparent that the cardiotoxic effects of both daunorubicin and doxorubicin are primarily dose-dependent [108–110]. However, advancing age and the presence of underlying heart disease or hypertension remain major risk factors for cardiac injury and subsequent anthracycline-induced congestive heart failure.

## 4. CHEMOTHERAPY OF ACUTE NONLYMPHOCYTIC LEUKEMIA IN THE ELDERLY

The major impact of age on the longevity of adults who have acute non-lymphocytic leukemia treated with chemotherapy arises from the adverse influence of advanced age on the opportunity to achieve complete remissions. This fact emerged as induction chemotherapy increased in intensity and toxicity without a corresponding improvement in efficacy, and the available techniques of supportive care were insufficient to sustain patients through the hazardous period of treatment. When treatment improved and the elderly more regularly entered remissions, it became apparent that the benefits received by the responders with respect to duration of remission and prolongation of life were similar to those enjoyed by younger patients. Since attaining remission status was, and still remains, the primary determinant of life expectancy for all patients regardless of age, induction chemotherapy became the focus of investigations in the management of acute nonlymphocytic leukemia.

The modern clinical era in the treatment of patients who have acute non-lymphocytic leukemia commenced with trials of agents such as vincristine, prednisone, 6-mercaptopurine, 6-thioguanine and methotrexate that are relatively innocuous and ineffective. Utilization of these drugs alone did not often induce remissions or significantly alter the clinical course for most patients treated [4, 8, 9, 11, 14, 28]. Thus, it is not unexpected that the minor differences conferred by age on the length of survival in untreated patients were not further exaggerated by inconsequential therapy. However, once these drugs were combined into more intensive and toxic multi-drug regimens, an effect on survival became apparent. The initial combinations of drugs produced complete remission in 20–25% of young adults, but responses were rarely observed in patients over 50 or 60 years of age [17, 19, 43, 111]. The improvements observed in the survival of young patients with leukemia were absent in the elderly. Whether these early treatment programs actually accelerated the rate of deaths in the elderly is uncertain, but median survival times as short as 19 days were reported [43]. There certainly were no improvements in the overall length of survival for the elderly as there were in the young and the disparity in the prognoses of younger and older patients was increased.

The introduction of cytosine arabinoside [1, 2, 7, 18] and the anthracycline antibiotic, daunorubicin [7, 20, 112, 113], made single chemotherapeutic agents available that could reliably yield complete remissions in 25–50% of the younger patients. However, response rates and survival in elderly patients remained substantially inferior to those achieved in young adults. In one of the first large studies employing cytosine arabinoside in the treatment of patients who had acute nonlymphocytic leukemia, 16% overall achieved a complete remission [7]. Although response rates were not specifically reported by age cohorts, it was noted that survival decreased with age. Patients over 50 years of age had a median survival of approximately seven weeks compared to 12 weeks for the younger patients. In other studies of cytosine arabinoside as a single agent, the actual rates of response to treatment also fell with advancing age [1, 2, 18].

The Southwest Oncology Group undertook a series of studies with cytosine arabinoside as a single agent and in patients under 50 years of age determined that the infusion of cytosine arabinoside continuously for 120 hours results in higher response rates than treatment for only 48 hours (46% versus 31%) [1, 18]. As the ages of the patients increased, the rates of response with either treatment schedule declined. However, the complete remission rate observed in patients over 50 years of age who received the prolonged infusion was still more than twice that in those treated for only 48 hours (22% versus 10%). This demonstrated that, although elderly patients as a group may not profit from a given treatment program at the same rate as younger patients, therapeutic advances that primarily benefit younger patients may also increase the response rate in the elderly. The intensification of treatment actually increased the response rate, but apparently at the expense of additional early deaths. The median survival time of the elderly was only three weeks compared to 10–20 weeks for the younger patients.

Similar findings of age-related decreases in response were reported following the introduction of daunorubicin. In a study of the Cancer and Leukemia Group B, regardless of whether daunorubicin was administered on each of three, five, or seven successive days, the complete remission rate decreased progressively with increasing age [20]. Overall, 40% of the patients who were less than 50 years of age entered complete remission compared to only 5% (3 of 56 patients) of those over 50 years. The median survival time for patients over 55 years was only four weeks. In part, these dismal results reflect the lack of effective supportive care available at the time these patients were treated. However, a more recent report of daunorubicin administered alone on three consecutive days and supplemented by more advanced supportive care indicated that remissions were obtained in 50% of patients less than 60 years of age, but only 22% (2 of 9 patients) of those over 60 years of age [114].

In a study at the University of Minnesota, we found that the complete remission rate with daunorubicin plus prednisone was 38% in 51 patients under 60 years of age, but in 21 patients who were 60 years of age and over it was only 10% [115]. All patients received intensive supportive care with empiric broad-spectrum antibiotics, and platelet and white blood cell transfusions as necessary. The number of deaths occurring during or immediately after induction chemotherapy was clearly related to age. Nearly 50% of the patients over 60 years of age died within 30 days of the induction attempt compared to 25% of the younger patients. Although improvements in supportive care are important in the overall management of patients, neither these advances nor the most efficacious drugs available used as single agents are sufficient to provide an adequate opportunity for the elderly to achieve remission.

It is in this context of disappointing results with single agents and ineffective combinations that opposition to the further exploration and use of intensive induction treatment in elderly patients arose. There was genuine concern over making the last days of any patient with acute nonlymphocytic leukemia more intolerable than if chemotherapy were simply withheld. Several authorities suggested that older patients either not receive treatment at all, or be treated only with conservative measures [43, 116–123]. Others felt that problems associated with the management of the aged patient with acute leukemia deserved further exploration [31, 52, 107, 111, 124–126]. Although the questions raised on both sides of this issue were valid and important, conclusions were often supported by anecdotal experience.

In reaction to the growing tendency to explore increasingly intensive chemotherapy for patients of all ages with acute nonlymphocytic leukemia, Burge et al. adopted a conservative approach in hopes of improving both the quality of life for their patients and the quantity of survival [118]. The intention was to reduce bone marrow suppression and, consequently, the morbidity and mortality of anti-leukemic chemotherapy. A group of 51 patients, 13–88 years of age, were treated with relatively conservative chemotherapy. Twenty-one of the patients were over 60 years of age. One 88-year-old patient refused any therapy and was excluded from the analysis. The other patients received primarily 6-mercaptopurine and allopurinol as treatment for acute nonlymphocytic leukemia. Seven patients, in addition, received daunorubicin and/or cytosine arabinoside.

Only one of the patients (5%) over 60 years of age achieved a complete remission with this conservative program specifically designed to reduce treatment-related morbidity and mortality. Three patients died before any treatment was instituted, three patients died during the treatment, and five additional patients spent the rest of their lives in the hospital. Thus, despite an earnest attempt to reduce morbidity and mortality and improve the quality of remaining life, median survival was 13 weeks and most of the patients (55%) died during their initial hospitalization. Although the survival time of the patients was not strikingly different from what had been achieved previously with more intensive chemotherapy, it does not represent a significant improvement compared to withholding treatment from elderly patients, nor does it compare favorably with therapeutic achievements since that time. Unfortunately, denying these patients effective chemotherapy does not prevent the morbidity associated with hemorrhagic and infectious complications that are part of the natural history of untreated leukemia. The low complete remission rate and high proportion of inpatient deaths make the routine adoption of conservative therapy, even in the elderly, currently unacceptable. With this approach, virtually all patients will die of their leukemia without being extended the potential benefits of treatment.

Most clinical investigators were determined to provide for their elderly patients with acute nonlymphocytic leukemia the same benefits they saw accruing to younger patients as a result of new therapeutic developments. Initially, attempts with intensive therapy directed at achieving remissions with combinations of the most effective drugs were also of marginal benefit to elderly patients. In a number of papers representing the experience of both single institutions and cooperative groups during the early 1970s, complete remission rates in patients over 60 or 65 years of age generally remained at less than 25% [2–4, 6, 21, 24, 31, 41, 114], and remissions in patients over 70 years of age were rare. Representative chemotherapeutic programs employed in these studies were combinations of cytosine arabinoside plus 6-thioguanine [4], cyclophosphamide, vincristine, cytosine arabinoside and prednisone (COAP) [44], and cytosine arabinoside in combination with daunorubicin [6, 21, 24]. The early results amply demonstrated the inability of the elderly to tolerate any treatment that induced prolonged periods of bone marrow hypoplasia without efficiently eradicating the leukemia and permitting rapid regeneration of normal hematopoietic tissue.

In 1973 elderly patients with acute nonlymphocytic leukemia who were fortunate enough to achieve complete remissions with chemotherapy were reported to benefit as greatly as younger patients in that the duration of remission and length of survival of the responders were comparable [31]. In a subsequent prospective study of intensive chemotherapy at the University of Minnesota utilizing identical treatment regimens for adults of all ages, the complete response rate in patients 60 to 70 years of age was 50%, similar to that in younger patients and, furthermore, the more intensive programs seemed to be most effective [52]. Overall survival in patients 60 to 70 years of age was over seven months and comparable to that seen in young patients. The median survival of those elderly patients achieving complete remission was 23 months. However, of the patients over 70 years of age only 8% achieved remission.

The benefits of remission-directed intensive chemotherapy in an elderly population with leukemia were also reported by Grann *et al.* [107]. Of 64 patients who were over 50 years of age and had acute nonlymphocytic leukemia treated with cytosine arabinoside plus 6-thioguanine, 28 (44%) achieved complete remission. Remission rates in these patients were nearly identical regardless of age over 50 years, and the median survival of all patients treated, responders plus nonresponders, was six months. For the first time, the median survival for an entire group of elderly patients with acute nonlymphocytic leukemia was substantially improved by the treatment they received. For the responders, alone, median survival was greater than 19 months. These results were better than those obtained with less intensive treatment programs by the same investigators and others [111] and clearly indicated that elderly patients with acute nonlymphocytic leukemia could benefit regularly by responding to combination chemotherapy and entering meaningful complete remissions.

Since these initial reports drew attention to the potential benefits of intensive chemotherapy in the elderly, the treatment of acute leukemia has been further refined. In almost every instance, the advances have resulted from raising the dosage of individual drugs, improving the schedule of administration, or adding additional effective agents to the therapeutic regimens and providing comprehensive supportive care. The contemporary treatment programs that developed from these changes are, in general, both more effective in producing high frequencies of response and more efficient in rapidly eradicating leukemic cells so that the bone marrow can be quickly repopulated by normal cells. The concurrent augmentation of supportive care programs has also resulted in a better opportunity for elderly patients to benefit from intensive induction treatment.

Investigators from the Southwest Oncology Group and the M. D. Anderson Hospital in Houston, Texas have explored a series of treatment programs for acute leukemia that have three drugs in common–vincristine, cytosine arabinoside and prednisone (OAP)– and in slight variations include additional drugs, such as cyclophosphamide (COAP) or daunorubicin (DOAP) [5, 13, 41, 44]. In a prospective randomized trial comparing the COAP, DOAP, and OAP schedules, overall complete remission rates of

Table 3. Results by age in acute nonlymphocytic leukemia treated with modifications of the OAP (vincristine, cytosine arabinoside, prednisone) regimen.

| Reference | Regimen | Age groups (years) | Number of patients | Complete remissions (%) | Median time to CR (weeks) | Patients receiving 'Adequate trials' (completed 2 cycles) |
|---|---|---|---|---|---|---|
| [5]* | OAP | | | | | |
| | Cytosine arabinoside 200 mg/m$^2$/day continuous infusion on days 1-5 | <50 | 53 | 30 (57%) | | 68% |
| | Vincristine 2.0 mg IV on day 1 | 50-64 | 19 | 7 (37%) | 7 weeks | 47% |
| | Prednisone 25 mg q.i.d. PO on days 1-5 | ≥65 | 19 | 3 (16%) | | 26% |
| | COAP | | | | | |
| | Cytosine arabinoside 100 mg/m$^2$/day continuous infusion on days 1-5 | <50 | 53 | 28 (53%) | | 68% |
| | Vincristine 2.0 mg IV on day 1 | 50-64 | 25 | 7 (28%) | 8 weeks | 48% |
| | Prednisone 25 mg q.i.d. PO on days 1-5 | ≥65 | 16 | 3 (19%) | | 25% |
| | Cyclophosphamide 100 mg/m$^2$/day IV on days 1-5 | | | | | |
| | DOAP | | | | | |
| | Cytosine arabinoside 100 mg/m$^2$/day continuous infusion on days 1-5 | <50 | 45 | 25 (56%) | | 76% |
| | Vincristine 2.0 mg IV on day 1 | 50-64 | 25 | 8 (32%) | 6.5 weeks | 48% |
| | Prednisone 25 mg q.i.d. PO on days 1-5 | ≥65 | 18 | 4 (22%) | | 28% |
| | Daunorubicin 60 mg/m$^2$ IV on day 1 | | | | | |

Table 3. (Continued).

| Reference | Regimen | Age groups (years) | Number of patients | Complete remissions (%) | Median time to CR (weeks) | Patients receiving 'Adequate trials' (completed 2 cycles) |
|---|---|---|---|---|---|---|
| [13] | ROAP, ADOAP, various schedules (see below) | <20 | 17 | 16 (94%) | | — |
| | | 20–50 | 96 | 65 (68%) | 6 weeks | — |
| | | 50–65 | 86 | 47 (55%) | | — |
| | | ≥65 | 46 | 14 (30%) | | — |
| [12]* | ROAP | | | | | |
| | Cytosine arabinoside 70 mg/m²/day continuous infusion on days 1–7 | 50–59 | 35 | 18 (51%) | | — |
| | Vincristine 2.0 mg IV on day 1 | 60–69 | 37 | 22 (59%) | 4 weeks | — |
| | Prednisone 25 mg q.i.d. PO days 1–5 | ≥70 | 24 | 8 (33%) | | — |
| | Rubidazone 200 mg/m² IV on day 1 | | | | | |
| | ADOAP | | | | | |
| | Cytosine arabinoside 70 mg/m²/day continuous infusion on days 1–7 | 50–59 | 34 | 14 (41%) | | — |
| | Vincristine 2.0 mg IV on day 1 | 60–69 | 32 | 19 (59%) | — | — |
| | Prednisone 25 mg q.i.d. PO days 1–5 | ≥70 | 26 | 7 (27%) | | — |
| | Adriamycin 40 mg/m² IV on day 1 | | | | | |

* Study also includes patients with acute lymphoblastic and acute undifferentiated leukemia.
† Some patients received rubidazone 150 mg/m² and cytosine arabinoside 55 mg/m²/day.

35–43% were obtained [5] (Table 3). In the patients less than 50 years of age, complete remission rates of 53–57% were established, but these rates declined to 28–37% in patients between 50 and 65 years and 16–22% for patients 65 years of age or older.

The response rates in the older patients might have been higher if it were not for the early deaths (21–24%) and the limited number of patients who were able to complete an adequate therapeutic trial. The median length of time it took for a complete remission to occur with these regimens was relatively long, ranging from 6.5 to 8 weeks, and resulted in an inability of many elderly patients either to survive or to tolerate the prolonged marrow aplasia. Slightly less than half of the patients between 50 and 65 years of age were able to complete two courses of chemotherapy and the percentage fell to 25–28% for patients 65 years of age and older. Similar decreases in the response rates for patients over 55 years of age have often been seen with other treatment schedules where the time to complete remission was long [4, 51, 127].

Results of studies with vincristine, cytosine arabinoside, and prednisone combined with either adriamycin (ADOAP) or rubidazone (ROAP) have recently been reported [13] (Table 3). Seventy-two percent of the adults under 50 years compared to 46% over 50 years of age achieved complete remission with these regimens. When patients over 50 years of age were subdivided further by age, complete remissions were obtained in 55% of patients 50–65 years and 30% of those over 65 years of age. Although the rates of response steadily decreased with advancing age, only in the group of patients who were over 65 years of age was the complete response rate less than 50%. The median time to complete remission with these two regimens was six weeks, and over half of the responders entered remission following only one course of therapy. In this study, patients with a preceding hematologic abnormality recognized for a period as brief as one month prior to the diagnosis of acute nonlymphocytic leukemia had a substantially reduced response rate. Most of these patients were over 50 years of age.

A more detailed analysis of the patients over 50 years of age treated specifically with ROAP has been undertaken [12]. The addition of rubidazone was studied because preliminary evidence suggested that it may be particularly effective as a single agent in elderly patients [128]. Treatment was initiated only when patients had more than a 50% leukemic infiltrate in the bone marrow or greater than $10.0 \times 10^9/l$ circulating myeloblasts. One-third of the patients had antecedent hematologic disorders. Of the 96 patients treated with ROAP, 50% obtained complete remissions [12]. The complete response rate was 56% in patients 50–69 years of age and 33% in patients over 70 years of age. Sixty-two percent of the responders entered remission after one course of therapy, and the median time to remission was only four weeks. When the results with ROAP were compared to the experience from earlier years with ADOAP, the rate of response in patients over 50 years of age with ROAP was slightly, but not significantly, higher.

The major problems during treatment with ROAP were infection and hemorrhage which could be attributed to myelosuppression. Of the 48 patients who failed to respond to chemotherapy, 32 (67%) died within the first six weeks. These deaths were most often related to infection and were only infrequently related to either refractory leukemia or prolonged marrow hypoplasia. Regeneration of the bone marrow occurred within 21 to 35 days (median 27 days) except in two patients both of whom had antecedent hematologic disorders and eventual regrowth of leukemia. Only 12 patients were considered refractory to the chemotherapy because they did not achieve a complete remission despite surviving an adequate trial of two or three courses of treatment. Most of these patients also had antecedent hematologic disorders. The median survival time for the entire group of patients was 20 weeks and for the responders, 60 weeks.

The Cancer and Leukemia Group B has investigated a series of therapeutic combinations which utilize cytosine arabinoside with either daunorubicin or adriamycin [16, 22] (Table 4). When cytosine arabinoside and daunorubicin were combined initially in a number of different dosages and schedules of administration, the complete remission rates were low, especially in patients over 60 or 70 years of age [16]. Most of these regimens used less than full doses of both drugs. However, since it was recognized that reducing doses in an attempt to lessen the risks of bone marrow aplasia and sepsis had the undesirable effect of compromising response rates and shortening survival [129], a logical strategy was to extend the infusion of cytosine arabinoside to seven days and administer three days of an anthracycline [130].

A prospective study examining these drugs together confirmed once again the earlier observations regarding the requirement of a certain degree of intensity in chemotherapy for success in patient management [16]. Three hundred and fifty-two patients with acute nonlymphocytic leukemia were randomized among four different schedules of treatment that employed cytosine arabinoside and daunorubicin (Table 4). The study was designed to determine whether the administration of cytosine arabinoside for seven days and daunorubicin for three days was superior to the same drugs given for five and two days, respectively, and whether giving cytosine arabinoside as a continuous infusion was superior to giving it intermittently. A prejudice concerning the ability of elderly patients to withstand aggressive chemotherapy was evident in the original study design since patients over 60 years of age were at first randomized to only the programs containing five and two days of drugs. However, when an interim analysis revealed the obvious

Table 4. Results in acute nonlymphocytic leukemia treated with cytosine arabinoside and an anthracyline.

| Reference | Regimen | Age groups (years) | Number of patients | Complete remissions (%) | Median time to CR (days) | Induction deaths |
|---|---|---|---|---|---|---|
| [16] | Cytosine arabinoside 100 mg/m² every 12 hours IV on days 1–5 Daunorubicin 45 mg/m²/day on days 1, 2 | 20–49 50–59 60–69 70–84 | 25 14 15 12 | 9 (36%) 5 (36%) 2 (13%) 1 ( 8%) | | 13 (33%) 17 (64%) |
| | Cytosine arabinoside 100 mg/m²/day by continuous infusion on days 1–5 Daunorubicin 45 mg/m²/day on days 1, 2 | 20–49 50–59 60–69 70–84 | 27 13 26 9 | 16 (59%) 2 (15%) 7 (27%) 0 | 47 days | 12 (30%) 24 (68%) |
| | Cytosine arabinoside 100 mg/m² every 12 hours IV on days 1–7 Daunorubicin 45 mg/m²/day IV on days 1–3 | 20–49 50–59 60–69 70–84 | 70 16 11 10 | 38 (54%) 6 (38%) 3 (27%) 5 (50%) | | 23 (27%) 9 (43%) |
| | Cytosine arabinoside 100 mg/m²/day by continuous infusion on days 1–7 Daunorubicin 45 mg/m²/day IV on days 1–3 | 20–49 50–59 60–69 70–84 | 63 19 12 10 | 39 (62%) 9 (47%) 6 (50%) 4 (40%) | 38 days | 16 (20%) 6 (28%) |
| [22] | Cytosine arabinoside 100 mg/m²/day by continuous infusion on days 1–7 Daunorubicin 45 mg/m²/day IV on days 1–3 | <60 60–69 ≥70 | 152 43 23 | 105 (69%) 16 (37%) 4 (17%) | — | 26 (17%) 23 (53%) 16 (70%) |
| | Cytosine arabinoside 100 mg/m²/day by continuous infusion on days 1–7 Daunorubicin 30 mg/m²/day IV on days 1–3 | <60 60–69 ≥70 | 132 44 26 | 76 (58%) 21 (48%) 11 (42%) | — | 29 (22%) 19 (43%) 11 (42%) |
| | Cytosine arabinoside 100 mg/m²/day by continuous infusion on days 1–7 Adriamycin 30 mg/m²/day IV on days 1–3 | <60 60–69 ≥70 | 124 63 20 | 69 (56%) 26 (41%) 4 (20%) | — | 40 (32%) 34 (54%) 13 (65%) |

Table 5. Complications of induction chemotherapy in acute nonlymphocytic leukemia treated with cytosine arabinoside and daunorubicin [16].

| | Treatment regimens | | | | Overall complications | |
|---|---|---|---|---|---|---|
| | Cytosine arabinoside (5 days) and daunorubicin (2 days) | | Cytosine arabinoside (7 days) and daunorubicin (3 days) | | | |
| | <60 years (n = 79) | >60 years (n = 62) | <60 years (n = 168) | >60 years (n = 43) | <60 years (n = 247) | >60 years (n = 106) |
| Hemorrhage | 15 (19%) | 15 (24%) | 22 (13%) | 6 (14%) | 15% | 20% |
| Infection | 32 (40%) | 41 (66%) | 76 (45%) | 23 (53%) | 44% | 61% |
| Hepatic dysfunction | 3 ( 4%) | 2 ( 3%) | 4 ( 2%) | 0 | 3% | 2% |
| Renal dysfunction | 3 ( 4%) | 6 (10%) | 4 ( 2%) | 4 ( 9%) | 3% | 10% |
| Cardiac toxicity | 0 | 3 ( 5%) | 1 (0.6%) | 1 ( 2%) | 0,4% | 4% |

superiority of the two regimens that employed seven days of cytosine arabinoside and three days of daunorubicin, all patients entering the study,
including those over 60 years of age, were subsequently distributed between
these regimens.

The treatment results for each of the four drug schedules in this study are
listed in Tables 4 and 5. Remission rates were consistently higher, regardless
of age, for patients who received the programs consisting of seven days of
cytosine arabinoside and three days of daunorubicin. Overall, 42% of the
patients who were over 60 years of age treated with these regimens attained
complete remissions compared to only 16% of those treated with the less
intensive five and two day programs. For patients over 70 years of age,
complete remission rates were 45% and 5%, respectively. In patients under
60 years, the complete remission rate with the seven and three day treatment programs was 57%.

Mortality in the time period immediately following treatment also varied
according to the treatment administered. Sixty-six percent of the patients
over 60 years of age who were treated with the less intensive five and two
day regimens died during the remission induction attempt compared to
35% with the more intensive treatment. This apparent paradox is related, in
part, to the time it took for remissions to occur. The time from the initiation of therapy to complete remission averaged 38 days for patients receiving the seven and three day programs and increased to 47 days for patients
receiving the abbreviated treatment. Only one course of the seven and three
day regimens was required to obtain the remission in 71% of the responders; only 36% of responders with the five and two regimens achieved
remission with one cycle. Presumably, the rapid and more complete elimination of leukemic cells after a single course of the more intensive therapy
permitted earlier regeneration and recovery of normal marrow function than
was seen with repetitive shorter courses of treatment. Thus, even in the
elderly more intensive and effective chemotherapy in the context of adequate supportive care can result in higher response rates and lower mortality
than relatively conservative therapy with the same drugs.

The preliminary results of an additional study exploring different dosages
of daunorubicin and the substitution of adriamycin for daunorubicin in
combination with cytosine arabinoside have been presented [22]. Patients of
all ages were randomized to receive daunorubicin at two dosage levels
($45 \text{ mg/m}^2$ and $30 \text{ mg/m}^2$) or adriamycin ($30 \text{ mg/m}^2$) on each of three consecutive days in addition to an infusion of cytosine arabinoside adminis-
tered continuously over seven days. The results with respect to age and
complete remission rates suggest there may be some advantage to a reduction in the standard dose of daunorubicin for elderly patients (Table 4).

Daunorubicin administered at $45 \text{ mg/m}^2\text{/day}$ proved superior to either the lower dose of daunorubicin or adriamycin (58% complete remissions versus 53% versus 48%) when all patients were considered. This result reflects primarily the higher rate of response with daunorubicin 45 mg/m$^2$/day in patients who were under the age of 60 years. Of the patients over 60 years of age, overall 37% entered complete remission. However, daunorubicin at the reduced dosage of 30 mg/m$^2$/day together with cytosine arabinoside resulted in a higher complete remission rate (46%) compared to either the standard dose of daunorubicin (30%) or adriamycin (36%). These variations in response were most striking in the oldest patients. Most of the differences can be attributed to the high frequencies of induction deaths, 57–59%, in the elderly treated with the two less effective regimens.

A number of other treatment programs that have been evaluated at various single institutions have resulted in higher overall complete remission rates than those reported from the cooperative groups, but the number of patients studied has been relatively small. The regimens investigated have all included cytosine arabinoside, an anthracycline, and either 6-mercapto-purine or 6-thioguanine [131–136]. In 1980, we reported the treatment results of a five-drug chemotherapeutic program for acute nonlymphocytic leukemia [134]. Eighteen of 22 newly-diagnosed patients (82%), including four of six patients over 60 years of age, entered complete remission. The median time to complete remission was 32 days and 72% of the responders required only one course of chemotherapy. We have now had an opportunity to treat a total of 19 consecutive patients over 60 years of age with this program and 11 (58%) have entered complete remission. Gale *et al.*, employing cytosine arabinoside, daunorubicin and 6-thioguanine, reported an 84% complete remission rate in a total of 70 patients [132, 137]. The age of patients did not influence response to treatment. Of the patients 60 years of age and older, 82% achieved a complete remission. The median time to remission was only 30 days. Others have reported comparable success with highly effective multi-drug regimens in small numbers of elderly patients [131, 133, 135, 136, 138]. Hopefully, when these newer regimens are examined in large-scale clinical studies, the results will substantiate these improvements in the complete remission rates of the elderly.

Although 40–50% of elderly patients treated intensively in cooperative group studies and even higher percentages treated at single institutions can now achieve complete remission and expect to have their lifetimes extended, there may be patients with acute nonlymphocytic leukemia who should have specific anti-leukemia therapy deferred. Initiating hazardous and potentially lethal treatment for any individual who is already severely compromised by concurrent chronic or acute disease requires cautious deliberation. Also, the responsiveness of the particular type of leukemia needs to be considered. Acute leukemias arising in patients who have had documented pre-leukemic states [69, 70] or appearing after treatment for other malignancies with cytotoxic drugs and/or irradiation [89] have generally proven difficult to successfully treat and meaningful responses are rarely seen. In these situations, a decision regarding the proper approach to be undertaken in an individual patient should be made by weighing the potential benefits and complications of treatment within the specific clinical context.

Delaying the induction chemotherapy of patients with smoldering leukemia has been suggested as a reasonable alternative to prompt therapeutic intervention, but the benefits of this approach have not yet been clearly established [53–57, 67, 68, 71, 72]. Patients who have smoldering leukemia comprise an estimated 6% to 10% of all adults with acute nonlymphocytic leukemia [55, 72]. The initial problem presented by the policy of deferring therapy is that it is difficult to identify at the time of diagnosis those patients with acute leukemia who are likely to have chronic indolent courses if left untreated. These patients can only be recognized with confidence after several months of close observation. Choosing observation without treatment may be an appropriate initial option for selected elderly patients who report a prolonged symptomatic interval preceding the diagnosis of leukemia or who have low percentages of myeloblasts and promyelocytes in the bone marrow, limited infiltration of the marrow by leukemia cells, and modest numbers of myeloblasts circulating in the peripheral blood. The relative merits of these criteria are unknown. It does not seem prudent, however, to delay treatment in someone who meets these criteria, but is already experiencing the consequences of leukemia, such as hemorrhage or infection, or is requiring frequent transfusions.

Whether waiting during a period of observation to initiate chemotherapy and possibly allowing the leukemia to progress will compromise the patients' subsequent opportunity to respond to treatment and experience extended survival is unknown. For patients selected to receive no immediate treatment by the preceding criteria at the time of diagnosis, median survival time is approximately nine months and the time to obvious progression of the leukemia, six months [57]. The complete remission rate in these patients following intensive chemotherapy initiated at the time of disease progression is only about 25%. Although this rate of response is lower than that generally attainable in elderly patients who have newly-diagnosed acute nonlymphocytic leukemia, the poor response rate may reflect biologic characteristics associated with the slowly progressive nature of the leukemia that makes it less susceptible to the effects of chemotherapy rather than the consequence of delaying effective therapy. Once the chronic or smoldering nature of the leukemia has been established by following patients closely for several months and eliminating those with progressive disease from consideration, the median length of survival for the remaining patients ranges from 16 to 29 months [55, 68]. The clinical status of these patients with untreated smoldering leukemia is highly variable. Some patients remain active and well, but others experience chronic discomfort, have low performance scores, and require frequent hospitalizations for the complications and consequences of untreated leukemia. For these reasons, careful consideration of each patient as a potential candidate for chemotherapy should be given before electing not to employ treatment.

Advanced age primarily influences the clinical course and survival of patients with acute nonlymphocytic leukemia through compromise of the ability to tolerate and respond to the intensive induction phase of chemotherapy rather than through any effect on the duration of response. When complete remissions occurred infrequently in the elderly and now as the response rates have improved, the duration of remission and survival time of the older responders have proven comparable to those observed in concurrently treated younger patients. Of all the factors that influence remission duration, none has been associated with aging, and age itself has little effect on the length of a complete remission once it has been achieved [26, 45]. The elderly are also among the increasing number of patients who have become long-term disease-free survivors and may be cured of acute nonlymphocytic leukemia [139–142]. Following relapse from complete remission, the elderly may survive for shorter periods of time than younger patients [15], but even at relapse they still have a comparatively good opportunity to achieve additional complete remissions and receive added months of life with intensive reinduction chemotherapy [143]. Thus, after successfully negotiating the hazards of initial induction chemotherapy and entering complete remission, the aged patient stands to benefit as much from the treatment received as the younger patient.

Significant therapeutic advances have been made in the management of adults of all ages with acute nonlymphocytic leukemia. Although there are certain biologic characteristics of the leukemia occurring in a few elderly patients that potentially make successful management more difficult, it is still primarily the inability of the aged to withstand the rigors and complications of leukemia and its chemotherapy that has limited the benefit they have received in the past from treatment. Since the rate of complete remissions in older patients continues to rise and survival continues to increase with improvements in treatment, the elderly now clearly benefit as a group from comprehensive supportive care and intensive chemotherapy. When at all possible, they should be afforded the same potential benefits of modern management as younger patients. This means that a decision to treat or not to treat an individual with acute nonlymphocytic leukemia should be made by considering the probable consequences of the choice and this will depend primarily upon specific features of the leukemia and the general underlying health status of the host rather than his chronological age.

REFERENCES

1. Bodey GP, Coltman CA, Freireich EJ, Bonnet JD, Gehan EA, Haut AB, Hewlett JS, McCredie KB, Saiki JH, Wilson HE: Chemotherapy of acute leukemia. Comparison of cytarabine alone and in combination with vincristine, prednisone, and cyclophosphamide. Arch Intern Med 133:260–266, 1974.
2. Carey RW, Ribas-Mundo M, Ellison RR, Glidewell O, Lee ST, Cuttner J, Levy RN, Silver R, Blom J, Haurani F, Spurr CL, Harley JB, Kyle R, Moon JH, Eagan RT, Holland JH: Comparative study of cytosine arabinoside therapy alone and combined with thioguanine, mercaptopurine, or daunorubicin in acute myelocytic leukemia. Cancer 36:1560–1566, 1975.
3. Clarkson BD: Acute myelocytic leukemia in adults. Cancer 30:1572–1582, 1972.
4. Clarkson BD, Dowling MD, Gee TS, Cunningham IB, Burchenal JH: Treatment of acute leukemia in adults. Cancer 36:775–795, 1975.
5. Coltman CA JR, Bodey GP, Hewlett JS, Haut A, Bickers J, Balcerzak SP, Costanzi JJ, Freireich EJ, McCredie KB, Groppe C, Smith TL, Gehan EA: Chemotherapy of acute leukemia: a comparison of vincristine, cytarabine, and prednisone alone and in combination with cyclophosphamide or daunorubicin. Arch Intern Med 137:1342–1348, 1978.
6. Crowther D, Powles RL, Bateman CJT, Beard MEJ, Gauci CL, Wrigley PFM, Malpas JS, Fairley GH, Scott RB: Management of adult acute myelogenous leukaemia. Br Med J 1:131–137, 1973.
7. Ellison RR, Holland JR, Weil M, Jacquillat C, Boiron M, Bernard J, Sawitsky A, Rosner F, Gussoff B, Silver RT, Karanas A, Cuttner J, Spurr CL, Hayes DM, Blom J, Leone LA, Haurani F, Kyle R, Hutchison JL, Forcier RJ, Moon JH: Arabinosyl cytosine: a useful agent in the treatment of acute leukemia in adults. Blood 32:507–523, 1968.
8. Ellison RR, Silver RT, Engle RL Jr,: Comparative study of 6-chloropurine and 6-mercaptopurine in acute leukemia in adults. Ann Intern Med 51:322–338, 1959.
9. Frei E, III, Freireich EJ, Gehan E, Pinkel D, Holland JF, Selawry O, Haurani F, Spurr CL, Hayes DM, James GW, Rothberg H, Sodee DB, Rundles RW, Schroeder LR, Hoogstraten B, Wolman IJ, Traggis DG, Cooper T, Gendel BR, Ebaugh R, Taylor R: Studies of sequential and combination antimetabolite therapy of acute leukemia: 6-mercaptopurine and methotrexate. Blood 18: 431–454, 1961.
10. Freireich EJ, Bodey GP, Harris JE, Hart JS: Therapy for acute granulocytic leukemia. Cancer Res 27:2573–2577, 1967.
11. Henderson ES: Treatment of acute leukemia. Ann Intern Med 69:628–632, 1968.
12. Keating MJ, McCredie KB, Benjamin RS, Bodey GP, Zander A, Smith TL, Freireich EJ: Treatment of patients over 50 years of age with acute leukemia with a combination of rubidazone and cytosine arabinoside, vincristine, and prednisone (ROAP). Blood 58:584–591, 1981.
13. Keating MJ, Smith TL, McCredie KB, Bodey GP, Hersh EM, Gutterman JU, Gehan E, Freireich EJ: A four-year experience with anthracycline, cytosine arabinoside, vincristine and prednisone combination chemotherapy in 325 adults with acute leukemia. Cancer (in press).

14. Medical Research Council: Treatment of acute leukaemia in adults: Comparison of steroid and mercaptopurine therapy, alone and in conjunction. Br Med J 1:1383–1389, 1966.

15. Medical Research Council: Treatment of acute myeloid leukaemia with daunorubicin, cytosine arabinoside, mercaptopurine, L-asparaginase, prednisone and thioguanine: results of treatment with five multiple drug schedules. Br J Haematol 27:373–389, 1974.

16. Rai KR, Holland JF, Glidewell OJ, Weinberg V, Brunner K, Obrecht JP, Preisler HD, Nawabi IW, Prager D, Carey RW, Cooper MR, Haurani F, Hutchison JL, Silver RT, Falkson G, Wiernik P, Hoagland HC, Bloomfield CD, James GW, Gottlieb A, Ramanan SV, Blom J, Nissen NI, Bank A, Ellison RR, King F, Henry P, McIntyre OR, Kaan SK: Treatment of acute myelocytic leukemia: a study by Cancer and Leukemia Group B. Blood (in press).

17. Rodriguez V, Hart JS, Freireich Ej, Bodey GP, McCredie KB, Whitecar JP Jr, Coltman CA Jr: POMP combination therapy of adult acute leukemia. Cancer 32:69–75, 1973.

18. Southwest Oncology Group: Cytarabine for acute leukemia in adults. Effect of schedule on therapeutic response. Arch Intern Med 133:251–259, 1974.

19. Thompson I, Hall TC, Moloney WC: Combination therapy of adult myelogenous leukemia. N Engl J Med 273:1302–1307, 1965.

20. Weil M, Glidewell OJ, Jacquillat C, Levy R, Serpick AA, Wiernik PH, Cuttner J, Hoogstraten B, Wasserman L, Ellison RR, Gailani S, Brunner K, Silver RT, Rege VB, Cooper MR, Lowenstein L, Nissen NI, Haurani F, Blom J, Boiron M, Bernard J, Holland JF: Daunorubicin in the therapy of acute granulocytic leukemia. Cancer Res 33:921–928, 1973.

21. Wiernik PH, Glidewell OJ, Hoagland HC, Brunner KW, Spurr CL, Cuttner J, Silver RT, Carey RW, DelDuca V, Kung FH, Holland JF: A comparative trial of daunorubicin, cytosine arabinoside, and thioguanine, and a combination of the three agents for the treatment of acute myelocytic leukemia. Med Pediatr Oncol 6:261–277, 1979.

22. Yates JW, Glidewell O, Wiernik P, Holland JF: A VALGB study of adriamycin vs daunorubicin induction and a four vs eight week maintenance in acute myelocytic leukemia. Proc Am Assoc Cancer Res Am Soc Clin Oncol 21:350, 1980.

23. Boggs DR, Wintrobe MM, Cartwright GE: The acute leukemias. Analysis of 322 cases and review of the literature. Medicine 41:163–225, 1962.

24. Crowther D, Beard MEJ, Bateman CJT, Sewell RL: Factors influencing prognosis in adults with acute myelogenous leukaemia. Br J Cancer 32: 456–464, 1975.

25. Ellison RR, Wallace HJ, Hoagland HC, Woolford DC, Glidewell OJ: Prognostic parameters in acute myelocytic leukemia as seen in the Acute Leukemia Group B. In: Advances in the Biosciences 14, Workshop on Prognostic Factors in Human Acute Leukemia, Reisensburg, Germany, October 1–3, 1973, Fliedner TM, Perry S (eds). New York: Pergamon Press, 1975, pp 51–69.

26. Freireich EJ, Keating MJ, Gehan EA, McCredie KB, Bodey GP, Smith T: Therapy of acute myelogenous leukemia. Cancer 42:874–882, 1978.

27. Gehan EA, Smith TL, Freireich EJ, Bodey G, Rodriguez V, Speer J, McCredie K: Prognostic factors in acute leukemia. Semin Oncol 3:271–282, 1976.

28. Gunz FW, Burns EW: Prognosis in acute leukaemia of adults. NZ Med J 64:555–561, 1965.

29. Reiffers J, Raynal F, Broustet A: Acute myeloblastic leukemia in elderly patients. Treatment and prognostic factors. Cancer 45:2816–2820, 1980.

30. Wiernik PH, Serpick AA: Factors effecting remission and survival in adult acute nonlymphocytic leukemia (ANLL). Medicine 49:505–513, 1970.

31. Bloomfield CD, Theologides A: Acute granulocytic leukemia in elderly patients. JAMA 226:1190–1193, 1973.

32. Cutler SJ, Axtell L, Heise H: Ten thousand cases of leukemia: 1940–62. J Natl Cancer Inst 39:993–1026, 1967.

33. Gunz FW, Hough RF: Acute leukemia over the age of fifty: a study of its incidence and natural history. Blood 11:882–901, 1956.

34. Roath S, Israëls MCG, Wilkinson JF: The acute leukaemias: a study of 580 patients. Q J Med 33:257–283, 1964.

35. Brandt L, Nilsson PG, Mitelman F: Trends in incidence of acute leukaemia. Lancet ii:1069, 1979.

36. Geary CG, Benn RT, Leck I: Incidence of myeloid leukaemia in Lancashire. Lancet ii:549–551, 1979.

37. Greenwald P, Burnett WS, Kirmss V, Brennan K: Cancer incidence and mortality in New York State. Bureau of Cancer Control, N Y State Dept. of Health, 1976.

38. Linos A, Kyle RA, Elveback LR, Kurland LT: Leukemia in Olmsted County, Minnesota, 1965–1974. Mayo Clin Proc 53:714–718, 1978.

39. Rowley JD: Chromosome abnormalities in human acute non-lymphocytic leukemia: relationship to age, sex, and exposure to mutagens. J Natl Cancer Inst (in press).

40. Bernard J, Jacquillat C, Weil M: Treatment of the acute leukemias. Semin Hematol 9:181–191, 1972.

41. Bodey GP, Coltman CA, Hewlett JS, Freireich EJ: Progress in the treatment of adults with acute leukemia. Review of regimens containing cytarabine studied by the Southwest Oncology Group. Arch Intern Med 136:1383–1388, 1976.

42. Gunz FW, Vincent PC: Towards a cure of acute granulocytic leukemia? Leukemia Res 1:51–66, 1977.

43. Husband RA, O'Neill BJ, Scamps RA: The treatment of adult acute leukaemia with modified VAMP therapy. Med J Aust 2:528–530, 1974.

44. Whitecar JP Jr, Bodey GP, Freireich EJ, McCredie KB, Hart JS: cyclophosphamide (NSC-26271), vincristine (NSC-67574), cytosine arabinoside (NSC-63878), and prednisone (NSC-10023) (COAP) combination chemotherapy for acute leukemia in adults. Cancer Chemother Rep 56:543–550, 1972.

45. Keating MJ, Smith TL, Gehan EA, McCredie KB, Bodey GP, Spitzer G, Hersh E, Gutterman J, Freireich EJ: Factors related to length of complete remission in adult acute leukemia. Cancer 45:2017–2029, 1980.

46. Berg J, Vincent PC, Gunz FW: Extreme leucocytosis and prognosis of newly diagnosed patients with acute non-lymphocytic leukaemia. Med J Aust: 580–482, 1979.

47. Freireich EJ, Gehan EA, Bodey GP, Hersh EM, Hart JS, Gutterman JU, McCredie KB: New prognostic factors affecting response and survival in adult acute leukemia. Trans Assoc Am Phys 87:298–305, 1974.

48. Holmes FF, Hearne E III, Conant M, Garlow W: Survival in the elderly with acute leukemia. J Am Geriatr Soc 27:241–243, 1979.

49. Medical Research Council: The relation between morphology and other features of acute myeloid leukaemia, and their prognostic signifiance. Br J Haematol 31 (Suppl):165–180, 1975.

50. Southam CM, Craver LF, Dargeon HW, Burchenal JH: A study of the natural history of acute leukemia with special reference to the duration of the disease and the occurrence of remissions. Cancer 4:39–59, 1951.

51. Mandelli F, Amadori S, Fabiani F, Grignani F, Liso V, Martelli M, Neri A, Petti MC, Tonato M: Treatment of acute nonlymphocytic leukemia (ANLL) in elderly patients. Results of a multicentric study. Haematologica 64:331–338, 1979.

52. Peterson BA, Bloomfield CD: Treatment of acute nonlymphocytic leukemia in elderly patients. A prospective study of intensive chemotherapy. Cancer 40:647–652, 1977.

53. Beard MEJ, Bateman CJT, Crowther DC, Wrigley PFM, Whitehouse JMA, Fairley GH, Scott RB: Hypoplastic acute myelogenous leukaemia. Br J Haematol 31:167–176, 1975.

54. Cohen JR, Creger WP, Greenberg PL, Schrier SL: Subacute myeloid leukemia. A clinical view. Am J Med 66:959–966, 1979.

55. Evensen SA, Stavem P: Smouldering acute myelogenous leukemia. Acta Med Scand 203:305–307, 1978.

56. Weil M, Jacquillat CI, Gemon-Auclerc MF, Chastang CL, Izrael V, Boiron M, Bernard J: Acute granulocytic leukemia. Treatment of the disease. Arch Intern Med 136:1389–1395, 1976.

57. Keating MJ, McCredie K, Freireich EJ: Prediction of progression and survival of untreated acute leukemia. Proc Am Assoc Cancer Res Am Soc Clin Oncol 19:340, 1978.

58. Bennett JM, Catovsky D, Daniel M-T, Flandrin G, Galton DAG, Gralnick HR, Sultan C: Proposals for the classification of the acute leukaemias. Br J Haematol 33:451–458, 1976.

59. Gralnick HR, Galton DAG, Catovsky D, Sultan C, Bennett JM: Classification of acute leukemia. Ann Intern Med 87:740–753, 1977.

60. Cuttner J, Conjalka MS, Reilly M, Goldberg J, Reisman A, Meyer RJ, Holland JF: Association of monocytic leukemia in patients with extreme leukocytosis. Am J Med 69:555–558, 1980.

61. Foon KA, Naiem F, Yale C, Gale RP: Acute myelogenous leukemia: morphologic classification and response to therapy. Leukemia Res 3:171–173, 1979.

62. Hetzel P, Gee TS: A new observation in the clinical spectrums of erythroleukemia. A report of 46 cases. Am J Med 64:765–772, 1978.

63. Mertelsmann R, Thaler HT, To L, Gee TS, McKenzie S, Schauer P, Friedman A, Arlin Z, Cirrincione C, Clarkson B: Morphologic classification, response to therapy, and survival in 263 adult patients with acute nonlymphoblastic leukemia. Blood 56:773–781, 1980.

64. Straus DJ, Mertelsmann R, Koziner B, McKenzie S, DeHarven E, Arlin ZA, Kempin S, Broxmeyer H, Moore MAS, Menendez-Botet CJ, Gee TS, Clarkson BD: The acute monocytic leukemias: multidisciplinary studies in 45 patients. Medicine 59:409–425, 1980.

65. Sultan C, Deregnaucourt J, Ko YW, Imbert M, Richard D'Agay MF, Gouault-Heilmann M, Brun B: Distribution of 250 cases of acute myeloid leukaemia (AML) according to the FAB classification and response to therapy. Br J Haematol 47:545–551, 1981.

66. Rubio F: Acute leukemia in patients past the age of 50. J Am Geriatr Soc 8:644–659, 1960.

67. Rheingold JJ, Kaufman R, Adelson E, Lear A: Smoldering acute leukemia. N Engl J Med 268:812–815, 1963.

68. Rheingold JJ: Acute leukemia. Its smoldering phase, or leukemia never starts on Thursday. JAMA 230:985–986, 1974.

69. Koeffler HP, Golde DW: Human preleukemia. Ann Intern Med 93:347–353, 1980.

70. Pierre RV: Preleukemic syndromes. Virchows Arch B Cell Path 29:29–37, 1978.

71. Knospe WH, Gregory SA: Smoldering acute leukemia. Clinical and cytogenetic studies in six patients. Arch Intern Med 127:910–918, 1971.

72. Speer JF, Freireich EJ, Hart JS, McCredie KB, Bodey GP, Rodriguez V, Burgess MA: Identification of smouldering leukemia by delaying chemotherapy. Proc Am Assoc Cancer Res Am Soc Clin Oncol 15:73, 1974.

73. Preisler HD, Bjornsson S, Henderson ES: Adriamycin-cytosine arabinoside therapy for adult acute myelocytic leukemia. Cancer Treat Rep 61:89–92, 1977.

74. Hart JS, George SL, Frei E Ill, Bodey GP, Nickerson RC, Freireich EJ: Prognostic significance of pretreatment proliferative activity in adult acute leukemia. Cancer 39:1603–1617, 1977.

75. Dosik GM, Barlogie B, Smith TL, Gehan EA, Keating MJ, McCredie KB, Freireich EJ: Pretreatment flow cytometry of DNA content in adult acute leukemia. Blood 55:474-482, 1980.

76. Buick RN, Minden MD, McCulloch EA: Self-renewal in culture of proliferative blast progenitor cells in acute myeloblastic leukemia. Blood 54:95-104, 1979.

77. Elias L, Greenberg P: Divergent patterns of marrow cell suspension culture growth in the myeloid leukemias: correlation of in vitro findings with clinical features. Blood 50:263-274, 1977.

78. Moore MAS, Spitzer G, Williams N, Metcalf D, Buckley J: Agar culture studies in 127 cases of untreated acute leukemia: the prognostic value of reclassification of leukemia according to in vitro growth characteristics. Blood 44:1-18, 1974.

79. Spitzer G, Dicke KA, Gehan EA, Smith T, McCredie KB, Barlogie B, Freireich EJ: A simplified in vitro classification for prognosis in adult acute leukemia: The application of in vitro results in remission-predictive models. Blood 48:795-807, 1976.

80. Greene W, Huffman D, Wiernik PH, Schimpff S, Benjamin R, Bachur N: High dose daunorubicin therapy for acute nonlymphocytic leukemia: correlation of response and toxicity with pharmacokinetics and intracellular daunorubicin reductase activity. Cancer 30:1419-1427, 1972.

81. Preisler HD, Rustum Y, Henderson ES, Bjornsson S, Creaven PJ, Higby DJ, Freeman A, Gailani S, Naeher C: Treatment of acute nonlymphocytic leukemia: use of anthracycline-cytosine arabinoside induction therapy and comparison of two maintenance regimens. Blood 53:455-464, 1979.

82. Rustum YM, Preisler HD: Correlation between leukemic cell retention of 1-$\beta$-D-arabinofuranosylcytosine 5'-triphosphate and response to therapy. Cancer Res 39:42-49, 1979.

83. Golomb HM, Vardiman JW, Rowley JD, Testa JR, Mintz U: Correlation of clinical findings with quinacrine-banded chromosomes in 90 adults with acute nonlymphocytic leukemia: an eight-year study (1970-1977). N Engl J Med 299:613-619, 1978.

84. Rowley JD, Golomb HM, Vardiman J, Fukuhara S, Dougherty C, Potter D: Further evidence for a non-random chromosomal abnormality in acute promyelocytic leukemia. Int J Cancer 20:869-872, 1977.

85. Kamada N, Okada K, Ito T, Nakatsui T, Uchino H: Chromosome 21-22 and neutrophil alkaline phosphatase in leukaemia. Lancet i:364, 1968.

86. Rowley JD: Identification of a translocation with quinacrine fluorescence in a patient with acute leukemia. Ann de Génét 16:109-112, 1973.

87. Rowley JD, Golomb HM, Vardiman J: Nonrandom chromosome abnormalities in acute nonlymphocytic leukemia in patients treated for Hodgkin's disease and non-Hodgkin's lymphomas. Blood 50:759-770, 1977.

88. Mitelman F, Brandt L, Nilsson PG: Relation among occupational exposure to potential mutagenic/carcinogenic agents, clinical findings, and bone marrow chromosomes in acute nonlymphocytic leukemia. Blood 52:1229-1237, 1978.

89. Casciato DA, Scott JL: Acute leukemia following prolonged cytotoxic agent therapy. Medicine 58:32-47, 1979.

90. Fernandez G, Schwartz JM: Immune responsiveness and hematologic malignancy in the elderly. Med Clin North Am 60:1253-1271, 1976.

91. Rowe JW: Clinical research on aging: strategies and directions. N Engl J Med 297:1332-1336, 1977.

92. Timiras PS: Biological perspective on aging. Am Sci 66:605-613, 1978.

93. Crooks J, Stevenson IH: Drugs and the elderly: perspectives in geriatric clinical pharmacology. Baltimore, Md: University Park Press, 1979.

94. Stevenson IH: Summary of workshops 1: drug metabolism in the elderly. Age Ageing 7 (Suppl):131-133, 1978.

95. Vestal RE: Drug use in the elderly: a review of problems and special considerations. Drugs 16:358–382, 1978.

96. Tobias JS, Wrigley PFM, O'Grady F: Bacterial infection and acute myeloblastic leukaemia: an analysis of two hundred patients undergoing intensive remission induction therapy. Eur J Cancer 14:383–391, 1978.

97. Kansal V, Omura GA, Soong S-J: Prognosis in adult acute myelogenous leukemia related to performance status and other factors. Cancer 38: 329–334, 1976.

98. Boyd NF, Clemens JD, Feinstein AR: Pretherapeutic morbidity in the prognostic staging of acute leukemia. Arch Intern Med 139:324–328, 1979.

99. Hartsock RJ, Smith EB, Petty CS: Normal variations with aging of the amount of hematopoietic tissue in bone marrow from the anterior iliac crest. A study made from 177 cases of sudden death examined necropsy. Am J Clin Pathol 43:326–331, 1965.

100. Freedman ML, Marcus DL: Anemia and the elderly: is it physiology or pathology? Am J Med Sci 280:81–85, 1980.

101. Giorno R, Clifford JH, Beverly S, Rossing RG: Hematology reference values: analysis by different statistical technics and variations with age and sex. Am J Clin Pathol 74:765–770, 1980.

102. Wolf NS: The haematopoietic microenvironment. Clin Haematol 8:469–500, 1979.

103. Smith IE, Powles R, Clink HM, Jameson B, Kay HEM, McElwain TJ: Early deaths in acute myelogenous leukemia. Cancer 39:1710–1714, 1977.

104. Chang H-Y, Rodriguez V, Narboni G, Bodey GP, Luna MA, Freireich EJ: Causes of death in adults with acute leukemia. Medicine 55:259–268, 1976.

105. Gurwith MJ, Brunton Jl, Lank BA, Ronald AR, Harding GKM: Granulocytopenia in hospitalized patients. I. Prognostic factors and etiology of fever. Am J Med 64:121–126, 1978.

106. EORTC International Antimicrobial Therapy Project Group: Three antibiotic regimens in the treatment of infection in febrile granulocytopenic patients with cancer. J Infect Dis 137:14–29, 1978.

107. Grann V, Erichson R, Flannery J, Finch S, Clarkson B: The therapy of acute granulocytic leukemia in patients more than fifty years old. Ann Intern Med 80:15–20, 1974.

108. Bristow MR, Thompson PD, Martin RP, Mason JW, Billingham ME, Harrison DC: Early anthracycline cardiotoxicity. Am J Med 65:823–832, 1978.

109. Von Hoff DD, Layard MW, Basa P, Davis HL Jr, Von Hoff AL, Rozencweig M, Muggia FM: Risk factors for doxorubicin-induced congestive heart failure. Ann Intern Med 91:710–717, 1979.

110. Von Hoff DD, Rozencweig M, Layard M, Slavik M, Muggia FM: Daunomycin-induced cardiotoxicity in children and adults. A review of 110 cases. Am J Med 62:200–208, 1977.

111. Crowell EB Jr. MacKinney AA, Pisciotta AV, Schloesser LL, Keimowitz RM: Age and treatment response in acute nonlymphoblastic leukemia, J Gerontol 33:52–56, 1978.

112. Bernard J, Jacquillat C, Weil M, Boiron M, Tanzer J: Present results on daunorubicin. Recent Results Cancer Res 30:3–8, 1970.

113. Boiron M, Jacquillat C, Weil M, Tanzer J, Levy D, Sultan C, Bernard J: Daunorubicin in the treatment of acute myelocytic leukaemia. Lancet i:330–333, 1969.

114. Wiernik PH, Schimpff SC, Schiffer CA, Lichtenfeld JL, Aisner J, O'Connell MJ, Fortner C: Randomized clinical comparison of daunorubicin (NSC-82151) alone with a combination of daunorubicin, cytosine arabinoside (NSC-63878), 6-thioguanine (NSC-752), and pyrimethamine (NSC-3061) for the treatment of acute nonlymphocytic leukemia. Cancer Treat Rep 60:41–53, 1976.

115. Peterson BA, Bloomfield CD, Theologides A, Kennedy BJ: Daunorubicin-prednisone in the treatment of acute non-lymphocytic leukemia. Cancer Treat Rep (in press).

116. Burge PS, Prankerd TAJ: Survival in acute myeloid leukaemia. Lancet ii:1091, 1975.

117. Burge PS, Prankerd TAJ, Richards JDM: Survival in acute myeloid leukaemia. Lancet i:85, 1976.

118. Burge PS, Prankerd TAJ, Richards JDM, Sare M, Thompson DS, Wright P: Quality and quantity of survival in acute myeloid leukaemia. Lancet ii:621-624, 1975.

119. Crosby WH: To treat or not to treat acute granulocytic leukemia. Arch Intern Med 122:79-80, 1968.

120. Crosby WH: Grounds for optimism in treating acute granulocytic leukemia. Arch Intern Med 134:177-180, 1974.

121. Crosby WH: Acute granulocytic leukemia (AGL) in the elderly. Arch Intern Med 136:493-494, 1976.

122. Jacobs P, Dubovsky D: Quality and quantity of survival in acute myeloid leukaemia. Lancet ii:1041, 1975.

123. Rose M: Survival in acute myeloid leukaemia. Lancet ii:1091, 1975.

124. Clink HM, Douglas IDC: Quality and quantity of survival in acute myeloid leukaemia. Lancet ii:988-989, 1975.

125. Johnson SAN, Beard MEJ, Lister TA, Wrigley PFM, Whitehouse JMA: Survival in acute myeloid leukaemia. Lancet ii:1254-1255, 1975.

126. Rosner F, Sawitsky A, Grünwald HW, Rai KR: Acute granulocytic leukemia in the elderly. Arch Intern Med 136:120, 1976.

127. Gee TS, Yu K-P, Clarkson BD: Treatment of adult acute leukemia with arabinosylcytosine and thioguanine. Cancer 23:1019-1032, 1969.

128. Benjamin RS, Keating MJ, McCredie KB, Bodey GP, Freireich EJ: A phase 1 and 2 trial of rubidazone in patients with acute leukemia. Cancer Res 37:4623-4628, 1977.

129. Holland JF, Glidewell O, Ellison RR, Carey RW, Schwartz J, Wallace HJ, Hoagland HC, Wiernik P, Rai K, Bekesi JG, Cuttner J: Acute myelocytic leukemia. Arch Intern Med 136:1377-1381, 1976.

130. Yates JW, Wallace HJ Jr, Ellison RR, Holland JF: Cytosine arabinoside (NSC-63878) and daunorubicin (NSC-83142) therapy in acute nonlymphocytic leukemia. Cancer Chemother Rep 57:485-488, 1973.

131. Arlin Z, Gee T, Fried J, Koenigsberg E, Wolmark N, Clarkson B: Rapid induction of remission in acute non-lymphocytic leukemia (ANLL). Proc Am Assoc Cancer Res Am Soc Clin Oncol 20:112, 1979.

132. Gale RP, Cline MJ: High remission-induction rate in acute myeloid leukaemia. Lancet i:497-499, 1977.

133. Glucksberg H, Buckner CD, Fefer A, Demarsh Q, Coleman D, Dobrow RB, Huff J, Kjobech C, Hill AS, Dittman W, Neiman PE, Cheever MA, Einstein AB Jr, Thomas ED: Combination chemotherapy for acute nonlymphoblastic leukemia in adults. Cancer Chemother Rep 59:1131-1137, 1975.

134. Peterson BA, Bloomfield CD, Bosl GJ, Gibbs G, Malloy M: Intensive five-drug combination chemotherapy for adult acute nonlymphocytic leukemia. Cancer 46:663-668, 1980.

135. Rees JKH, Sandler RM, Challener J, Hayhoe FGJ: Treatment of acute myeloid leukaemia with a triple cytotoxic regime: DAT. Br J Cancer 36:770-776, 1977.

136. Uzuka Y, Liong SK, Yamagata S: Treatment of adult acute non-lymphoblastic leukemia using intermittent combination chemotherapy with daunomycin, cytosine arabinoside, 6-mercaptoputine and prednisolone-DCMP two step therapy. Tohoku J Exp Med 118 (Suppl):217-225, 1976.

137. Gale RP, Zighelboim J, Foon KA, Cline MJ: Intensive chemoimmunotherapy in acute myelogenous leukemia. Blood 52 (Suppl):250, 1978.

138. Rees JKH, Hayhoe FGJ: D.A.T. (daunorubicin, cytarabine, 6-thioguanine) in acute myeloid leukaemia. Lancet i:1360-1361, 1978.

139. Coltman CA Jr, Freireich EJ, Savage RA, Gehan EA: Long-term survival of adults with acute leukemia. Proc Am Assoc Cancer Res Am Soc Clin Oncol 20:389, 1979.
140. Ellison RR, Glidewell O: Improved survival in adults with acute myelocytic leukemia (AML). Proc Am Assoc Cancer Res Am Soc Clin Oncol 20:161, 1979.
141. Keating MJ, Bodey GP, McCredie KB, Freireich EJ: Five year survival and remission duration in adult acute myelogenous leukemia (AML). Proc Am Assoc Cancer Res Am Soc Clin Oncol 20:416, 1979.
142. Peterson BA, Bloomfield CD: Long-term disease-free survival in acute nonlymphocytic leukemia. Blood 57:1144–1147, 1981.
143. Peterson BA, Bloomfield CD: Re-induction of complete remissions in adults with acute non-lymphocytic leukemia. Leukemia Res 5:81–88, 1981.
144. Bloomfield CD, Brunning RD, Theologides A, Kennedy BJ: Daunorubicin-prednisone remission induction with hydroxyurea maintenance in acute non-lymphocytic leukemia. Cancer 31:931–938, 1973.

# 8. Early Identification of Potentially Cured Patients with Acute Myelogenous Leukemia — A Recent Challenge

MICHAEL J. KEATING

## CONTENTS

## 1. INTRODUCTION

Historically, the treatment of adults with acute myelogenous leukemia (AML) has evolved through a number of phases. In the initial phase we saw the accumulation of information on the natural history of acute leukemia and study of the patterns of survival [1, 2]. Analysis of survival data in patients with acute leukemia who were treated with supportive care only was adequately documented and showed that half of all patients would die in less than four months and less than one patient in ten would live for one year. The early literature was concerned with documentation of spontaneous remissions, and up until 1960, there was no evidence that chemotherapy-induced remissions were of longer duration [1, 2] than those which occurred spontaneously. In addition, no accurate estimate of the response rate to chemotherapeutic agents was available, despite the fact that the 'chemotherapy era' in acute leukemia had been ushered in by Farber in 1949 [4].

In the period 1960–69, the beneficial effect of obtaining a complete remission (CR) with antimetabolites on survival was established and it was shown that the entire benefit of chemotherapy on survival was accounted for by the duration of response to the effective agent(s) [5]. Although the CR rate at this time was only of the order of 15%, data such as these encouraged physicians to pursue treatment with chemotherapy to induce remissions and publications during this period stressed CR rate with little emphasis on CR duration [6, 7, 8]. Active debate continued in some quarters as to the wisdom of treating AML. Crosby suggested that patients with blastic transformation of myeloproliferative disorders, smouldering leukemia, AML with megaloblastosis, myelomonocytic leukemia, progranulocytic leukemia and AML, if they were over 50 years of age, did not benefit from chemotherapy [9], demonstrating that an exploratory evaluation of the influence of prognostic factors on response and survival was ongoing at that time. Various reports supported or refuted the claims being made [6, 7]. Although the overall CR rate during this period was only 20–30%, promising new agents such as daunorubicin and cytosine arabinoside (ara-C) were actively being explored [10–14].

The first indication of the possibility of cure in adult acute leukemia came in 1967, when Burchenal published the results of a world-wide survey conducted in an attempt to find long-term survivors in Burkitt's lymphoma and acute leukemia [15]. However, only 16 adults of all morphologic subtypes of acute leukemia were recorded to be alive and free of disease more than five years from the time of diagnosis.

The decade of the seventies has been a period of major development and shift in emphasis in AML. The successful introduction of ara-C [11, 16, 17] and the anthracyclines, daunorubicin (DNR) [12, 13, 14, 18, 19], doxorubicin (adriamycin, ADR) [20], and zorubicin (rubidazone, RUB) [21] into wide-spread clinical practice has increased the overall CR rate to 60–80% [22–27, 70, 71].Previously reported adverse prognostic characteristics such as promyelocytic leukemia [28] and myelomonocytic leukemia [26] (see chapter by Bennett) and age [29-32] (see chapter by Peterson), have become much less significant. Many reports now describe in detail the duration of complete remission, the effect of pretreatment characteristics, maintenance chemotherapy and immunotherapy on CR duration [57] and the number of patients still in remission for two years or more are noted [26, 53, 57]. Reports of long-term survivors in AML have appeared with increasing frequency. Although early studies from Japan [33], France [34], and Argentina [35] suggested that 0.1-2.2% of patients with AML survive five years, more recently, Oliff reported that 4-5% of 211 patients with AML treated at the National Cancer Institute (N.C.I.) in the United States between 1973 and 1975 survived for more than four years [36].

In the last two years, our group at the M. D. Anderson Hospital [37], two large cooperative study groups [38, 39], and a French group [40] have reported their results of long-term follow-up studies on patients with AML. An update of the M. D. Anderson Hospital (MDAH) data will be presented in detail here, and used for comparison with these and other studies.

## 2. M. D. ANDERSON HOSPITAL DATA

From 1965 until September 1975, 396 previously untreated patients with AML received their initial remission induction treatment at the M. D. Anderson Hospital (Department of Developmental Therapeutics). Several different protocols were used during the time period being analyzed (Table 1). The first protocols were based on the principles of combination chemotherapy established in childhood acute lymphoblastic leukemia and incorporated mercaptopurine combined either with methyl-mecaptopurine riboside (MP+MMPR) [41] or methotrexate, vincristine, and prednisone (POMP) [42]. All subsequent protocols incorporated ara-C used alone or in combination with other agents such as cyclophosphamide [43, 44], daunorubicin [45], and adriamycin [20] in an attempt to achieve a clinical synergistic or at least additive cytoreductive effect. Most of the programs also included the administration of vincristine and prednisone (VP) because of the minimal toxicity of these drugs, especially myelosuppression, and their potential clinical usefulness. Most patients received maintenance treatment with the same chemotherapy which was used for remission induction. In one study conducted in 1970-71 POMP was compared to COAP as a remission induction program [46]. Patients were randomized to receive one or the other induction program and complete responders received a cyclical chemotherapy maintenance program (CYCLE) consisting of three additional

*Table 1.* Chemotherapy programs used at the M.D. Anderson Hospital 1965–1975.

| Remission induction drugs | No. of patients | V.P. [‡] | | Abbreviation | Maintenance chemotherapy |
|---|---|---|---|---|---|
| | | Yes | No | | |
| Adriamycin + Ara-C [†] | 144 | 144 | — | AD-OAP * | OAP * |
| Daunorubicin + Ara-C [†] | 17 | 17 | — | DOAP | OAP (COAP, 2 pts.) |
| Ara-C [†] | 63 | 41 | 22 | OAP * Ara-C | OAP * [† 16 pts.] Ara-C |
| Cyclophosphamide + Ara-C († 15 pts.) | 88 | 70 | 18 | COAP Cyclo + Ara-C | COAP Cyclo + Ara-C 'cycle' |
| Mercaptopurine + methotrexate | 27 | 27 | — | POMP | POMP cycle |
| Mercaptopurine + methyl mercapto- purine riboside | 32 | — | 32 | MP + MMPR | MP + MMPR |
| Miscellaneous | 25 | 1 | 24 | Misc. | Misc. |

* BCG also administered.
[†] Continuous in infusion.
[‡] Vincristine—prednisone.

courses of their remission induction program, then three courses of the alternate program, followed by three courses of daunorubicin and L-aspar-aginase, after which they received further therapy with their original com-bination program until two years of complete remission had been reached.

Nine patients whose remission was induced with OAP were given three intensive courses of chemotherapy with OAP after achieving remission (ear-ly intensification) [47]. From late 1970 most patients who remained in re-mission for at least one year were entered on a late intensification program and received intensive chemotherapy with agents to which they had not been previously exposed, usually POMP [48]. Chemotherapy was then dis-continued and patients received only treatment with BCG (Bacillus Cal-mette Guerin) by scarification [49]. From 1971 until 1975 BCG was given together with chemotherapy during maintenance programs and following late intensification chemotherapy.

## 3. FIVE-YEAR SURVIVAL – OVERALL AND CHEMOTHERAPY EFFECT

The survival curves for all patients, complete responders, and failing patients are shown in Figure 1. The impact of achieving complete remission

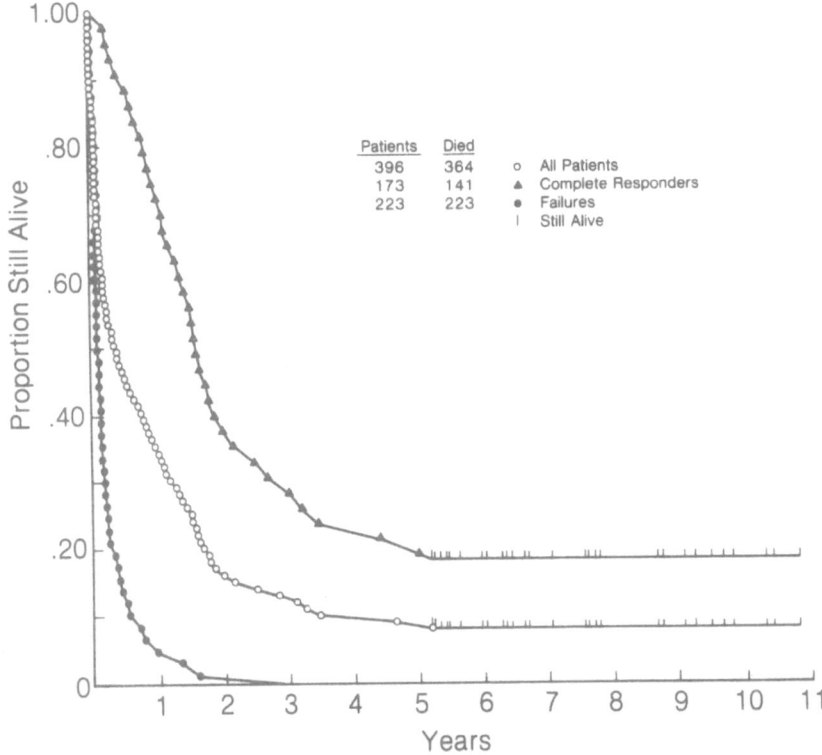

*Figure 1.* Survival of AML patients 1965–1975 – all, complete responders, and failures.

is obvious. While 19% of the CR patients survived five years, none of the 223 patients failing to obtain a CR did so. In fact, none of these patients survived three years and only nine (4%) lived longer than one year. The survival curve for failing patients is almost identical to that of patients receiving supportive care only, confirming the observation of Freireich that obtaining a remission is the only way to significantly affect survival. As recently as 1975, there was still discussion as to the need to achieve CR to affect survival. Burge *et al.* [50] compared the survival data of the patients who received 'less-aggressive' treatment with patients treated with intensive chemotherapy in one of the Medical Research Council trials. The CR rate was only 6.5%. While the overall survival data are comparable to the M.R.C. trial only 2/51 (4%) of these patients survived two years and thus are far inferior to published data from several other cooperative studies.

Although the overall five-year survival rate from 1965 to 1975 is 33/396 (8.3%), marked differences with date of entry on study and the different protocols used are noted (Table 2). The most recent studies have combined ara-C by continuous infusion, vincristine, and prednisone with an anthracy-

*Table 2.* Overall results according to remission induction program at the M.D. Anderson Hospital 1965–1975.

| Chemotherapy program | No. of patients | CR | | 5-yr survivors | | % CRs lasting 5 years | |
|---|---|---|---|---|---|---|---|
| | | No. | (%) | No. | (%) | No. | (%) |
| ADOAP* | 144 | 81 | (56) | 18 | (13) | 16 | (20) |
| DOAP* | 17 | 11 | (65) | 3 | (18) | 3 | (27) |
| ARA-C + OAP* | 63 | 24 | (38) | 10 | (17) | 9 | (38) |
| CYCLO + ARA-C, | | | | | | | |
| COAP (15 pts) | 88 | 31 | (35) | 1 | ( 1) | 1 | ( 3) |
| POMP | 27 | 15 | (56) | 1 | ( 4) | 1 | ( 7) |
| MP + MMPR | 32 | 7 | (22) | 0 | (−) | 0 | (−) |
| MISC | 25 | 4 | (16) | 0 | (−) | 0 | (−) |
| Total | 396 | 173 | (44) | 33 | ( 8) | 30 | (17) |

* Continuous infusion Ara-C in remission induction.

cline (either adriamycin-ADOAP or daunorubicin-DOAP). The five-year survival rate for the anthracycline-ara-C group is 21/161 (13%). Most current chemotherapy regimens include an anthracycline and continuous infusion ara-C. With improved supportive care and increasing expertise in the use of these agents, the CR rates now being reported are 70–90%, so that the figure of 13% is probably a minimal estimate of the 'potentially cured' fraction for adult AML.

An intriguing observation is that although the CR rate for the ara-C and OAP groups of patients was substantially lower (38%) than the anthracycline-ara-C group (57%) the five-year survival figure is similar (16%). One feature common to these studies and the anthracycline-ara-C studies is the heavy reliance on ara-C in remission induction (by continuous IV infusion) and during maintenance (sub-cutaneously). The CR duration of the ara-C and OAP group of patients is longer, possibly related to the use of continuous infusion ara-C in maintenance (Figure 2). Nine of the OAP patients received three courses of ara-C during the early part of their maintenance therapy as early intensification. All seven of the ara-C patients alone who achieved a CR received five-day continuous IV infusions of ara-C each month during the maintenance phase of their chemotherapy.

Our highest proportion of long-term survivors is noted in the ara-C and OAP groups of patients. The contribution of anthracyclines to long-term survival (L.T.S.) is arguable. Studies using daunorubicin as a remission induction agent, without the concomitant use of ara-C, have produced satisfactory CR rates but short remission durations.

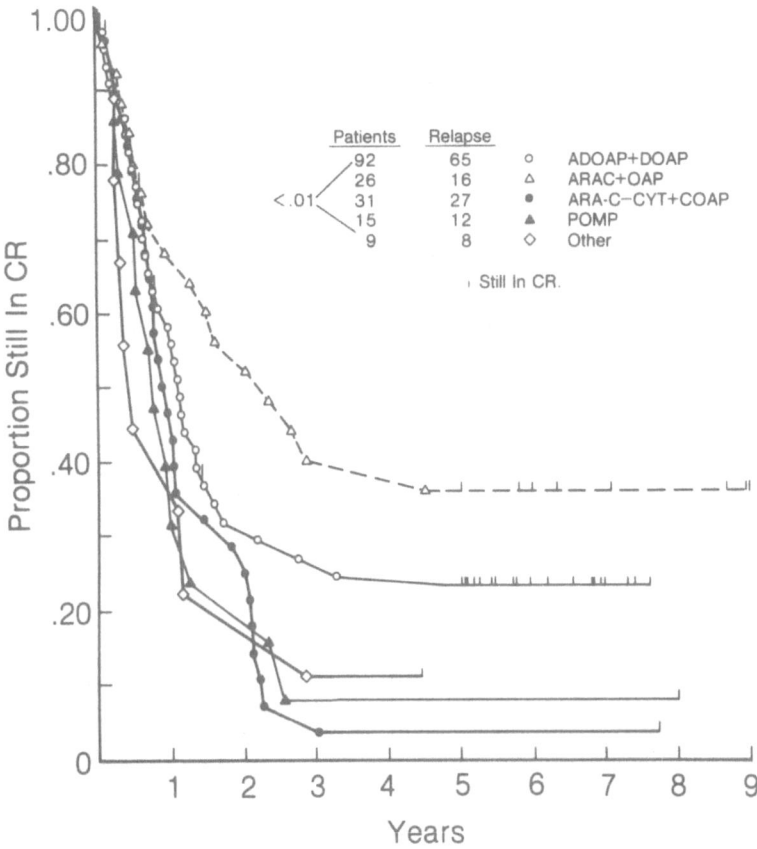

*Figure 2.* Remission duration according to chemotherapy used, 1965–1975.

Several studies have reported CR rates of 35–56% for daunorubicin or rubidazone as a single agent [13, 14, 18, 19, 21]. However, if patients are maintained on programs not including substantial ara-C therapy the CR duration is short and less than 10% of patients stay in remission for more than two years [18, 19, 21]. However, 20% of patients who achieved CR

*Table 3.* Recent analyses of long-term survival (L.T.S.) in adult AML.

| Study group | Period | No. of patients | L.T.S. No. | (%) | Disease free No. | (%) | Analysis point |
|---|---|---|---|---|---|---|---|
| M.D.A.H. | 1965–75 | 396 | 33 | (8.3) | 30 | (7.6) | 5 yrs. |
| SWOG | 1967–75 | 524 | 30 | (5.7) | 28 | (5.3) | 5 yrs. |
| Hôpital-St-Louis | 1967–76 | 815 | – | | 55 | (6.7) | 3 yrs. |
| CALGB | 1967–75 | 2201 | 129 | (5.9) | 81 | (3.7) | 3 yrs. |

with rubidazone and who received substantial amounts of ara-C remained in CR for more than two years [21].

The shorter CR duration of the anthracycline-ara-C patients may be caused by the early omission during maintenance (3 months) of the anthracycline which formed a significant part of their remission induction program. It is possible that the leukemic cells of a significant fraction of these patients were sensitive primarily to the anthracycline and not ara-C. Hence, maintenance programs which rely heavily on ara-C would not be expected to be very effective for these patients. Another possible contributing factor in the longer CRs in the DOAP, ADOAP, and OAP patients compared to other regimens is the addition of immunotherapy with BCG given by scarification to these patients.

The results for the cyclophosphamide + ara-C programs are disappointing with only one of 88 patients surviving for five years. The inferior results for these programs could occur for several reasons. In contradistinction to

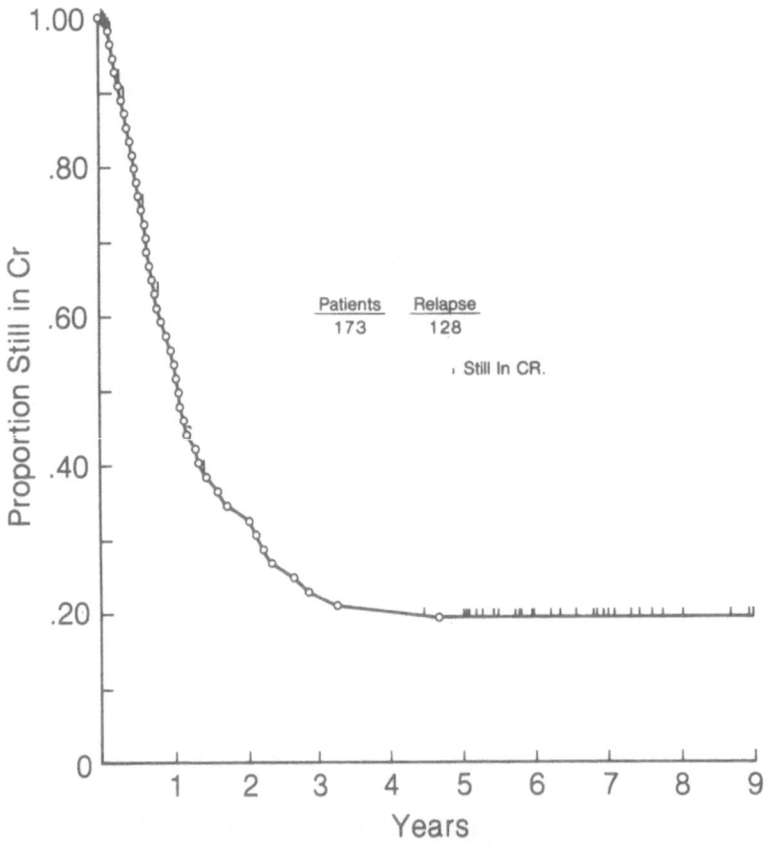

*Figure 3.* CR duration of all AML patients 1965–1975.

the other remission induction programs described above which included ara-C and in which all patients received ara-C by continuous intravenous infusion, 73/88 of the cyclophosphamide + ara-C patients received ara-C by rapid intravenous infusion over 15–30 minutes each eight hours. The majority of the cyclophosphamide-ara-C patients received both cyclophosphamide and ara-C in their maintenance regimens whereas the anthracycline + ara-C and ara-C groups received OAP or ara-C. The continued use of cyclophosphamide during maintenance effectively reduced the amount of ara-C administered by 50%, compared with the patients maintained on ara-C alone or OAP, as both ara-C and cyclophosphamide have dose-limiting myelosuppression. Third, as opposed to most of the anthracycline + ara-C and the OAP groups of patients, none of these patients received immunotherapy with BCG by scarification during the maintenance phase of their treatment.

The only other five-year survivor was a patient who received a complete remission on POMP and was maintained on the cyclic maintenance program. None of the MP+MMPR or miscellaneous groups survived beyond five years although one elderly patient who obtained a complete remission on guanazole died at the age of 82 years, of natural causes, while still in his first CR of four and one-half years' duration.

None of our patients have relapsed after five years and only three of thirty-three after three years (Figure 3). All patients now have been off chemotherapy for more than three years. One of the five-year survivors has died. He was still in CR at the time of his death which occurred as a result of a motor vehicle accident. The rate of relapse appears to decrease sharply at three years.

Three of the 33 five-year survivors have experienced one relapse while off chemotherapy, at 2.1, 3.3, and 4.7 years. All three received ADOAP as reinduction therapy and achieved a second CR. They were maintained on an OAP maintenance program with POMP late intensification. Two patients are again off all chemotherapy after a second late intensification. The duration of chemotherapy for the 30 patients in continuous complete remission (CCR) for five years was 16–18 months in 19 patients, 18–30 months in nine and longer than 30 months in two patients.

## 4. COMPARISON WITH OTHER STUDIES

Three other major studies of long-term survivals have recently been published, in abstract form. The French group from Hôpital-Saint-Louis reported on 815 patients with AML treated between 1967 and 1976 [40]. The three-year relapse-free survival for various morphologic categories was

34/697 (4.9%) for acute myeloblastic leukemia (A.M.L.), 17/64 (26.5%) for acute promyelocytic leukemia (A.P.L.), and 4/54 (7.4%) for acute monocytic leukemia (A.Mo.L.). The respective percentages of remissions lasting three years were A.M.L. 10%, A.P.L. 51% and A.Mo.L. 12%. The probability of relapse after three years of CCR was projected to be 20% for A.M.L. and 11% for A.P.L. There was no comment on the duration of maintenance therapy or longest time to relapse after discontinuation of treatment.

For a subset of 73 patients with acute myeloblastic leukemia who were treated with daunorubicin and ara-C and maintained on an intermittent ara-C regimen, 44 patients (60%) obtained a CR and 10/44 (23%) were still in remission for three years. Thus the three-year survival was 14% and three-year CCR rate was 23% compared to our five-year figures of 13% and 21%, respectively.

The Southwest Oncology Group data for adult acute leukemia (including acute lymphoblastic leukemia (ALL) and acute undifferentiated leukemia (AUL) treated during the period from 1967 to 1973, shows that 28/524 patients (5.3%) were alive and free of disease at five years [38]. Four of their patients have relapsed after five years. Again no comment was published on duration of maintenance or time to relapse after discontinuation of treatment. Analysis of hazard function statistics suggests that the risk of death approaches zero after seven years of survival. The chemotherapy programs included ara-C-continuous infusion, COAP, OAP, and DOAP. M. D. Anderson Hospital patients were included in this analysis.

Three-year survival data are also available from Cancer and Leukemia Group B for patients treated between 1967 and 1975 [39]. Overall 129/2201 patients (5.9%) survived three years. The three year CCR number is 81 patients (8.7% of complete responders). Fifteen of these 81 patients had subsequently relapsed. Twelve percent of patients entered on a daunorubicin + ara-C study are alive at three years and CRs have lasted for three years in 24% of these patients. The authors suggest that the use of daunorubicin and/or ara-C during the maintenance phase of therapy is an important factor in the more recent increase in three-year CCR.

Other smaller studies of patients who received ara-C and thioguanine as maintenance therapy have reported CR durations of three years in 8 of 40 (20%) [51] and five years in 7 of 26 (27%) [52]. Other single institution studies using ara-C-containing maintenance programs confirm that 20% of CRs will last for three or more years [53, 54].

The improving prospects for long-term survival are supported by several other studies. Fevre has reported that six of 276 patients with AML (2.2%) treated between 1964 and 1971 survived three years compared with six of 96 patients (6%) treated in 1972–73 [55]. The Hôpital-Saint-Louis group reported in 1973 that 2% of their patients with AML survived four years whereas the three-year relapse-free survival of their most recently treated group of patients is 14% [34, 40].

A report on a nation-wide study of five-year survival in acute leukemia from Japan in 1974 suggested that only 0.1% of patients treated prior to 1970 survived five years [33]. The same group has reported in 1980 that while only 13 patients were identified as five-year survivors prior to 1970, another 43 patients were identified who were treated between January 1970 and July 1973 [56]. Only 2/41 adults whose first remission lasted for more than five years have relapsed. The dramatic increase in survival was associated with increased use of regimens containing ara-C and daunorubicin. Approximately 75% of the more recent five-year survivors were treated with such combinations.

No significant increase in L.T.S. occurred in a report from Argentina. The four-year survival rate prior to and after 1971 was 1–2%. None of the reported protocols used ara-C extensively.

## 5. SUMMARY OF PUBLISHED DATA

A consensus opinion is, therefore, that 60–70% of all patients with AML will achieve a CR on current anthracycline-ara-C combinations ± thioguanine or vincristine and prednisone and that 20–25% of these patients will stay in CR for five or more years.

The increased long-term survival fraction being reported in patients treated after 1970 appears to be related to several factors. A major impact on survival has resulted from the high CR rate associated with anthracycline-ara-C combinations. It appears that it is essential that a patient achieve a CR to have a possibility of long-term survival. In our study, despite having CR rates equivalent to the ara-C and OAP programs, the POMP and cyclophosphamide-ara-C programs produced many fewer long-term suvivors. The ara-C, OAP, and anthracycline OAP programs each incorporated the use of continuous infusion ara-C during remission induction and rely on maximally-tolerated doses of ara-C during maintenance. There are no reports in AML of a substantial proportion of long-term survivors using programs which do not rely heavily on ara-C during maintenance.

## 6. FACTORS AFFECTING LONG-TERM SURVIVAL

As has been mentioned earlier the major factor influencing survival is whether or not a patient obtains a complete remission (Figure 1). Thus, factors which are associated with response rate are of major importance in analyzing survival. However, the classic features associated with CR rate such as age, temperature elevation, presence of an antecedent hematologic disorder, etc., have not been found to influence remission duration [57]. Therefore we have analyzed our data separately according to factors influencing CR rate and factors influencing remission duration.

## 7. PROGNOSTIC FACTORS INFLUENCING CR RATE

In our study, in addition to treatment, the major factors found to influence CR rate and, as a consequence, the probability of long-term survival in AML are age, temperature elevation, hemoglobin level, serum blood urea nitrogen level, presence of Auer rods, and a history of an antecendent hematologic disorder (AHD—defined as a documented abnormality in the peripheral blood for more than one month prior to the start of treatment) (Table 4). There was no significant influence of sex, platelet count, white blood cell count, hepatomegaly, splenomegaly, lymph node enlargement, serum calcium, serum lactic dehydrogenase (LDH), % blasts in the bone marrow, differentiation ratio (% Blast + Pros.)/Myelocytic + Metas.

*Table 4.* Prognostic factors affecting CR rate and 5-year survival in AML 1965–1974.

| Characteristics | | No. | CR | % | P value | 5-yr survival No. | (%) | P value |
|---|---|---|---|---|---|---|---|---|
| Age (years) | <20 | 35 | 25 | (71) | | 4 | (11) | |
| | 20–49 | 157 | 88 | (56) | < 0.01 | 19 | (12) | 0.03 |
| | 50–64 | 125 | 44 | (33) | | 9 | ( 7) | |
| | ≥65 | 79 | 19 | (24) | | 1 | ( 1) | |
| Temperature | <101 °F | 265 | 133 | (50) | < 0.01 | 25 | ( 9) | 0.35 |
| | ≥101 °F | 131 | 40 | (31) | | 8 | ( 6) | |
| Hemoglobin | <12G% | 336 | 138 | (41) | 0.02 | 27 | ( 8) | 0.01 |
| | ≥12G% | 60 | 35 | (58) | | 6 | (10) | |
| B.U.N (MG%) | <23 | 327 | 153 | (47) | 0.02 | 32 | (10) | 0.09 |
| | ≥23 | 55 | 16 | (29) | | 1 | ( 2) | |
| Auer rods | Negative | 259 | 94 | (36) | < 0.01 | 15 | ( 6) | 0.02 |
| | Positive | 137 | 79 | (58) | | 18 | (13) | |
| Antecedent hematologic disorder | No | 310 | 148 | (47) | | 32 | (10) | |
| | Yes | 86 | 25 | (29) | < 0.01 | 1 | ( 1) | 0.01 |
| Morphologic diagnosis | Promyelocytic | 22 | 8 | (36) | 0.62 | 5 | (23) | 0.03 |
| | Other | 374 | 165 | (44) | | 28 | ( 7) | |

+ Polys.) in the bone marrow or % marrow eosinophils on response rate. Several of these factors will be shown later to have an effect on remission duration.

The stepwise decline in response rate with age, as expected, was associated with fewer older patients surviving for five years. The higher response rates noted in patients with a normal hemoglobin and Auer rods present in the bone marrow supports our earlier data and the conclusions of others regarding the influence of these factors on survival [58, 59]. The low response rate and five-year survival of patients with marked liver enlargement (19%, 3%) and elevated BUN (29%, 2%) suggest that leukemic infiltration of organs other than blood and bone marrow is an adverse factor in such patients' response to chemotherapy.

The patients with an AHD, many of whom present with a smouldering acute leukemia initially, had a low but definite response rate. There is, however, only one long-term survivor in this category. The exceptions to the rule of low response rate being associated with a low chance of five-year survival is acute promyelocytic leukemia. Although the CR rate with chemotherapy was slightly lower than for the other patients, the remission duration of responders is very long and only three of eight complete responders have relapsed. All were treated with an anthracycline-ara-C combination initially and maintained on OAP + BCG.

Thus, when the patient is first seen there are several pretreatment characteristics which provide prognostic information regarding long-term survival, in so far as they provide information for the probability of obtaining a CR and achievement of CR status appears to be a prerequisite to have prospects for long-term survival.

## 8. PROGNOSTIC FACTORS INFLUENCING REMISSION DURATION

Once the patient has survived the remission induction phase and has achieved a CR, the new threat which looms is the risk of relapse. The survival from the time of relapse for patients in this study is short. The probability of long-term survival after relapse is approximately 2%.

The factors which predict for long remission duration and thus the chance of long-term survival from the time of CR are different from those predicting for probability of CR. When the influence of various pretreatment factors on CR duration is examined, no significant effect of the age of the patient, pretreatment temperature status, presence of Auer rods, hemoglobin level and history of an antecedent hematologic disorder, liver size or BUN level was noted. Major factors affecting remission duration were the treatment received, a diagnosis of acute promyelocytic leukemia, white blood

*Table 5.* Factors with an influence on remission duration and 5-year CCR in AML 1965–1974.

| Characteristic | Favorable | Remission duration | 5-year CCR |
|---|---|---|---|
| L.D.H. | <400 | +++ | ++ |
| Differentiation ratio | High | +++ | ++ |
| Acute promyelocytic leukemia | Yes | +++ | +++ |
| Marrow eosinophilia | >4% | +++ | 0 |
| Serum calcium | Low | +++ | +++ |
| White blood cell count | Low | 0 | ++ |
| % Decrease in marrow infiltrate/day | >5% | +++ | 0 |
| Courses to CR | 1–2 | ++ | 0 |
| Halving time peripheral blasts | Short | ++ | 0 |
| Consolidation hepatitis | Yes | +++ | ++ |
| Treatment | Anthracycline +ARA-C or ARA-C | ++ | +++ |

+++  −  $P<0.01$
 ++  −  $P<0.01$
  +  −  $P = 0.05–0.10$
  0  −  $P>0.10$

cell count, the serum lactic dehydrogenase level, serum calcium, presence of >4% eosinophils in the pretreatment bone marrow and lack of differentiation or immaturity of the marrow myeloid series which is expressed as a high differentiation ratio of (Blasts + Promyelocytes)/(Myelocytes + Metamyelocytes + Neutrophils) (Table 5). None of these factors which affect CR duration influence the probability of obtaining CR. An effect of rate of response to treatment on CR duration was noted in so far as patients whose bone marrow leukemic infiltrate and peripheral blood blasts cleared quickly had longer remission and a higher five-year CCR fraction than patients whose rate of cytoreduction was slower.

In the three months following the achievement of CR status (consolidation phase), 38% of patients developed an elevation of the SGOT level to greater than twice normal which persisted for more than one month. Patients who develop this 'consolidation hepatitis' have significantly longer CR duration and higher probability of five-year CCR than patients who do not develop SGOT elevation.

## 9. PROGNOSTIC FACTORS FOR LONG-TERM SURVIVAL IN OTHER STUDIES

In addition to the primary effect of achieving CR on long-term survival, and the effect of age on CR rate, few other factors have been noted. The advent of newer chemotherapy combinations, especially the effect of the anthracyclines and ara-C, as mentioned earlier, is cited as the major reason for the improved L.T.S. fraction in several studies [37–40, 51, 52, 55, 56]. The recent French data support their early data on the long duration of remission in acute promyelocytic leukemia [28, 40]. Fevre reported that their long-term survivors were characterized by a low white blood cell count and minimal evidence of extramedullary disease [55], supporting our observation of the adverse effect of marked liver enlargement, a high white blood cell count, and elevated BUN.

## 10. COMMENTS ON SPECIFIC PROGNOSTIC FACTORS

### 10.1. Acute Promyelocytic Leukemia

Weil reported that half of the 33 patients with acute promyelocytic leukemia (A.Pro.L.) were in CCR at >3 years, confirming the early reports from their group [28]; similarly, only three of our eight patients have relapsed (Figure 4). Recently, a specific chromosome alteration has been described in A.Pro.L., a translocation of chromosomal material from a No. 15 to a No. 17 chromosome t(15;17) [60]. All the reports of L.T.S. are from the era prior to banding studies. Golomb in this volume and elsewhere has described a 'microgranular' variant of A.Pro.L. in which the t(15;17) is present but in which the cells lack the usual morphologic characteristics of A.Pro.L. [61]. Whether the 'microgranular' variant of A.Pro.L. has the same prognosis for L.T.S. as the classical variety is unknown.

### 10.2. The 8;21 Translocation

Another chromosome pattern associated with a favorable prognosis is a translocation between a No. 8 and a No. 21 chromosome t(8;21), initially reported before banding studies were available as being a complex rearrangement $46XX, -C, +D, +D, -G$ [63] (see chapter by Golomb). Twenty-one of our 396 patients have had this pattern, either alone or associated with other abnormalities. The CR rate was 15/21 (71%). The remission duration was not longer than that of the remaining 158 patients (median 55 weeks). Three patients are five-year survivors, two being in CCR at 9.1+ and 5.2+ years and one relapsing at 4.7 years. The major benefit of this translocation on survival thus appears to be due to the high CR rate although continued follow-up of a greater number of patients is needed for a more precise estimate of remission duration in patients treated with current chemotherapy regimens.

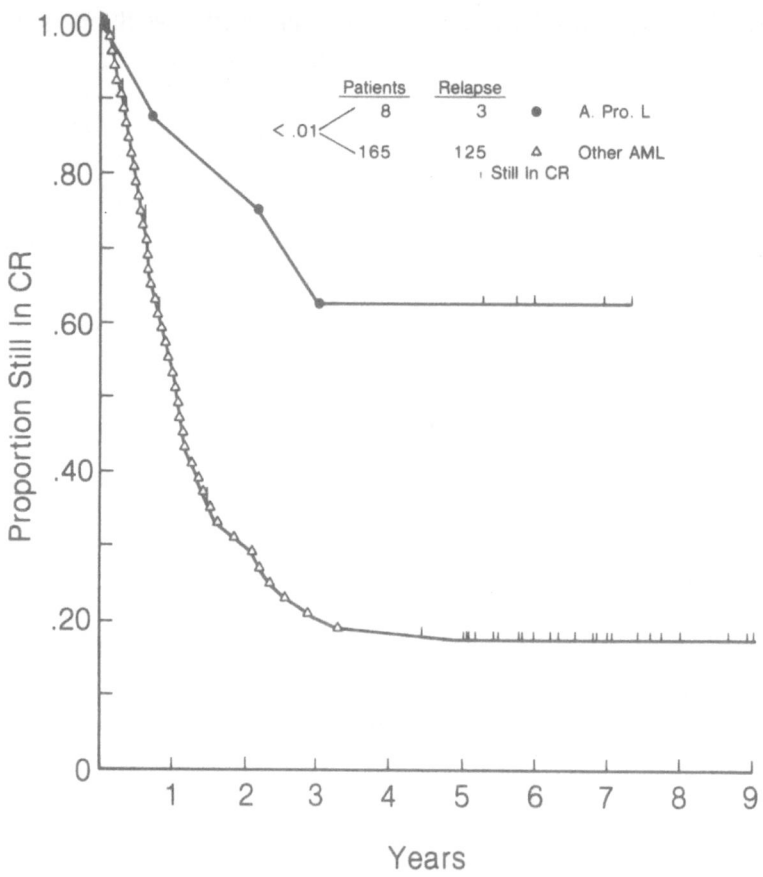

*Figure 4.* CR duration, 1965–1975. Acute promyelocytic leukemia vs. other AML.

## 10.3. Degree of Differentiation

Although the degree of differentiation of the tumor has no effect on CR rate, it has a major influence on remission duration and probability of L.T.S. (Figure 5). It is possible, in view of the maturation present in the initial bone marrow, that the leukemic cells of these patients are capable of differentiation and that the normal bone marrow and peripheral blood represent 'mature' leukemic cells. Ample evidence exists for maturation of human leukemia cell lines *in vitro* under the influence of a variety of agents [63]. Thus a number of 'CRs' may, indeed, be 'pseudo-remissions.' In the case of differentiated leukemia, prolongation of survival may be accomplished by using drugs which cause differentiation rather than cytocidal agents.

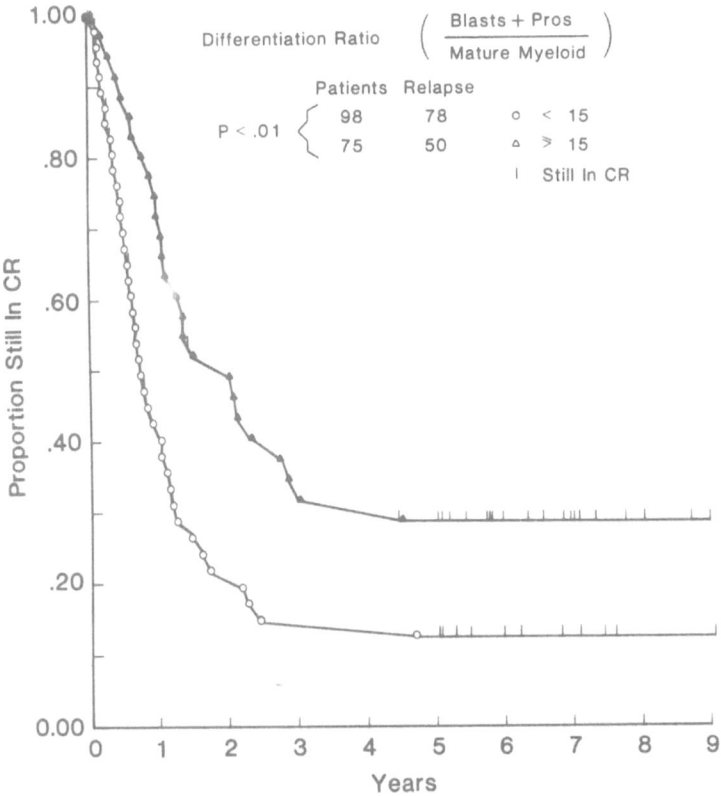

*Figure 5.* CR duration according to differentiation of leukemia, 1965–1975.

## 10.4. Serum Lactic Dehydrogenase

The serum lactic dehydrogenase (LDH) level is strongly predictive for remission duration (Figure 6). The LDH level is negatively correlated with the differentiation ratio, i.e., patients with differentiated leukemia tend to have markedly elevated LDH levels. The LDH is elevated more frequently in patients with a high white blood cell count, extramedullary disease, and with a high labelling index in the leukemic blast cells [57]. The white blood cell count as reported by us and others [53, 57, 64] has an effect on CR duration (Figure 7). We found that the white blood cell count did not predict for CR duration as strongly as did the serum LDH level [57].

## 10.5. Eosinophilia

Eosinophilia (>4%) in the initial bone marrow, while not associated with a higher CR rate, is associated with prolonged CR duration (Figure 8). Of interest, the three patients who have survived five years despite relapsing

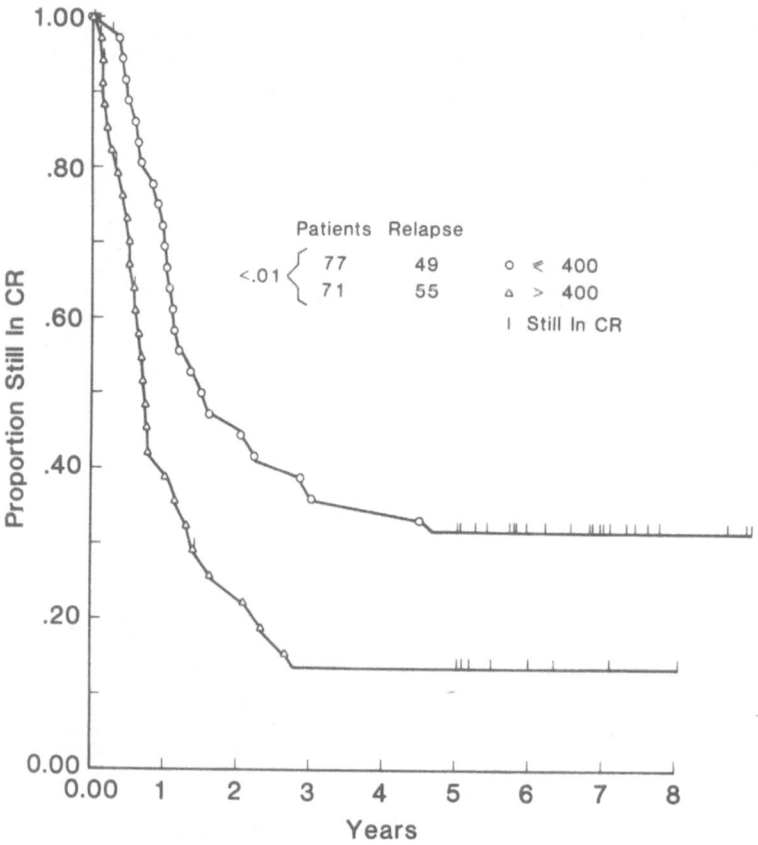

*Figure 6.* Effect of serum LDH on CR duration, 1965–1975.

before that time had significant eosinophilia in their pretreatment bone marrow (6%, 14%, and 8%). All three have had prolonged second remission. Whether the eosinophilia is a sign of immune reaction to the tumor or whether the eosinophils are leukemic cells is uncertain. Most of the patients with eosinophilia have evidence of maturation in the neutrophil and occasionally the basophil series.

### 10.6. Tumor Sensitivity to Chemotherapy

The sensitivity of the patient's tumor to chemotherapy can be evaluated by the time to hypoplasia (<10% marrow infiltrate), the number of courses to CR, time to CR, or % decrease in marrow infiltrate/day following the first course of chemotherapy [27]. Similarly, the time to halving of the peripheral blast cells after chemotherapy can be measured. The values for each of these characteristics indicating rapid cytoreduction are all significantly associated

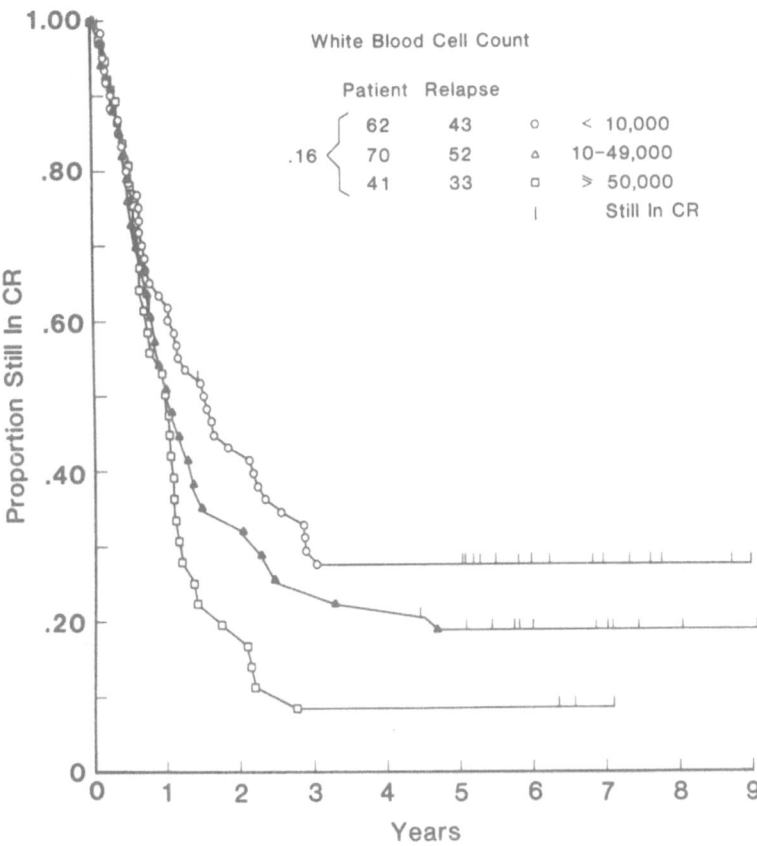

*Figure 7.* Duration of CR according to pretreatment white blood cell count, 1965–1975.

with longer CR duration than for values suggesting a slower rate of cytore-duction.

## 10.7. Development of 'Hepatitis'

Barton and Conrad suggested in 1979 a beneficial effect on survival of 'hepatitis' in patients with acute leukemia [64]. This was noted in the first three months of therapy. Our results support this observation although the effect was examined only in patients achieving CR (Figure 9). The effect appears to influence risk of relapse throughout the period of remission. Wiernik has reported data supporting the concept of SGOT elevation favorably influencing survival [65]. The reason for this effect is difficult to define. It is known that the severity of hepatitis B is correlated with T-cell function with immunoincompetent patients having mild disease and vice versa [66, 67]. Possibly, the elevation of SGOT is an indication of the ability of

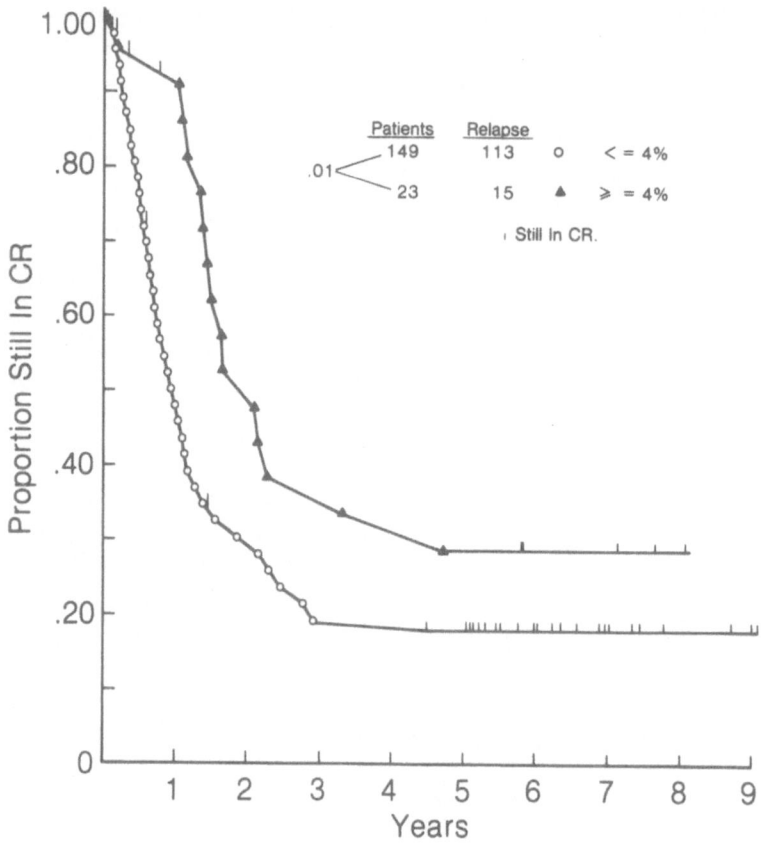

*Figure 8.* Influence of pretreatment marrow eosinophilia on CR duration, 1965–1975.

the patient to react to a transfused liver pathogen, i.e., immunocompetence. Alternatively the hepatic dysfunction may be a sign of drug toxicity with an alteration in drug metabolism accounting for the improved remission duration.

The effect of a low pretreatment serum calcium on CR duration is also difficult to understand, although patients with a low serum calcium tend to have more rapid cytoreduction. This factor requires further evaluation.

## 11. FUTURE APPLICATION OF PROGNOSTIC FACTOR ANALYSIS

Increasingly, physicians caring for patients with AML are addressing the problem of remission induction and remission maintenance separately. The validity of this approach is enforced by the findings of different sets of

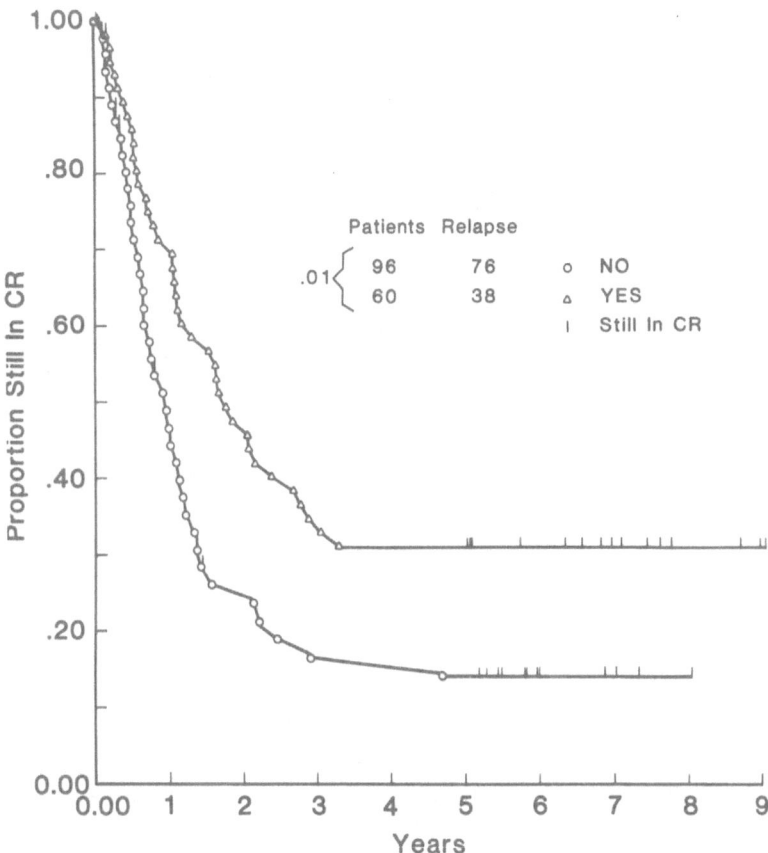

*Figure 9.*

factors influencing the probability of obtaining a CR and of staying in CR. The first step towards long-term survival is to obtain a CR. Analysis of prognostic factors has identified groups of patients with inferior results, such as patients who are elderly, infected, have Auer rod negative disease, have a history of smouldering leukemia or iatrogenic leukemia [26], or 100% abnormal metaphases [68]. Many of the adverse factors for response and survival are interrelated. By the use of logistic regression analysis techniques, these factors can be quantitated and predictive models for response developed [58, 69]. Similarly, models to predict for remission duration can be developed [57] and used to predict for long-term remission. With further refinement of these techniques it may be possible to identify groups of patients at high risk of failing remission induction therapy or of relapsing on maintenance therapy so that innovative treatment can be offered to these patients.

## 12. TREATMENT PROSPECTS – CHEMOTHERAPY AND TRANSPLANTATION

Although many groups are now reporting CR rates of 70–80% in AML [22, 23, 24, 70, 71, 72], patients with a poorer prognosis need new treatment approaches. The most promising new agent in this regard is m-AMSA [73], which has a CR rate of 30% in relapsing patients. A major remaining problem in AML is remission maintenance. Despite the emphasis in this chapter on improved prospects for long-term survival, we must emphasize that 75–80% of all complete responders relapse. New chemotherapy approaches are required. Recently, Weinstein has reported that a sequential program of adriamycin + ara-C, adriamycin and 5-azacytidine, POMP, and ara-C has achieved a median CR duration of 2 years with >40% of their patients predicted to be in CR at 3+ years [74].

Another approach is to use allogeneic bone marrow transplantation in first remission of AML [75, 76] (see chapter by Kay). The basis of this approach is in the observation that 7/47 adults with AML transplanted by the Seattle Group in relapse (35 pts) or in partial remission (12 pts) were still alive from 335 to 1598 days post-transplant. Three patients were still alive and free of leukemia more than three years post-transplant. All three had graft versus host disease. Of 14 adult patients recently reported who were transplanted in first remission, 57% were still alive more than one year post-transplant, and three for more than two years. Four of 12 patients with AML transplanted in first complete remission by the City of Hope group [76] were still alive more than one year post-transplant, and three for more than two years. All four had 100% performance status on the Karnofsky scale. If these early results persist an alternative form of maintenance therapy to chemotherapy will be available.

## 13. CRITERIA OF CURABILITY OF AML

Whilst the achievement of five-year CCR in a significant proportion of patients is a considerable accomplishment in its own right, is it possible to state that these patients are cured? Certainly, we cannot state that patients are cured if they are still receiving cytoreductive chemotherapy. Our longest relapse occurred 3.4 years after discontinuation of chemotherapy. The cytogenetic pattern in this patient at relapse was identical to the initial pattern. Thus, patients still appear to be at risk for 3.4 years after stopping chemotherapy. It is important that in future reports of long-term survival, the time off chemotherapy should be mentioned. Late relapses need thorough study to ascertain whether the relapse is of the initial AML or a second disease. It appears likely that with an increasing number of patients available for analysis, better estimates of curability should soon be available.

## 14. CONCLUSIONS

The improved response rate and longer survival, with a potentially-cured fraction of patients with AML, create new challenges for the oncologist. Each failure in induction therapy due to failure of supportive care rather than chemotherapy failure is the possible loss of a 'cured' patient. Continued emphasis on improving the CR rate to 100% including the 'poor-risk' groups is a challenge of the 1980s. Development of better maintenance programs is likely to have the greatest impact on long-term survival. The incorporation of new active agents such as AMSA and innovative maintenance programs such as allogeneic transplantation in remission, into the overall treatment program is a task requiring ingenuity and skillful analysis of results to measure the overall impact of these strategies. It is of great importance that we preserve the good results that we have already achieved for a small proportion whilst improving the results for those in whom we are currently failing.

## REFERENCES

1. Tivey H: The natural history of untreated acute leukemia. Ann NY Acad Sci 60:322–358, 1954.
2. Southam CM, Craver LF, Dargeon HW, et al.: A study of the natural history of acute leukemia with special reference to the duration of the disease and the occurrence of remissions. Cancer 4:39–59, 1951.
3. Boggs DR, Wintrobe MM, Cartwright GE: To treat or not to treat acute granulocytic leukemia. II. Arch Intern Med 123:568–570, 1969.
4. Farber S: Some observations on the effect of folic acid antagonists on acute leukemia and other forms of cancer. Blood 4:160, 1949.
5. Freireich EJ, et al.: The effect of chemotherapy on acute leukemia in the human. J Chronic Dis 14:593–607, 1961.
6. Boggs DR, Wintrobe MM, Cartwright GE: The acute leukemias: an analysis of 322 cases and review of the literature. Medicine 41:163–225, 1962.
7. Freireich EJ, Bodey GP, Harris JE, Hart JS: Therapy for acute granulocytic leukemia. Cancer Res 27:2573–2577, 1967.
8. Levin RH, Henderson E, Karon M, Freireich EJ: Treatment of acute leukemia with methyl-glyoxal-bis-guanylhydrazone (methyl GAG). Clin Pharmacol Ther 6:31–42, 1964.
9. Crosby WH: To treat or not to treat acute granulocytic leukemia. Arch Intern Med 122:79–80, 1968.
10. Ellison RR, Holland JF, Weil M, Jacquillat C: Arabinosyl cytosine: a useful agent in the treatment of acute leukemia in adults. Blood 32: 307–523, 1968.
11. Bodey GP, et al.: Cytosine arabinoside (NSC-63878) therapy for acute leukemia in adults. Cancer Chemother Rep 53:59–65, 1969.
12. Boiron M, Jacquillat C, Weil M, Tanzier J, Levy D, Sultan C, Bernard J: Daunorubicin in the treatment of acute myelocytic leukemia. Lancet i:330, 1969.

260

13. Jacquillat C, Boiron M, Weil M, Tanzer J, Najean Y, Bernard J: Rubidomycin, a new agent active in the treatment of acute lymphoblastic leukaemia. Lancet ii:27, 1966.

14. Burgess MA, Garson OM, De Gruchy GC: Daunorubicin in the treatment of adult acute leukaemia. Med J Aus 1:629–635, 1970.

15. Burchenal JH: Formal discussion: Long-term survival in Burkitt's tumor and in acute leukemia. Cancer Res 27:2616–2618, 1967.

16. Southwest Oncology Group: cytarabine for acute leukemia in adults: effects of schedule on therapeutic response. Arch Intern Med 133:251–259, 1974.

17. Goodell B, Leventhal B, Henderson E: Cytosine arabinoside in acute granulocytic leukemia. Clin Pharmacol Ther 12:599–606, 1971.

18. Wiernik PH, Schimpff SC, Schiffer CA, Lichtenfeld JL, Aisner J, O'Connell MJ, Fortner C: Randomized clinical comparison of daunorubicin (NSC-82151) alone with a combination of daunorubicin, cytosine arabinoside (NSC-63878), 6-thioguanine (NSC-752), and pyrimethamine (NSC-3061) for the treatment of acute nonlymphocytic leukemia. Cancer Treat Rep 60:41–53, 1976.

19. Weil M, Glidewell OJ, Jacquillat C, Levy R: Daunorubicin in the therapy of acute granulocytic leukemia. Cancer Res 33:921–928, 1973.

20. McCredie KB, Bodey GP, Freireich EJ, Hester JP: Chemoimmunotherapy of adult acute leukemia. Cancer (in press).

21. Jacquillat CL, Weil M, Gemon-Aucler MF, Izrael V: Clinical study of rubidazone (22 050 R.P.), a new daunorubicin-derived compound, in 170 patients with acute leukemias and other malignancies. Cancer 37:653–659, 1976.

22. Gale RP, Cline MJ: High remission-induction rate in acute myeloid leukaemia. Lancet i:497–499, 1977.

23. Peterson BA, Bloomfield CD, Bosl GJ, Gibbs G, Malloy M: Intensive five-drug combination chemotherapy for adult acute nonlymphocytic leukemia. Cancer 46:663–668, 1980.

24. Preisler HD, Rustum Y, Henderson ES, Bjornsson S, et al.: Treatment of acute nonlymphocytic leukemia: use of anthracycline-cytosine arabinoside induction therapy and comparison of two maintenance regimens. Blood 53:455–464, 1979.

25. Glucksberg H, Buckner CD, Fefer A, DeMarsh Q, Coleman D, et al.: Combination chemotherapy for acute nonlymphoblastic leukemia in adults. Cancer Chemother Rep 59:1131–1137, 1975.

26. Keating MJ, Smith TL, McCredie KB, Bodey GP, et al.: A four-year experience with anthracycline, cytosine arabinoside, vincristine and prednisone combination chemotherapy in 325 adults with acute leukemia. Cancer (in Press).

27. Ohno R, Hirano M, Imai K, Katsuo K, et al.: Daunorubicin, cytosine arabinoside, 6-mercaptopurine riboside, and prednisolone (DCMP) combination chemotherapy for acute myelogenous leukemia in adults. Cancer 36:1945–1949, 1975.

28. Bernard J, Weil M, Boiron M, et al.: Acute promyelocytic leukemia. Blood 41:489–496, 1973.

29. Reiffers J, Raynal F, Broustet A: Acute myeloblastic leukemia in elderly patients. Treatment and prognostic factors. Cancer 45:2816–2820, 1980.

30. Grann V, Erichson R, Flannery J, Finch S, Clarkson B: The therapy of acute granulocytic leukemia in patients more than 50 years old. Ann Intern Med 80:15–20, 1974.

31. Peterson BA, Bloomfield CD: Treatment of acute non-lymphocytic leukemia in elderly patients. A prospective study of intensive chemotherapy. Cancer 40:647–652, 1977.

32. Keating MJ, Benjamin RS, McCredie KB, Bodey GP, Freireich EJ: Remission induction therapy with a rubidazone-containing combination (ROAP) in acute leukemia. Proc Am Assoc Cancer Res 18:180, 1977 (Abst. #719).

33. Yamada K, Uetani T: Five-Year survivors with acute leukemia in Japan. Acta Haematol Jap 37:99–107, 1974.

34. Jacquillat CI, Weil M, Gemon M-F, *et al.*: Evaluation of 216 four-year survivors of acute leukemia. Cancer 32:286–293, 1973.

35. Pavlovsky S, Muriel FS: Long-term survival in acute leukemia in Argentina. Cancer 40:1402–1409. 1977.

36. Oliff A, Poplack D: Characteristics of long-term survivors in AML. Med Pediatr Oncol 5:219–223, 1973.

37. Keating MJ, Bodey GP, McCredie KB, Freireich EJ: Five-year survival and remission duration in adult acute myelogenous leukemia. Proc Am Soc Clin Oncol 20:416, 1979 (Abstract).

38. Coltman CA, Jr, Freireich EJ, Savage RA, Gehan EA: Long term survival of adults with acute leukemia. Proc Am Soc Clin Oncol 20:389, 1979 (Abstract).

39. Ellison RR, Glidewell O: Improved survival in adults with acute myelocytic leukemia (AML). Proc Am Assoc Cancer Res 20:161, 1979 (Abstract).

40. Weil M, Auclerc MF, Jacquillat CL, *et al.*: Long term relapse free survivals (R.F.S.) in 815 patients (pts) with acute granulocytic leukemias (A.G.L.). Proc Am Soc Clin Oncol 21:444, 1980 (Abstract C-494).

41. Hewlet JS, Bodey GP, Wilson HE: Combination 6-mercaptopurine and 6-methylmercaptopurine riboside in the treatment of adult acute leukemia: a Southwest Oncology Group study. Cancer Treat Rep 63:156–158, 1979.

42. Rodriguez V, Hart JS, Freireich EJ, *et al.*: POMP combination chemotherapy of adult acute leukemia. Cancer 32:69–75, 1973.

43. Bodey GP, Rodriguez V, Hart J, *et al.*: Therapy of acute leukemia with the combination of cytosine arabinoside (NSC-63878) and cyclophosphamide (NSC-26271). Cancer Chemother Rep 54:255–262, 1970.

44. Whitecar JP, Jr, Bodey GP, McCredie KB, *et al.*: Cyclophosphamide, vincristine, arabinosyl cytosine and prednisone (COAP) combination chemotherapy for adult acute leukemia. Cancer Chemother Rep 56:543–550, 1972.

45. Rogriguez V, Bodey GP, Gutterman JU, *et al.*: Combination chemotherapy of adult acute leukemia for remission induction and maintenance. In: Therapy of acute leukemias, Mandelli F, Amadori S, Mariani E (eds). Rome: Minerva Medica, 1973, pp 569–577.

46. McCredie KB, Freireich EJ, Bodey GP, Burgess MA, *et al.*: A study of intermittent alternating drug program reinduction therapy on the frequency and duration of response in adult acute leukemia. Med Pediatr Oncol 2:309–318, 1976.

47. Bodey GP, Rodriguez V, McCredie KB, *et al.*: Early consolidation chemotherapy for adults with acute leukemia in remission. Med Pediatr Oncol 2:299–307, 1975.

48. Bodey GP, Freireich EJ, Gehan E, *et al.*: Late intensification therapy for acute leukemia in remission. Chemotherapy and Immunotherapy. JAMA 235:1021–1025, 1976.

49. Gutterman JU, Hersh EM, Rodriguez V, *et al.*: Chemoimmunotherapy of adult acute leukaemia: prolongation of remission in myeloblastic leukemia with B.C.G. Lancet ii:1405–1409, 1974.

50. Burge PS, Richards JDM, Thampson DS, *et al.*: Quality and quantity of survival in acute myeloid leukaemia. Lancet 621–624, 1975.

51. Armitage JO, Burns CP: Long term results of maintenance therapy in adult acute nonlymphoblastic leukemia (ANLL) using cytosine arabinoside and thioguanine: the effect of FAB subtype on outcome. Proc Am Soc Clin Oncol 21:439, 1980 (Abstract C-477).

52. Peterson BA, Bloomfield CD: Long-term disease-free survival in acute non-lymphocytic leukemia. Blood 57:1144–1147, 1981.

53. Clarkson BD, Dowling MD, Gee TS, Cunningham IB, Burchenal JH: Treatment of acute leukemia in adults . Cancer 36:775–795, 1975.

54. Vaughan WP, Karp JE, Burke PJ: Long chemotherapy-free remissions after single-cycle times-sequential chemotherapy for acute myelocytic leukemia. Cancer 45:859–865, 1980.

262

55. Fiere D, Martin C, Van H-Vu, *et al.*: Leucémies myéloides aiguës survie supérieure à 3 ans chez 16 malades. La Nouvelle Pres Medicale 7:899–902, 1978.
56. Kawashima K, Suzuki H, Yamada K, *et al.*: Long-term survival in acute leukemia in Japan. A study of 304 cases. Cancer 45:2181–2187, 1980.
57. Keating MJ, Smith TL, Gehan EA, *et al.*: Factors related to length of complete remission in adult acute leukemia. Cancer 45:2017–2029, 1980.
58. Gehan EA, Smith TL, Freireich EJ, *et al.*: Prgnostic factors in acute leukemia. Semin Oncol 3:271–282, 1967.
59. Henderson ES, Wallace HJ, Yates J, Scharlaw C *et al.*: Factors influencing prognosis in adult acute myelocytic leukemia. In: Advances in the biosciences, workshop on prognostic factors in human acute leukemia, Vol. 14, Fliedner TM, Perry S (eds). New York: Pergamon Press, 1975, pp 71–82.
60. Golomb HM, Rowley JD, Vardiman JW, Testa JR, Butler A: 'Microgranular' acute pro-myelocytic leukemia: a distinct clinical, ultra-structural, and cytogenetic entity. Blood 55:253–259, 1980.
61. Golomb HM, Rowley JD, Vardiman JW, Baron MM, Locker G, Krasnow S: Partial delec-tion of long arm of chromosome 17: a specific abnormality in acute promyelocytic leuke-mia? Arch Intern Med 136:825–828, 1976.
62. Trujillo JM, Cork A, Ahearn MJ, Youness EL, McCredie KB: Hematologic and cytologic characterization of 8/21 translocation acute granulocytic leukemia. Blood 53:695–706, 1979.
63. Hoelzer D, Kurrle E, *et al.*: Evidence for differentiation of human leukemic blood cells in diffusion chamber culture. Blood 49:729–744, 1977.
64. Barton JC, Conrad ME: Beneficial effects of hepatitis in patients with acute myelogenous leukemia. Ann Intern Med 90:188–190, 1979.
65. Wade JC, Wiernik PH, Schimpff SC, Schiffer CA: Hepatitis prolongation of complete re-mission and survival in acute nonlymphocytic leukemia (ANLL) patients. Proc Am Soc Clin Oncol 21:439, 1980 (Abstract C-474).
66. Dudley FJ, Fox RA, Sherlock S: Cellular immunity and hepatitis-associated, Australia antigen liver disease. Lancet i:723–726, 1972.
67. Werner B, London WT: Host responses to hepatitis B infection: hepatitis B surface antigen and host proteins (editorial). Ann Intern Med 83:113–114, 1975.
68. Sakurai M, Sandberg AA: Chromosomes and causation of human cancer and leukemia. Correlation of karyotypes with clinical features of acute myeloblastic leukemia. Cancer 37:285–299, 1976.
69. Freireich EJ, Keating MJ, Gehan EA, McCredie KB, Bodey GP, Smith T: Therapy of acute myelogenous leukemia. Cancer 42:874–882, 1978.
70. Rees JKH, Sandler RM, Challener J, Hayhoe FGJ: Treatment of acute myeloid leukaemia with a triple cytotoxic regimen: DAT. Br J Cancer 36:770–776, 1977.
71. Uzuka Y, Liong SK, Yamagata S: Treatment of adult acute non-lymphoblastic leukemia using intermittent combination chemotherapy with daunomycin, cytosine arabinoside, 6-mercaptopurine and prednisolone DCMP two step therapy. Tohoku J Exp Med 118:217–225, 1976.
72. Bodey GP, McCredie KB, Keating MJ, Freireich EJ: Treatment of acute leukemia in pro-tected environment units. Cancer 44:431–436, 1979.
73. Legha SS, Keating MJ, Zander AR, McCredie KB, Bodey GP, Freireich EJ: 4'-(9-acridinyl-amino) methanesulfon-m-anisidide (AMSA): a new drug effective in the treatment of adult acute leukemia. Ann Intern Med 93:17–21, 1980.
74. Weinstein HJ, Mayer RJ, Rosenthal DS, Camitta BM, *et al.*: Treatment of acute myelogen-ous leukemia in children and adults. N Engl J Med 303:473–478, 1980.

75. Thomas ED, Buckner CD, Clift RA, *et al.*: Marrow transplantation for acute nonlympho-blastic leukemia in first remission. N Engl J Med 301:597–599, 1979.
76. Blume KG, Beutler E, Bross KJ, *et al.*: Bone-marrow ablation and allogeneic marrow trans-plantation in acute leukemia. N Engl J Med 302:1041–1046, 1980.

# 9. The Clinical Relevance of Lymphocyte Surface Markers in Adult Acute Lymphoblastic Leukemia

CLARA D. BLOOMFIELD *

## CONTENTS

* Supported by the Coleman Leukemia Research Fund, and National Cancer Institute grant CA-26273.

Immunologic classification based on lymphocyte surface markers of the leukemic cells has been widely applied in childhood acute lymphoblastic leukemia [1–3]. Multiple studies suggest the clinical importance of such classification. However, relatively little data are available regarding immunologic classification of adult ALL. This article summarizes current knowledge regarding the clinical utility of classifying adult ALL according to the immunologic phenotype of the neoplastic cell as defined by surface markers. The major immunologic classes that have been identified in adult ALL are first described. The biological and clinical characteristics of the major immunologic classes are then presented. Finally, the therapeutic and prognostic implications of these classes are considered. The data in this article come from three major sources: the published literature, the University of Minnesota series, and the Third International Workshop on Chromosomes in Leukemia.

## 1. IMMUNOLOGIC CLASSES

A large number of lymphocyte surface markers have been used to classify ALL. These are reviewed in references [1–3] and the more common markers are listed in Table 1. In this article we will focus on those markers that have been studied in sufficient numbers of patients that some indication of their clinical utility is apparent.

The two markers that have been most widely studied in adult ALL are the receptor for unsensitized sheep erythrocytes (E) by spontaneous rosette formation and surface associated immunoglobulin (SIg) of intrinsic origin using direct immunofluorescence. Several studies assaying leukemic cells in adults with ALL have demonstrated that 63 to 85% of cases lack receptors for E and SIg; these have been designated non-T, non-B (E-, SIg-) ALL. In 8 to 27% of cases, the leukemic blasts demonstrate E and are designated T (E+) ALL, and in 2 to 17% of cases the leukemic blasts demonstrate SIg and are designated B (SIg+) ALL (Table 2).

More recently, antisera raised against the common-ALL associated antigen (cALL), human B lymphocyte antigens or the Ia-like antigen and T-

*Table 1.* Selected cell surface markers in acute lymphoblastic leukemia.

| SURFACE RECEPTORS | SURFACE ANTIGENS | |
|---|---|---|
| | *Detected by xenoantisera* * | *Detected with monoclonal antibodies* † |
| Intrinsic surface immunoglobulin (SIg) | *B-Cell antigens* <br> Ia-like (HLA-DR; p23, 30; p28, 33) [6–8, 10, 13–16, 19] | *B-Cell antigens* <br> 'Pan-B' <br> BA-1 [25], P1153/3 [26, 27] FMC1 (HC11A) [28], B1 [29] |
| Complement receptors (C') [9, 13, 15, 52, 53, 55, 61] | BDA (60) | B subset <br> A689 [30], FMC7 [31] |
| Ig-Fc receptors (Fc) [9, 13, 52, 55, 56] | *T-Cell antigens (T)* [6–10, 12–14, 17–19] | HLA-DR <br> DA2 [32], 7.2 [33] OKI1 [34] |
| Unsensitized erythrocyte receptors | *Common-ALL antigens (cALL)* [3–13, 19] | *T-Cell antigens* <br> 'Pan-T' <br> 9.6 [35], OKT11 [36] T101 [37], 17F12 [38] ‡ Leu 1 [39] |
| Sheep (E) <br> Mouse (mE) [9, 55, 61] | | T subset <br> Helper: OKT4 (T4) [40, 41] Cytotoxic-suppressor: OKT8 (T8) [40, 41] |
| Peanut agglutinin (PNA) receptor [54, 170] | | Mature T <br> OKT3 (T3) [42] |
| | | Thymic <br> NA 1/34 (anti-HTA-1, HLK) [43–45], 127E7 [46], IG11 [38], OKT6 (T6) [40–42] |
| | | *Common-ALL antigens* <br> J5 (anti-gp100) [47], BA-2 (anti-p24) [48] |

* Reviewed in references [1, 2]. Listed in parentheses are selected more recent articles describing these markers in ALL.
† Names of antibodies (with synonyms in parentheses) are followed by a reference in brackets. See reference [163] for a review of monoclonal antibodies in human leukemia and lymphoma.
‡ Leu 1 is the designation given by Wang *et al.* [39] to describe the cell surface structure recognized by the antibody.

Table 2. Frequency of major immunologic classes of adult ALL. Selected representative series.

| Series* | No. Pts. | Non-T, Non-B (E-, SIg-) ALL | | | | | | | | T (E+) | | B (SIg+) | |
|---|---|---|---|---|---|---|---|---|---|---|---|---|---|
| | | Common-ALL | | Null-ALL | | Pre-T | | Total E-, SIg- | | No. | % | No. | % |
| | | No. | %‡ | No. | %‡ | No. | %‡ | No. | % | | | | |
| Thiel et al. [9] | 113 | 50 | 54 | 23 | 25 | 19 | 21 | 92 | 81 | 19 | 17 | 2 | 2 |
| TIWCL [71] | 93 | — | | — | | — | | 63 | 68 | 20 | 22 | 10 | 11 |
| Brouet & Seligmann [57] | 57 | — | | — | | — | | 39 | 68 | 14† | 25 | 4 | 7 |
| Greaves et al. [4] | 54 | 33 | 72 | 13 | 28 | — | | 46 | 85 | 5† | 9 | 3 | 6 |
| Catovsky et al. [49] | 50 | 20 | 50 | 20 | 50 | — | | 40 | 80 | 4† | 8 | 6 | 12 |
| University MN [76] | 35 | — | | — | | — | | 24 | 69 | 8 | 23 | 3 | 9 |
| Borgström et al. [112] | 24 | — | | — | | — | | 15 | 63 | 5 | 21 | 4 | 17 |
| Liso et al. [100] | 22 | — | | — | | — | | 16 | 73 | 6 | 27 | 0 | 0 |
| Ruggero et al. [70] | 16 | — | | — | | — | | 11 | 69 | 3 | 19 | 2 | 13 |
| Total | 464 | | | | | | | 346 | 75 | 84 | 18 | 34 | 7 |

* All series consist of patients studied at diagnosis except [49] where time of study is not specified.
† Some cases may be T based on T+ rather than E+.
‡ Percent of non-T, non-B ALL.

lymphocyte antigens (T) have been used to further define immunologic sub-sets of ALL [1–19]. Similarly, cytoplasmic immunoglobulin (CIgM) has been studied to identify pre-B lymphoblasts [9, 13, 19–24]. The use of these multiple immunologic markers has resulted in the classification of ALL into at least six groups (common-ALL, pre-B ALL, null-ALL, pre-T ALL, T-ALL, B-ALL). Most recently, extensive monoclonal antibody libraries de-rived by cell hybridization have been developed for leukemic cell character-ization. Some of the more widely used monoclonal antibodies with selected references are listed in Table 1. Almost no data regarding their clinical util-ity in adult ALL are available. They are listed in the table because they are almost certain to be extensively applied to the study of adult leukemia in the next few years.

### 1.1. Non-T, Non-B ALL

The largest immunologic group is non-T, non-B ALL. This group, which is defined by the absence on the blast cells of receptors for E and SIg, is heterogeneous with respect to other immunologic markers. The most com-monly studied additional surface markers have been the cALL, T and Ia antigens. Antigenic determinants to cALL have been most frequently stud-ied. In children, approximately 80% of cases of non-T, non-B ALL demon-strate cALL antigens; such cases are frequently termed 'common-ALL.' The cALL antigen has not been extensively studied in adults, but 58% of adults with non-T, non-B ALL appear to demonstrate this antigen (Table 2). Blasts from patients with common-ALL generally also demonstrate Ia-like antigens.

Blasts from some patients with common-ALL also demonstrate T-anti-gens [1, 9], suggesting that these cases arise from T-cell progenitors. In the largest study in adults to date, Thiel et al. [9] found that 34% of adults with common-ALL had T-antigens on their blasts. Blasts from other patients with common-ALL demonstrate CIgM and thus presumably arise from B-cell progenitors [9, 13, 20, 22–24, 51]. Such cases have been designated pre-B ALL (E–, SIg–, cALL+, CIgM+, Ia+, T–). In the largest study reported in adults, Greaves et al. [23, 24] found 26% of common-ALL to be pre-B. Further study is required to determine with confidence what percen-tage of adult common-ALL is pre-T, what percentage pre-B, and what frac-tion neither (lymphoid stem cell).

The second major subgroup in non-T, non-B ALL, lacks the cALL anti-gen but demonstrates a T-antigen. This group has also been designated as pre-T ALL and has been reported in 19 of 92 cases of adult non-T, non-B ALL [9]. This group is included in T-ALL by many authors and care must be taken to note whether T-ALL refers to cases that are only E+ or also those that are E− but T+. The usual phenotype of pre-T ALL is E−, SIg−, cALL−, T+, Ia−, CIgM−.

Blasts from patients with non-T, non-B ALL may have as their only immunologic marker the Ia-like antigen [1, 10], or may be totally negative when assayed for the usual immunologic markers (E, SIg, CIgM, cALL, Ia, T). It has been suggested that approximately 90% of E−, SIg−, cALL−, T−, ALL are Ia+ [3]. However, an insufficient number of adult cases have been studied for multiple markers to know how many demonstrate Ia and how many demonstrate none of the above markers.

Non-T, non-B ALL has been found to be heterogeneous with respect to a number of other lymphocyte surface markers including complement receptors (C′) [1, 9, 13, 15, 52], Ig-Fc receptors [1, 9, 13], peanut agglutinin (PNA) receptors [1, 54, 170], mouse erythrocyte receptors (mE) [1, 9], and some of the monoclonal antibodies [38, 62, 163, 173, 174]. Unfortunately, in few instances have multiple immunologic markers been studied simultaneously and in few cases have adults been studied.

The terminology in the literature for non-T, non-B ALL is quite varied. Many reports refer to this group as 'null', cell ALL, i.e., E−, SIg−. However, investigators who routinely use the cALL antigen in immunologically classifying patients with ALL, frequently use the term 'null' cell ALL to refer to cases where the lymphoblasts do not demonstrate receptors for E, SIg, or the cALL antigen. Those patients with non-T, non-B ALL with cALL+ lymphoblasts, they call common-ALL. Consequently, when reading the literature the criteria for designating a case as non-T, non-B, and 'null' must be carefully observed. In this review null-ALL is used for cases that are E−, SIg−, cALL−.

## 1.2. T-ALL

T-ALL, as defined by the ability of the lymphoblasts to form rosettes with E, accounts for about 18% of adult ALL (Table 2). The incidence of T-ALL varies depending upon the criteria used to consider the case E+. It is clear that in some patients only a small percentage of the lymphoblasts form E rosettes. Most investigators require at least 10% of the malignant cells to form E rosettes before they will call the case E+. However, we [1] and others [13, 17, 18, 40] prefer to see at least 20% E-rosetting neoplastic cells.

Although T-ALL is most commonly defined by the presence of receptors for E on leukemic blasts, with the increasing use of antisera to detect T-cell surface antigens, some authors now include cases which are T+ but E− in the T-ALL group. When reviewing the literature, the criteria for the designation of T-ALL must be carefully noted. Unfortunately, in some articles the criteria are not clearly defined.

T-ALL, even when defined based on the presence of E receptors, is clearly heterogeneous. Reinherz *et al.* [40] using seven T-cell monoclonal antibodies demonstrated nine different subgroups among 25 patients tested. Using a xenoantiserum (anti-TH$_2$), the same investigators have divided E+ ALL into two groups [17, 18]. Interestingly, seven of seven adults (>20 years of age) studied were TH$_2$− in contrast to 13 of 18 (72%) children [18].

Using various xenoantisera for surface antigens, E+ ALL has been found to be heterogeneous with regard to the cALL antigen [13] and the Ia antigen [13, 10] although most cases are cALL−, Ia−. E+ ALL is also heterogeneous for complement receptors [1, 9, 15, 52, 55] and PNA receptors [54]. T-cell lymphoblasts have been found to express receptors for the Fc fragment of both IgG and IgM [1, 9, 55]. A greater number of T lymphoblasts appear to have IgG Fc receptors (FcγR) than IgM Fc receptors (FcμR). T-ALL appears to be negative for CIgM and mE [9]. These markers have not been separately studied in adult T-ALL.

### 1.3. B-ALL

B-ALL, as defined by the production by the leukemic cells of monotypic SIg, accounts for only about 2% of childhood ALL [1] and perhaps 7% of adult ALL (Table 2). This higher frequency among adults with ALL may be accounted for by the inclusion of some patients with peripheralizing lymphoma who have no apparent lymphadenopathy [1, 58]. Since B-ALL accounts for such a small fraction of ALL, relatively few cases have been studied.

The lymphoblasts in B-ALL usually synthesize SIgM with little or no SIgD [57]. There is usually a high density of SIgM. The majority of cases appear to synthesize μλ. Among 31 cases reported in the literature, 20 (65%) synthesized μλ, eight (26%) μκ, and three (10%) γκ [1]. B-ALL lymphoblasts are generally cALL− [1, 3, 9], Ia+ [50, 3, 10, 1], CIgM− [9, 13, 61], often FcγR+ (in about half the cases [130]) and occasionally C′+ [1, 9] and PNA+ [54]. However, cALL+ cases [9, 10] and CIgM+ cases [13] have been reported. Too few cases in adults have been studied to precisely assign the relative frequency of various phenotypes to them.

### 1.4. Phenotypic Stability

Relatively few sequential studies of ALL have been reported. Most cases appear to remain in the same broad immunological class (i.e., non-T, non-B, T or B). Among 150 patients (121 non-T, non-B, 26T, 3B) studied sequentially at diagnosis and first relapse, shifts among major immunologic classes occurred in two [4, 63–64]. In both patients, the phenotype changed from T-ALL (E+, T+, cALL−, Ia−) to non-T, non-B ALL (cALL+, Ia+ in one patient [4] and E−, T+, SIg−, cALL− in the other [64]).

Shifts in surface antigens rather than receptors appear to be more common. Greaves *et al.* [4] studied the cALL and Ia antigens in 119 patients at diagnosis and first relapse. In 19 (16%), there was a change in cALL status. In 11 patients, there was a loss of the cALL antigen; in six, there was acquisition of the cALL antigen. In all 17 of these patients the Ia antigen persisted. Two patients (one T as noted above and one non-T, non-B ALL) of the 119 acquired both the cALL and Ia antigens. In a separate study of the cALL antigen in 11 adult patients (ten cALL+, one cALL−), there were changes in cALL antigen status in three (27%) at relapse [4]. Two patients lost the cALL antigen and one gained it. Changes in the status of T-cell antigens may also not be uncommon. Borella *et al.* [64] studied the T antigen in 18 patients sequentially; in one patient, the T antigen was absent at diagnosis and present at relapse (E−, T−, SIg−, cALL− → E−, T+, SIg−, cALL−). Preliminary studies using multiple monoclonal T-cell antibodies suggest that changes in phenotype at relapse, often to a less mature T-cell phenotype, are not uncommon (Reinherz, personal communication).

B-ALL has not been extensively studied sequentially. However, among three cases reported by Borella *et al.* [64], there was a change in the heavy chains in one, with IgM and IgD present at diagnosis but only IgM present at relapse.

Few adults with ALL have been studied sequentially for multiple immunologic markers. Clearly, more studies are needed. Moreover, the clinical relevance of a change in immunologic phenotype following treatment is unknown. Many studies evaluating the clinical features of ALL immunologic classes combine phenotypes from patients studied at relapse following therapy with those from patients studied at diagnosis. Results from such studies must be viewed with caution. How inclusion of cases which have changed their phenotype might bias a study is currently unclear.

## 2. CLINICOPATHOLOGIC FEATURES OF ALL IMMUNOLOGIC CLASSES

Information regarding the morphologic, cytochemical, enzymatic, cytogenetic, hormone receptor, and clinical characteristics of the various immunologic types of ALL is beginning to accumulate. We will first review these data and then consider the therapeutic and prognostic significance of immunologic classification.

### 2.1. Morphology

*2.1.1. FAB Classification.* In recent years several groups have classified ALL on the basis of cytomorphology in order to identify subgroups having different prognoses. The classification that has been most widely adopted is that of the French-American-British Cooperative Group (FAB classification) [65, 66]. This classification divides ALL into three groups (L1, L2, and L3) based on cell size, nuclear cytoplasmic ratio, presence, prominence and frequency of nucleoli, and regularity of nuclear membrane outline (see Table 1 in chapter by Esterhay and Wiernik). The majority of children have the L1 morphologic form. The Children's Cancer Study Group (CCSG) evaluated 566 children with ALL and found the following frequencies of the FAB classes: L1−84%, L2−15%, L3−1% [67]. However, several studies in adults suggest that FAB L2 is most common. Among 324 adult patients (≥15 years of age), 29% were L1, 64% L2, and 7% L3 [1, 68–71]. In its most recent study, the FAB group classified 39 adults (>15 years) and found 44% L1, 49% L2, and 8% L3 [66].

In most studies, patients with L2 cytology have been shown to survive a significantly shorter period than those with L1 cytology [66, 67, 69, 72, 73, 74]. Patients with L3 leukemia have particularly dismal survivals. Several studies evaluating the prognostic significance of the FAB system in a multivariate fashion suggest that FAB class is an independent prognostic factor in childhood ALL [67, 73, 74]. The prognostic significance of the FAB classification in adult ALL is currently unclear [68, 69, 75].

The distribution of FAB morphologic types within the various immunologic classes has only recently begun to be evaluated. In a large CCSG study, among children with non-T, non-B ALL, 78% of cases were L1; the rest were L2 [73]. Among 136 adults with non-T, non-B ALL, 35% of cases were reported to be L1, 64% L2, and 1% L3 (Table 3). At least two additional cases of non-T, non-B ALL have been reported to be L3 [77, 130]. One was an adult with Fc receptors [77].

Data on most of the immunologic subtypes of non-T, non-B ALL are limited. However, among 111 children with common-ALL, 71% were L1,

*Table 3.* FAB classification of ALL in adults by immunologic phenotype.

| | Non-T, Non-B ALL | | | | T (E+) ALL | | | | B (SIg+) ALL | | | |
|---|---|---|---|---|---|---|---|---|---|---|---|---|
| Reference | No. of patients | L1 % | L2 % | L3 % | No. of patients | L1 % | L2 % | L3 % | No. of patients | L1 % | L2 % | L3 % |
| [68] | 33 | 33 | 67 | 0 | 5 | 20 | 80 | 0 | 1 | 0 | 0 | 100 |
| [70] | 11 | 18 | 82 | 0 | 3 | 33 | 67 | 0 | 2 | 0 | 100 | 0 |
| [71] | 58 | 26 | 72 | 2 | 16 | 31 | 69 | 0 | 10 | 0 | 30 | 70 |
| [76] | 34 | 59 | 41 | 0 | 8 | 75 | 25 | 0 | 5 | 0 | 60 | 40 |
| Total | 136 | 35 | 64 | 1 | 32 | 41 | 59 | 0 | 18 | 0 | 44 | 56 |

28% L2, and 0% L3 [3]. Among 21 adults with common-ALL, 33% were L1 and 67% L2 [68]. L3 morphology has only occasionally been reported in common-ALL [9]. Among 19 children with pre-B ALL, 18 were L1 and 1 L2 [13]. At least one child with pre-B ALL and L3 morphology has been reported [78]. Data in adult pre-B ALL are not available. Among 12 children with null-ALL (E−, SIg−, cALL−), 58% were L1 and 41% L2 [3]. Among 12 adults with null-ALL, 33% were L1 and 67% L2 [68].

T-ALL appears to have a distribution of L1 and L2 similar to that of non-T, non-B ALL in both children [73] and adults. Among 32 adults, 41% were reported to be L1 and 59% L2 (Table 3). At least one case of adult T-ALL (E+) with L3 morphology has been reported [77].

Using different cytologic classifications than the FAB, others have also noted no difference in morphology between T and non-T, non-B ALL [1]. Recently, however, McKenna *et al.* [79] have reported morphologically distinctive cells in the blood and marrow of 10 of 11 T-ALL patients. These cells were characterized by markedly hyperchromatic nuclei which often demonstrated prominent nuclear convolution. Nucleoli could not be identified. Cytoplasm was generally sparse or absent. The cells were best demonstrated in well-prepared finger-stick blood smears or direct bone marrow smears. These cells were also ultrastructurally distinctive, exhibiting nuclear membrane reduplication, nuclear blebs and splits. Similar cells were found in only four of 47 cases of non-T, non-B ALL. Confirmation of these findings in a larger series is needed.

B-ALL in children commonly demonstrates L3 morphology [3, 72]. However, in adult patients who may be presenting in the leukemic phase of malignant lymphoma, L2 morphology is often seen (Table 3). Cases of L1 have been reported [13].

*2.1.2. Acute Undifferentiated Leukemia (AUL).* A fraction of acute leukemia in adults is classified on morphologic and cytochemical criteria as AUL. The proportion of AUL varies from center to center. Immunologic markers offer the opportunity to more precisely classify these cases. Thiel *et al.* [9] studied 59 adults diagnosed as AUL based on morphological and cytochemical criteria (negative for peroxidase, naphthol-AS-acetate esterase, and coarse granular periodic acid–Schiff). An immunologic diagnosis of ALL (cALL+, T+, E+ or SIg+) was made in 38 (64%). Gordon *et al.* studied 13 cases of adult AUL with heterologous and monoclonal antisera; seven exhibited lymphoid antigens, five myeloid antigens, and one was unclassifiable [175]. Similarly, Greaves and his colleagues studied 12 adults with AUL: six were cALL+, one was mixed lymphoid-myeloid, one was immunologically myeloid, and four were unclassifiable but nonlymphoid with respect to hexosaminidase isoenzymes and lymphoid antigens [3]. Greaves *et al.* suggested that patients with AUL who were lymphoid immunologically had a better prognosis. Certainly, for selecting therapy, it may be helpful to differentiate the lymphoid cases from the myeloid cases among AUL. The new monoclonal antibodies may be helpful in this respect.

## 2.2. Cytochemistry

Few large studies have reported the cytochemical characteristics of the various immunologic classes of ALL in children, let alone adults. The cytochemical stains which have been most frequently evaluated are periodic acid-Schiff, acid phosphatase, acid alpha naphthyl esterase, and beta glucuronidase. Although further study is needed, it appears that none of these enzyme markers correlate precisely with immunologic markers.

### 2.2.1. Periodic Acid–Schiff (PAS).

Among the various cytochemical stains, PAS has been most extensively studied in ALL. The degree of PAS positivity has been suggested in many studies to correlate with survival [80]. A recent multivariate analysis of children with ALL identified the percentage of lymphoblasts with PAS positive coarse granules in blocks as an independent prognostic variable for predicting duration of initial complete remission [74]. Patients with more PAS positive blasts had longer remissions. Unfortunately only 78 of the 209 cases in this study were phenotyped immunologically.

The PAS stain is positive in 56 to 77 % of cases of non-T, non-B ALL [1]. PAS positivity may be somewhat more frequent in common-ALL than in null-ALL (Table 4). The number of cases of pre-B and pre-T ALL studied is still very small. However in recent studies, of 20 cases of pre-B ALL only four were PAS positive [13] while none of 12 cases of pre-T ALL were PAS positive [9]. It has been suggested that among patients with non-T, non-B ALL, those with low PAS scores have a poorer prognosis [72, 81].

T-ALL has been reported to be PAS positive in 9 to 91 % of cases [1] (Table 4). All series reported have been relatively small (<25 cases), and this variability may result from differences in interpretation of positivity or from the heterogeneity of T-ALL patients included in these small series [40, 176]. Several groups have found PAS positivity to be less frequent in T-ALL than in non-T, non-B ALL [1, 9, 3, 13, 50, 55]. However, we [72] and others [81, 82] have found no differences. In our series there were no appreciable differences in percent PAS positive cells, their staining intensity, nor the cytoplasmic distribution of PAS between the two immunologic groups.

B-ALL lymphoblasts appear to generally be PAS negative [1] (Table 4).

*Table 4.* Cytochemical reactivity according to ALL immunologic class.

| | Non-T, Non-B (E-, SIg-) | | | | | | | | T (E+) | | B (SIg+) | |
| | COMMON-ALL | | NULL-ALL | | PRE-B | | PRE-T | | | | | |
| | Percent positive | No. pts. ‡ | Percent positive | No. pts. | Percent positive | No. pts. | Percent positive | No. pts. | Percent positive | No. pts. | Percent positive | No. pts. |
|---|---|---|---|---|---|---|---|---|---|---|---|---|
| **PERIODIC ACID-SCHIFF (PAS)** | | | | | | | | | | | | |
| Pesando et al. [8] | 69 | 93 | 53 | 19 | — | 0 | — | 0 | — | 0 | — | 0 |
| Thiel et al. [9] | 39 | 33 | — | 0 | — | 0 | 0 | 12 | 13 | 15 | — | 0 |
| Pullen et al. [13]* | — | 0 | — | 0 | 20 | 20 | — | 0 | 9 | 11 | 0 | 1 |
| Greaves [3]* | 68 | 140 | 45 | 20 | — | 0 | — | 0 | 40 | 20 | 0 | 4 |
| Lister et al. [50]† | 57 | 23 | 55 | 11 | — | 0 | — | 0 | 40 | 5 | — | 0 |
| Total | 64 | 289 | 50 | 50 | 20 | 20 | 0 | 12 | 25 | 51 | 0 | 5 |
| **ACID PHOSPHATASE (AcP)** | | | | | | | | | | | | |
| Thiel et al. [9] | 30 | 33 | — | 0 | — | 0 | 83 | 12 | 87 | 15 | 0 | 0 |
| Greaves [3]* | 2 | 97 | 9 | 23 | — | 0 | — | 0 | 90 | 20 | 0 | 2 |
| Pullen et al. [13]* | — | 0 | — | 0 | 28 | 18 | 0 | 4 | 44 | 18 | 0 | 1 |
| Total | 9 | 130 | 9 | 23 | 28 | 18 | 63 | 16 | 73 | 53 | 0 | 3 |
| **ACID ALPHA NAPHTHYL ESTERASE (ANAE)** | | | | | | | | | | | | |
| Kulenkampff et al. [87] | 11 | 9 | 0 | 3 | — | 0 | — | 0 | 80 | 5 | — | 0 |
| Thiel et al. [9] | 25 | 28 | — | — | — | 0 | 83 | 12 | 50 | 14 | — | 0 |
| Knowles et al. [88] | — | 0 | — | — | — | 0 | — | 0 | 0 | 3 | — | 0 |
| Total | 22 | 37 | 0 | 3 | — | 0 | 83 | 12 | 50 | 22 | — | 0 |

\* Children.
† Adults.
‡ Represents number of patients studied.

*2.2.2. Acid Phosphatase (AcP).* The cytochemical stain most frequently suggested to discriminate immunologic classes of ALL is AcP. Cases where the lymphoblasts demonstrate strong focal positivity in a paranuclear distribution have been thought to be T-cell. However, as larger numbers of cases have been studied for AcP and surface markers, it has become clear that the correlation between T-cell phenotype and AcP is not as high as initially thought.

In most series less than 15% of cases of non-T, non-B ALL demonstrate characteristic AcP positivity [1, 3, 13, 80]. However, Thiel *et al.* [9] found AcP positivity in 10 of 33 cases of common-ALL (cALL+, T−, E−, SIg−) and Pullen *et al.* [13] found positivity in five of 18 cases of pre-B ALL. There may be considerable differences among immunologic subtypes of non-T, non-B ALL. Greaves [3] found AcP positivity more frequently in null than common-ALL (Table 4). Thiel *et al.* [9] found AcP positivity more frequent in pre-T than common-ALL, but Pullen *et al.* [13] studied four cases of pre-T ALL and found none to be positive (Table 4). Whether these differences relate to problems in interpretation of the positivity or differences in populations of patients studied is unclear. Determination of AcP positivity is somewhat subjective. Even using the standard method of Goldberg and Barka [83] up to 30% of cells may demonstrate a weak or moderate reaction in cases that Goldberg and Barka would call AcP negative. Using the method of Li *et al.* [84] almost 90% of cases will demonstrate some AcP positivity, though rarely in a focal paranuclear distribution. To try to avoid these problems some authors have tried to quantitate AcP positivity [85]. Application of the hybridoma monoclonal antibodies may resolve the question of patient population heterogeneity in small series.

The AcP stain has been reported to be positive in 44 to 90% of T(E+) ALL (Table 4). Of 79 cases, 73% were positive [3, 9, 13, 55, 72, 80]. Few cases of B-ALL have been studied but they have generally been reported to have lymphoblasts that are negative for focal paranuclear AcP reactivity [3, 13, 72].

*2.2.3. Acid Alpha Naphthyl Esterase (ANAE).* The ANAE reaction was initially reported to be useful in distinguishing non-T, non-B ALL from T-ALL [87]. Lymphoblasts from eight of nine cases of common-ALL and three of three cases of null-ALL were negative. T-ALL lymphoblasts in four of five cases showed a strongly positive reaction characteristic of that of thymocytes and different from that of mature peripheral blood T lymphocytes. However, more recently Thiel *et al.* [9] have found positivity in seven of 28 cases of common-ALL and Knowles *et al.* [88] have reported negativity in three cases of T-ALL (Table 4). Results in B-ALL have not been reported. Obviously more cases must be studied before the utility of this reaction can be determined. It is important to emphasize that the widely used alpha naphthyl *acetate* esterase stain of Yam *et al.* [89] is not useful for differentiating immunologic groups of ALL [72].

*2.2.4. Beta Glucuronidase (βG).* βG reactivity has been proposed as another useful cytochemical approach for separating non-T, non-B ALL and T-ALL. Normal peripheral blood T lymphocytes are more often βG positive than normal B lymphocytes or non-T, non-B lymphocytes and often demonstrate a strong focal paranuclear pattern [90]. Normal B lymphocytes and non-T, non-B lymphocytes, when positive, usually manifest a pattern of multiple small scattered granules.

There have been two large studies of βG activity in ALL [72, 82]. In the study of Brouet *et al.* [82] approximately two-thirds of both non-T, non-B ALL and T-ALL cases had βG positive leukemic cells; no mention is made of the portion of cells with βG activity, their staining pattern, or intensity. Recently similar results were reported in six cases of non-T, non-B ALL by Machin *et al.* [91]. In the study of McKenna *et al.* [72], βG activity was demonstrated in the leukemic cells in 89% of the non-T, non-B cases and in 100% of the T-ALL cases. However, 63% of the T cases exhibited a strong focal paranuclear pattern of βG activity in more than 75% of the cells. Only 16% of the non-T, non-B ALL cases manifested this βG staining pattern. The remaining positive cases manifested a scattered granule pattern similar to that described for normal blood B lymphocytes and non-T, non-B lymphocytes.

The βG staining profile in the non-T, non-B ALL and T-ALL cases was similar to that of AcP. The interpretation of βG reactivity, however, was more difficult. Although focal paranuclear βG staining is suggestive of T-ALL, it appears to be a less reliable indicator than the characteristic AcP stain [72].

βG activity has been reported in the lymphoblasts of one of two cases of B-ALL studied; however, its distribution was not paranuclear [72].

*2.3. Biochemical Enzymology*

As noted above, cytochemical studies of the immunologic classes of ALL have demonstrated differing, although not unique, cellular distributions of a number of enzymes. Studies using biochemical techniques suggest that the total specific activity of several enzymes [92–109] also differ among immunologic classes (Table 5). The enzymes most studied to date are terminal deoxynucleotidyl transferase, adenosine deaminase, and hexosaminidase isoenzymes.

Table 5. Biochemical profiles according to ALL immunologic class.

| | NON-T, NON-B (E−, SIg−) ALL | | | | | | | | T (E+) ALL | | B (SIg+) ALL | | |
| --- | --- | --- | --- | --- | --- | --- | --- | --- | --- | --- | --- | --- | --- |
| | COMMON-ALL | | NULL-ALL | | Pre-B | | PRE-T | | | | | | |
| | Percent positive* | No. pts | Percent positive | No. pts | Percent positive | No. pts | Percent positive | No. pts | Percent positive | No. pts | Percent positive | No. pts | Relative level of activity |
| **TERMINAL DEOXYNUCLEOTIDYL TRANSFERASE (TdT)** | | | | | | | | | | | | | |
| Janossy et al. [95] | 93 | 96 | 100 | 19 | — | — | 100 | 9 | 87 | 23 | — | 0 | Common-ALL>Null-ALL |
| Greaves et al. [23] | 93 | 57 | — | 0 | 91 | 22 | — | 0 | — | 0 | 0 | 4 | Common-ALL>Pre-B |
| Thiel et al. [9] | 100 | 9 | — | 0 | — | 0 | 71 | 7 | 100 | 9 | 0 | 1 | Common-ALL>T>Pre-T>B |
| Strivastava et al. [96]† | 100 | ~14 | — | 0 | — | 0 | — | 0 | 100 | 3 | 0 | 1 | |
| Catovsky et al. [49]† | 89 | 9 | 75 | 8 | — | 0 | — | 0 | 100 | 3 | — | 0 | T>Common-ALL>Null-ALL |
| Total | ‡ | | ‡ | | 91 | 22 | 88 | 16 | 92 | 38 | 0 | 6 | |
| **ADENOSINE DEAMINASE (ADA)** | | | | | | | NON-T, NON-B *Unspecified Type* | | | | | | |
| Liso et al. [100]† | | | | | | | 65 | 17 | 50 | 6 | — | 0 | Non-T, Non-B>T |
| Smyth et al. [99] | | | | | | | ~43 | 14 | 89 | 9 | — | 0 | T>Non-T, Non-B |
| Coleman et al. [171] | | | | | | | 92 | 13 | 100 | 7 | 0 | 3 | T>Non-T, Non-B>B |
| Chechik et al. [102] | | | | | | | 56 | 9 | 100 | 9 | 0 | 1 | |
| Ben-Bassat et al. [101]§ | | | | | | | 1.7-107 | 13 | 4.9-64 | 10 | 0-5 | 6 | T>Non-T, Non-B>B |
| **HEXOSAMINIDASE I** | | | | | | | | | | | | | |
| Greaves et al. [23] | 65 | 37 | 33 | 9** | 42 | 19 | | | 0 | 9 | 0 | 2 | T>Non-T, Non-B>B |
| Broadhead et al. [106] | 82 | 11 | 100 | 1 | — | 0 | | | 0 | 2 | 0 | 1 | |
| Muchi et al. [172] | | | | | 100 | 2 | 89 | 9 | — | 0 | | | |

\* % of cases with elevated levels.
† Adult series.
‡ Unclear number of patients reported several times in references [23, 49, 95].
§ Range of activity in μmol/h per 10⁸ cells.
** From references [103 and 104].

*2.3.1. Terminal Deoxynucleotidyl Transferase (TdT).* TdT has been the enzyme most extensively studied in ALL. It is a unique DNA polymerase which copies deoxynucleotidyl sequences but does not require nucleic acid template information. In normal tissues, TdT is found only in the cortex of the thymus and in rare small bone marrow cells of lymphoid appearance [92]; it is not present in normal peripheral T or B lymphocytes. In the marrow, the TdT positive cells are usually Ia positive and in children 40 to 60% express the cALL antigen [93]. In adults the cells are usually cALL antigen negative [94].

TdT has been studied most extensively in leukemia with a biochemical assay. The recent development of a highly specific antibody to TdT has allowed the development of an indirect immunofluorescent (IF) assay which detects TdT in individual cells [92]. Preliminary studies suggest an excellent correlation between the enzyme assay and immunocytochemical staining (the IF assay) when there are more than 5% TdT positive cells as determined by IF [94].

Elevated levels of TdT have been reported in most cases of non-T, non-B ALL and T-ALL [1] (Table 5). TdT is elevated in most cases of all subgroups of non-T, non-B ALL, including pre-B ALL [23]. The levels found by biochemical assay have varied widely among immunologic classes. In most series common-ALL has had a higher level of TdT activity than pre-B, pre-T, null-ALL or T-ALL (Table 5).

Elevated TdT levels have not been reported in any well-documented case of B-ALL. One unusual case of ALL with SIgG on the leukemic cells, a mediastinal mass, and elevated TdT levels has been published [97]. However, the synthesis of monotypic IgG by the lymphoblasts was not demonstrated and the B-cell nature of this case remains in doubt.

Several groups have reported TdT levels in adult ALL [49, 95, 96, 98]. To date obvious differences between childhood and adult leukemia have not emerged.

*2.3.2. Adenosine Deaminase (ADA).* ADA is a polymorphic enzyme which catalyzes the deamination of adenosine to inosine. ADA activity is high in normal mitogen-stimulated peripheral T lymphocytes and thymocytes and low in normal peripheral B lymphocytes. Several recent studies have correlated ADA activity with the immunologic class of ALL (Table 5). Most cases of both non-T, non-B ALL and T-ALL have had elevated levels. However, the activity of ADA per cell was significantly higher in T-ALL in three of the studies. In one study the levels were similar for non-T, non-B ALL and T-ALL. ADA activity was low in all nine cases of B-ALL. Recently a radioimmunoassay has been developed which has shown good correlation with the enzymatic method in one study of normal and leukemic cells [102]. With the radioimmunoassay, cells from all 9 cases of T-ALL, five of eight cases of common-ALL, none of one case of pre-B ALL and none of one case of B-ALL demonstrated increased quantities of ADA [102]. Confirmation of the utility of this radioimmunoassay to detect ADA in cells is necessary.

*2.3.3. Hexosaminidase Isoenzymes.* Hexosaminidase (N-acetyl β gluco-saminidase) is one of the lysosomal acid hydrolases. Three major isoen-zymes (A, I, and B) have been identified and found to have characteristic profiles in normal granulocytes, lymphocytes, and thymocytes. The isoen-zyme pattern, determined either by automated ion-exchange chromatogra-phy [23, 103, 104] or isoelectric focusing [105, 106], has been reported by two groups to be useful in distinguishing immunologic types of ALL. In particular the intermediate isoenzymes (hexosaminidase I) appear to be greatly increased primarily in common-ALL (Table 5). Elevated levels have been found in only eight of 19 cases with pre-B ALL. Elevated levels have also been reported in some cases of null-ALL but not in T-ALL or B-ALL.

Recently other lysosomal enzymes (α-D-mannosidase, α-D-galactosidase, α-fucosidase, β-glucuronidase, acid phosphatase) have also been found to have unusual isoenzyme forms (or a greatly raised activity of forms present in normal cells at very low levels) in most cases of common-ALL [104, 106]. Preliminary results suggest that there is an almost exact correspondence between the expression of raised late peaks of α-D-mannosidase and α-D-galactosidase and raised hexosaminidase I irrespective of the nature of other cell markers [104]. However, studies for hexosaminidase at the current time appear to give the most consistent and sensitive results [104, 106].

## 2.4. Cytogenetics

Cytogenetic analysis with banding techniques has demonstrated clonal chromosome abnormalities in the majority of cases of ALL. In the largest series reported to date, abnormalities were found in 66% of 330 newly diagnosed patients [71]. Smaller studies have found clonal abnormalities in over 80% of patients [75, 110, 111]. A number of specific chromosomal subgroups of ALL have been recognized including $Ph^1+$ (22q−) ALL, t(4; 11) ALL, 8q− ALL, 14q+ ALL, and 6q− ALL. Other chromosome abnormalities have been grouped by modal number (i.e., the predominent number of chromosomes in cells with a range of chromosome numbers). Some of these karyotypic subgroups appear to have distinctive clinical and hematologic features and response to treatment. Karyotype has also been demonstrated to be an independent prognostic variable [71].

*Table 6.* Clonal chromosome abnormalities according to ALL immunologic class: results from unselected banded series.

| | Non-T, Non-B (E−, SIg−) | | T (E+) | | B (SIg+) | |
|---|---|---|---|---|---|---|
| | Percent abnor- mal [‡] | No. pts. [§] | Percent abnor- mal [‡] | No. pts. | Percent abnor- mal [‡] | No. pts. |
| ADULTS | | | | | | |
| * Borgström *et al.* [112] | 40 | 15 | 20 | 5 | 100 | 4 |
| * TIWCL [71] | 71 | 63 | 45 | 20 | 100 | 10 |
| * Arthur *et al.* [111] | 88 | 17 | 43 | 7 | 100 | 2 |
| Kaneko & Rowley [113] | 67 | 3 | − | 0 | 100 | 1 |
| Total adults | 69 | 98 | 41 | 32 | 100 | 17 |
| CHILDREN | | | | | | |
| * TIWCL [71] | 68 | 65 | 27 | 11 | 100 | 5 |
| * Brodeur *et al.* [114] | 68 | 102 | 61 | 23 [†] | 100 | 2 |
| * Arthur *et al.* [111] | 85 | 33 | 100 | 1 | − | 0 |
| Kaneko & Rowley [113] | 65 | 17 | 33 | 3 | − | 0 |
| Total children | 70 | 217 | 50 | 38 | 100 | 7 |
| ADULTS and CHILDREN | | | | | | |
| Oshimura *et al.* [115] | 49 | 37 | 25 | 4 | 100 | 1 |
| Total | 68 | 352 | 45 | 74 | 100 | 25 |

* Studied at diagnosis.
[†] T = E+ and T+.
[‡] Percentage of patients with clonal chromosome abnormalities.
[§] Represents number of patients studied.

Several studies have recently correlated karyotype with immunologic phe-notype (Table 6). Significant differences in frequency of clonal chromosomal abnormalities have been found among ALL immunologic classes. All cases of B-ALL have had abnormalities identified compared with 68 % of non-T, non-B ALL and only 45 % of T-ALL. Striking differences between children and adults have not been seen. Among 92 children with common-ALL, 67 % had clonal abnormalities compared with 7 of 10 with null-ALL [114].

The most common specific chromosomal abnormality in non-T, non-B ALL is a Philadelphia chromosome (Ph$^1$), most commonly t(9; 22) (q34; q11) (Table 7). Among adults with non-T, non-B ALL, as many as 30 % have been found to have Ph$^1$+ lymphoblasts [116]. The next most

Table 7. Types of chromosome abnormalities according to ALL immunologic class. Results from the Third International Workshop on Chromosomes in Leukemia [71].

| Clonal chromosome abnormality | Non-T, Non-B (E−, SIg−) | | | | T (E+) | | | | B (SIg+) | | | |
|---|---|---|---|---|---|---|---|---|---|---|---|---|
| | Adults | | Children | | Adults | | Children | | Adults | | Children | |
| | % | No. pts. | % | No. pts. | % | No. pts. | % | No. pts. | % | No. pts. | % | No. pts. |
| None | 29 | 18 | 32 | 21 | 55 | 11 | 73 | 8 | – | 0 | – | 0 |
| Ph[1] | 24 | 15 | 8 | 5 | – | 0 | – | 0 | – | 0 | – | 0 |
| t(8;14) | – | 0 | – | 0 | – | 0 | – | 0 | 60 | 6 | – | 0 |
| t(4;11) | 5 | 3 | 6 | 4 | 5 | 1 | – | 0 | – | 0 | – | 0 |
| 14q+ | 6 | 4 | 2 | 1 | – | 0 | – | 0 | 40 | 4 | 100 | 5 |
| 6q− | – | 0 | 5 | 3 | – | 0 | 9 | 1 | – | 0 | – | 0 |
| <46 | 10 | 6 | 3 | 2 | 10 | 2 | – | 0 | – | 0 | – | 0 |
| 46 Abnl | 14 | 9 | 12 | 8 | 20 | 4 | 18 | 2 | – | 0 | – | 0 |
| 47–50 | 8 | 5 | 12 | 8 | 10 | 2 | – | 0 | – | 0 | – | 0 |
| >50 | 5 | 3 | 20 | 13 | – | 0 | – | 0 | – | 0 | – | 0 |

common recurring chromosome abnormality is t(4; 11) (q21; q23). The only other recurring translocation that has been noted is t(11; 14) (q23; q32) [110]. Among the nonspecific chromosome abnormalities, the only one usually restricted to non-T, non-B ALL is a modal number >50. ALL with a modal number >50 may constitute as much as 20% of childhood non-T, non-B ALL and appears to carry an unusually good prognosis [71].

Data on most of the immunologic subtypes of non-T, non-B ALL are limited. Among three cases of pre-B ALL reported, one had the Ph[1] [117], one was 46,XY, − 8,del(3)(q12q25), t(8; 14)(q24; q32), + der(8)t(1q; 8q) (cen; cen) [118] and one had t(16; 17) [113].

Recurring specific chromosome abnormalities have rarely been reported in T-ALL. Most cases of T-ALL have had a modal number of 46. Six of 12 cases with abnormalities in the Third International Workshop fell into the 46 abnormal group (Table 7). Rare cases with the Ph[1] [114, 119] or the t(4; 11) [71] have been reported.

All the completely banded cases of B-ALL reported to date have demonstrated an 8q− or a 14q+.

## 2.5. Hormone Receptors

Hormone receptors have recently begun to be studied in ALL and correlated with immunologic class. Glucocorticoid receptors have been most extensively studied (Table 8). These are cytoplasmic binding proteins that are specific for glucocorticoids and appear to be required for hormone action in all glucocorticoid sensitive tissues. Several groups have found that response to glucocorticoids in lymphoproliferative disorders correlates well with glucocorticoid receptor level [120–122]. Moreover, one group has found that within immunologic classes (non-T, non-B and T-ALL) glucocorticoid receptor number has prognostic significance in childhood ALL [123]. The duration of complete remission was longer in patients with higher receptor levels. These results have yet to be confirmed by other groups.

Several studies have correlated glucocorticoid receptor level with ALL immunologic class at diagnosis (Table 8). Among patients with non-T, non-B ALL, three groups have found median numbers of glucocorticoid receptor sites per cell of approximately 7 000 [120, 122, 127]. Results have been comparable in children and adults. Few patients have been studied among the immunologic subtypes of non-T, non-B ALL. However, common-ALL may have higher receptor levels than null-ALL. One study suggests that pre-B ALL may have particularly high levels [129].

T-ALL in children has been reported to have lower glucocorticoid receptor levels than non-T, non-B ALL, with median levels of approximately 2 000–2 500 [127, 129]. Few cases of adult T-ALL have been studied but some cases with quite high levels have been reported [122, 126]. Studies

Table 8. Glucocorticoid receptor level according to ALL immunologic class.

| | NON-T, NON-B (E−, SIg−) ALL | | | | T(E+) ALL | | B(SIg+) ALL | |
| | Common-ALL | Null-ALL | Pre-B ALL | Not subclassified | | | | |
| | Median* (n)† | Median (n) | Median (n) | Median (n) | Median | (n) | Median | (n) |
|---|---|---|---|---|---|---|---|---|
| ADULTS | | | | | | | | |
| Bloomfield et al. [122] | | | | 6956 (11) | 8150 | (3) | | |
| Nakao et al. [124] | | | | High (5) | Low | (3) | | |
| | | | | | | | | |
| ALL AGES | | | | | | | | |
| Bell et al. [125] | ~11 000 (15) | ~1500 (2) | | | ~1500 | (6) | | |
| Ho et al. [126] | 19 392 (6) | | | | 5899 | (3) | | |
| | | | | | | | | |
| CHILDREN | | | | | | | | |
| Yarbro et al. [127, 128] | | | | 6700 (27) | 2200 | (18) | | |
| Crist et al. [129] | 14 000 (14) | | 21 000 (10) | | 2500 | (9) | <1000 | (8) |
| Mastrangelo et al. [120] | | | | 7072 (11) | | | | |

* Glucocorticoid receptor sites per cell.
† (n) is the number of patients studied.

with hybridoma antibodies suggest that adult T-ALL may be immunologically considerably more heterogeneous than childhood T-ALL. It is possible that T-ALL when of the same immunologic subtypes would have comparable glucocorticoid receptor levels in children and adults.

Only one study of B-ALL has been reported. Glucocorticoid receptor levels were very low, but half of the patients had had prior therapy [128].

### 2.6. Clinical Characteristics

Although the clinical features of the ALL immunologic classes in adults have not been fully delineated, clear differences among immunologic types have emerged (Table 9). A detailed comparison has not been made, but the presenting clinical and hematologic features are not strikingly different from those recorded for children.

*2.6.1. Non-T, Non-B ALL.* Detailed data regarding the clinical characteristics of adults with non-T, non-B ALL are now available from five series of at least 15 patients [70, 71, 76, 100, 112]. Adults with non-T, non-B ALL appear to be intermediate in age between those with T-ALL and B-ALL (Table 9). In four different series of 15 to 63 patients the median age ranged from 26 to 34 years [71, 76, 100, 112]. In one small series of 11 patients the median age was 44 years [70]. A slight male predominance has been reported (55% of 129 cases) but nowhere near the predominance seen in B- and T-ALL (Table 9). Organomegaly has been less frequent at diagnosis than in B- and T-ALL, being present in less than half the patients. Splenomegaly has been reported in 47%, lymphadenopathy in 39%, and hepatomegaly in 30%. Similarly, involvement of the mediastinum (3%) and the CNS (8%) has been much less frequent than in T- and B-ALL.

Hematologic parameters at diagnosis in non-T, non-B ALL have also differed from those of B-ALL and T-ALL. The median presenting hemoglobin has been lower (8–10 g per dl in different series). The initial WBC tends to be low (medians of $7–15 \times 10^9/l$). The frequency of presenting leukocyte counts of more than 50 000 is intermediate between that of B- and T-ALL, as are the median initial platelet counts and percent circulating blasts (Table 9).

The clinical features of the immunologic subtypes of adult non-T, non-B ALL have been rarely reported. The median age for common-ALL was 20 years in one series [9] and 31 in the other [50]. A slight male predominance for common-ALL has been reported (57%) [9]. The median age for null-ALL has been reported in one small series as 21 years [50]. In the same series, mediastinal masses were found in 18% of patients with null-ALL, but in no adults with common-ALL. Both groups had similar frequencies of splenomegaly and hepatomegaly [50]. Pre-T ALL in one adult series has

*Table 9.* Clinical features at diagnosis according to ALL immunologic class in adults.

| | NON-T, NON-B | T (E+) ALL | B (SIg+) ALL |
|---|---|---|---|
| Series * | 70, 71, 76, 100, 112 | 70, 71, 76, 100, 112 | 70, 71, 76, 112, 130 |
| Number of patients | 129 | 42 | 28 |
| Median age (yrs.) | 26–44 [†] | 20, 23 [‡] | 34–47 |
| Sex (% Male) | 55 | 74 | 82 |
| Presenting signs (%) | | | |
|   Lymphadenopathy | 39 | 72 | 46 |
|   Splenomegaly | 47 | 72 | 70 |
|   Hepatomegaly | 30 | 31 | 56 |
|   Mediastinal mass | 3 | 48 | 17 |
|   CNS leukemia | 8 | 25 | 48 |
| Hematologic parameters at diagnosis | | | |
|   Median hemoglobin (g/dl) | 8–10 | 11 | 10–11 |
|   Median WBC ($\times 10^9$/l) | 7–15 | 40, 42 [‡] | 5–14 |
|    % 50–100 $\times 10^9$/l | 11 | 15 | 4 |
|    % >100 $\times 10^9$/l | 9 | 23 | 4 |
|   Median platelets ($\times 10^9$/l) | 43–76 | 80, 82 [‡] | 23–90 |
|   Median % circulating blasts | 26–62 | 70, 75 [‡] | 4–21 |
|   Median % blasts in marrow | 90, 96 [‡] | 91, 99 [‡] | 83, 93 [‡] |

* Numbers refer to references from which data obtained.
[†] When medians are presented they represent the range from several series.
[‡] Medians from only two series.

been reported to have a median age of 21 years and a male predominance (68%). The one series available suggests that pre-B ALL may occur in younger adults [23]. Among nine adults a median age of 23 was reported with the oldest patient being 32; there was a slight female (55%) predominance as has been reported in children [13, 23]. In children the presenting WBC has been somewhat higher in pre-B ALL but no data are available in adults.

Although a characteristic clinical and hematologic pattern at presentation appears to exist for non-T, non-B ALL, as shown in Table 9, this is a large group of ALL and within it are subgroups that are quite distinctive, both in terms of clinical and hematologic features at presentation and response to treatment. Some of these groups are beginning to be defined by cytogenetic analysis [71]. Examples of this include non-T, non-B ALL with the Philadelphia chromosome and non-T, non-B ALL with a t(4; 11) [131, 132, 71].

*2.6.2. T-ALL.* As in children, the clinical features of adult T-ALL are quite different from those of adult non-T, non-B ALL (Table 9). When adult patients from the same institutions are compared, those with T-ALL tend to be younger, more frequently male, and more frequently demonstrate lymphadenopathy and splenomegaly [70, 71, 76, 100, 112]. Almost half of the patients have had a mediastinal mass and 25% have had CNS leukemia at diagnosis.

The initial hematologic parameters have also differed. The presenting hemoglobin, platelet count, WBC and percent circulating blasts are higher in T-ALL than in non-T, non-B ALL. Almost 25% of adults with T-ALL have presented with leukocyte counts of more than $100 \times 10^9/l$, in comparison to less than 10% of patients with non-T, non-B ALL (Table 9).

*2.6.3. B-ALL.* The limited data in adult B-ALL also suggest a quite characteristic and distinctive clinical pattern (Table 9). These patients tend to be older than those with non-T, non-B or T-ALL. They have the highest male:female ratio. As in T-ALL, splenomegaly is particularly common and hepatomegaly is more frequent than in other types of adult ALL. Almost half of the patients present with CNS leukemia, a substantially higher fraction than in any other type of adult ALL. With regard to hematologic parameters, these patients more frequently present with low leukocyte counts and usually have a low percentage of circulating blasts.

Although the clinical features summarized in Table 9 are quite different from those seen in non-T, non-B ALL or T-ALL it is important to note that within the spectrum of adult B-ALL there appear to be two quite different subgroups—those with Burkitt's leukemia with the characteristic 8q—chromosome abnormality and other patients (who may usually cytogenetically have a 14q+ with material from a chromosome region other than the long arm of No. 8). Most of the cases summarized in Table 9 are Burkitt's leukemia; the clinical spectrum of the non-Burkitt group, which may represent peripheralizing malignant lymphoma, has not been well defined.

## 3. RESPONSE TO TREATMENT AND SURVIVAL ACCORDING TO ALL IMMUNOLOGIC CLASSES

Data are beginning to accumulate in adult ALL on the response to treatment and survival of patients according to general immunologic class. Results must be considered preliminary since the first large prospective trials including immunologic phenotype are still ongoing. In this section, data will be considered in four areas. First, response to treatment will be considered from two aspects—the achievement of complete remission and the duration of first remission. Survival according to immunologic class is then discussed. Finally, response to treatment and survival are considered relative to other known prognostic factors in ALL.

## 3.1. Achievement of Complete Remission

A number of recent studies have reported complete remission rates according to immunologic phenotype in adult ALL. For adult non-T, non-B ALL response rates of 67% to 86% have been noted (Table 10). In the one series of adults which evaluated common-ALL and null-ALL separately, the

Table 10. Response to therapy and survival according to immunologic classes in adult ALL.

|  | NON-T, NON-B | | T(E+)ALL | | B(SIg+)ALL | |
|---|---|---|---|---|---|---|
| **COMPLETE REMISSION RATE** | | | | | | |
| TIWCL [71] | 70% | (61) * | 79% | (19) * | 44% | (9) * |
| Lister et al. [50] | 79% | (34) | 60% | (5) | (0) | (1) |
| Baccarani et al. [135] | 81% | (31) | 88% | (8) | (1) † | (4) |
| University MN [76] | 67% | (24) | 75% | (8) | (0) | (3) |
| Liso et al. [100] | 69% | (16) | 33% | (6) | 43% | (7) ‡ |
| Borgström et al. [112] | 73% | (15) | 60% | (5) | (3) | (4) |
| Burns et al. [133] | 67% | (9) | 100% | (7) | – | (0) |
| Bitran [134] | 86% | (7) | 40% | (5) | (1) | (1) |
| Total | 74% | (197) | 71% | (63) | 41% | (29) |
| **MEDIAN DURATION FIRST REMISSION (Mos.)** | | | | | | |
| TIWCL [71] | 15 § | (42) | 7 | (14) | 4 | (4) |
| Lister et al. [50] | No Data | | 5, 10, 48+ | | No CR | |
| Baccarani et al. [135] | 15 | (25) | Not Reached | | No Data | |
| University MN [76] | 8+ | (16) | 17+ | (6) | No CR | |
| Borgström et al. [112] | 11+ | (11) | 2, 2, 7 | (3) | 3, 3, 7 | (3) |
| Burns et al. [133] | Not Reached | | 5 § | (7) | – | (0) |
| Bitran [134] | 18 | (6) | No Data | | 2 | (1) |
| **MEDIAN SURVIVAL (Mos.)** | | | | | | |
| TIWCL [71] | 15 § | (62) | 12 | (19) | 6§ | (9) |
| Baccarani et al. [135] | 26 | (31) | Not Reached | | No Data | |
| University MN [76] | 15 | (24) | 17 | (8) | 2 | (3) |
| Borgström et al. [112] | 14+ | (14) | 12 | (5) | 9 | (4) |
| Bitran [134] | 24 § | (7) | 9 | (5) | 1 | (8) ‡ |

* No. pts. studied.
† No. pts. achieving CR.
‡ Series from reference [130].
§ Projected from life table analysis.

response rates were comparable (78 % and 82 % respectively) [50]. Results in the other immunologic subclasses of non-T, non-B ALL have not been reported for adults. Among the few children studied, the remission rate for pre-B ALL appears comparable to that for other common-ALL patients [23, 75]. One small study of 13 children suggests a slightly lower response rate for pre-T ALL (77 % vs. 92 % for 91 children with common-ALL) [9]. Obviously more patients need to be studied.

Complete remission rates of 33 % to 100 % have been reported in adult T-ALL (Table 10). A review of eight series suggests that there are no significant differences in response rates between non-T, non-B ALL and T-ALL. This also appears to be the case for children [75]. In the four series with the largest numbers of cases of adult T-ALL, the response for T-ALL has been slightly higher than for non-T, non-B ALL [71, 133, 135, 76]. However, this comparison of response rates between immunologic groups must be viewed with caution since treatment has not always been the same for all patients [71, 76, 135] and in some reports treatment is not adequately indicated [100, 112]. It is quite likely that with some regimens the response rates will be comparable for non-T, non-B ALL and T-ALL and that for others a given immunologic group will respond better.

Remission rates in relatively few adults with B-ALL have been reported. The frequency of response in very small series has varied from 0 to 44 % (Table 10). More cases obviously need to be studied, but similar low remission rates in B-ALL relative to non-T, non-B or T-ALL have been reported in children [75].

Even though rates of remission induction have been similar in patients with non-T, non-B and T-ALL, medical complications arising during induction have been different. Metabolic problems may be more common in patients with T-ALL [116, 136]. These problems have included hyperkalemia, hypocalcemia, hyperphosphatemia, hyperuricemia and disseminated intravascular coagulation. Significant problems of this nature, for example, occurred in four of our eight adults with T-ALL and resulted in death within 48 hours in two of them. The reasons for the increased frequency of metabolic complications in T-ALL are unknown. The problems may be related to total tumor burden but do not appear to be solely related to high initial leukocyte counts. In two of our T-ALL patients with metabolic problems the initial WBC were 7 and $24 \times 10^9/l$, respectively. The acute tumor lysis syndrome has also been noted in B-ALL where the initial leukocyte count is usually low [137–139], although again the total tumor burden may be very high. Because of such metabolic problems, many oncologists start patients with T-ALL on low doses of prednisone initially and then escalate the intensity of therapy. Leukopheresis on admission should be considered for all patients who present with a WBC greater than $100.0 \times 10^9/l$ regardless of immunologic class since the cell lysis syndrome has also been reported in non-T, non-B ALL [140].

Other differences in medical complications during remission induction arise as a result of the large tumor masses frequently seen in patients with T- and B-ALL. Thus the superior vena caval syndrome is primarily seen in patients with T-ALL who have large mediastinal masses, and bowel obstructions are most common in patients with B-ALL who have large cecal masses. Similarly the high frequency of CNS involvement at diagnosis in T- and B-ALL create clinical problems that are rare in patients with non-T, non-B ALL.

## 3.2. Duration of Initial Complete Remission

Limited data are available on remission duration according to immunologic phenotype in adult ALL. Among patients with non-T, non-B ALL, projected median durations of first remission from 15 to 24 months have been reported (see Figure 1 and Table 10). In contrast, among children with non-T, non-B ALL median remissions of two to four years have been suggested in those few large series of children followed for median periods of at least several years [2, 7]. In those studies of children where projections of median remission duration are not possible, presumably because observation periods are short, more than 70% of patients remain in remission at 18 to 24 months [13, 57]. Although a more definitive answer will not be forthcoming until a number of large on-going studies have median follow-up periods of three to five years, it appears that among non-T, non-B ALL, adults have significantly shorter remissions than children.

Almost no data are available on remission duration for the immunologic subclasses of adult non-T, non-B ALL. In the one series which compared remission duration of common-ALL and null-ALL (in patients who lacked the Philadelphia chromosome), adults with common-ALL had significantly longer remissions (approximate medians of 44 vs. 10 months, $p = 0.01$) [141]. These results are comparable to those reported by three groups in children [3, 11, 142]. One group, however, has not found a significant difference in remission duration in children between those with and without the common-ALL antigen [7]. Obviously more data are required to confirm that remission duration is longer in common-ALL than in null-ALL.

Data regarding remission duration for pre-B or pre-T ALL in adults are not available. The Southwest Oncology Group has recently suggested that children with pre-B ALL may have shorter durations of complete remission than other children with non-T, non-B ALL, though the difference is not yet significant and a comparison with other children with common-ALL has not been reported [13]. Children with pre-T ALL have been suggested by two groups to have a poor prognosis compared to other children with non-T, non-B ALL [3, 9]. Many more patients must be studied before definite conclusions can be drawn regarding the significance of the pre-T and pre-B immunologic subtypes of non-T, non-B ALL relative to remission duration.

Remission duration in T-ALL in adults can only be evaluated in the four series in which six to 14 patients obtained a complete remission [71, 76, 133, 135]. Median remissions of five to more than 17 months were reported. Too few cases have been studied to compare remission duration for adult T-ALL with that of childhood T-ALL. In two of four series of adult ALL, the remission duration was longer in non-T, non-B ALL than in T-ALL [71, 133], though the difference was significant in only one series [133]. In two series the remission duration was comparable for non-T, non-B and T-ALL [76, 135]. Similar conflicting results have been reported in children. In most early reports remissions were significantly longer in children with non-T, non-B ALL [3, 7, 13, 57], but recently no significant differences have been seen between non-T, non-B ALL and T-ALL in a number of childhood series [71, 142, 143]. Whether these differences in results represent a change in therapy in recent years, differences in criteria for the diagnosis of T-ALL, or the confounding effects of other prognostic factors awaits multivariate analysis of large numbers of patients. Large studies prospectively evaluating multiple prognostic factors are now on-going in the large cooperative cancer study groups in the United States and England.

In addition to the differences in remission duration between non-T, non-B ALL and T-ALL seen in some series, several groups have suggested differences in the sites of relapse. Thus, among children, relapse in the central nervous system appears to be more frequent [7, 57, 144] and occur earlier [57, 144] in T-ALL than in non-T, non-B ALL. Relapse in the central nervous system has been reported in spite of central nervous system prophylactic therapy and has been more commonly associated with facial palsies [144]. CNS relapse has occurred even in the absence of high initial leukocyte counts [144]. In one study, testicular relapses were reported to be more common in T-ALL [7]. These results need to be confirmed in larger studies. It is unknown whether results will be similar in adult ALL.

Few remissions have been reported in adult B-ALL (Table 10). In almost all instances they have been of very short duration, usually in the range of two to four months. Results have been similar in children [130].

### 3.3. Survival

Fewer data are available on survival according to immunologic phenotype than on remission duration in adult ALL. In children it has been found that

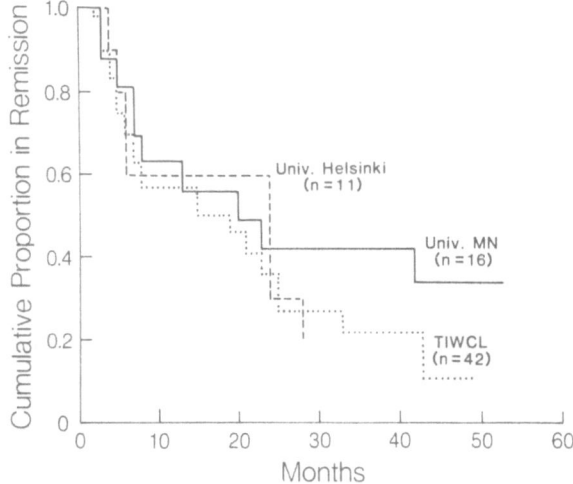

*Figure 1.* Remission duration in adult non-T, non-B ALL. Results from the University of Minnesota [76], the Third International Workshop on Chromosomes in Leukemia [71], and the University of Helsinki [112].

duration of survival tends to parallel duration of first remission. The limited information available suggests that such will also be the case for adults.

Among adults with non-T, non-B ALL, median survivals of 15 to 26 months have been reported (Table 10). These survivals are much shorter than those reported for children, in whom essentially all series have reported median survivals in excess of three years [63, 71, 145, 146]. In one

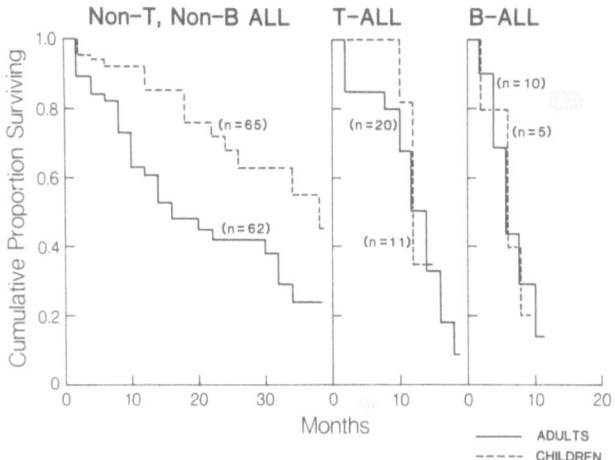

*Figure 2.* Survival according to immunologic phenotype; a comparison of children and adults with ALL. Data from the Third International Workshop on Chromosomes in Leukemia [71].

study, the median survival was suggested to be more than five years [146]. No data are available on survival among immunologic subgroups of non-T, non-B ALL in adults or children.

Among adults with T-ALL median survivals of nine to 17 months have been reported (Table 10). These results are similar to those published for children [63, 71, 145] (see Figure 2). In some series, survival for adults with T-ALL has been shorter than for those with non-T, non-B ALL [71, 112, 134] (Figure 3), but the difference has been statistically significant in only one small series [134]. In other series, survival among adults with T-ALL has been longer [76, 135], though the differences have not been significant. Among children, survival has almost always been longer for those with non-T, non-B ALL, although significance testing has not always been performed. Occasional groups have reported no differences in survival in children [143, 148].

Among adults with B-ALL, median survivals of one and six months have been reported in the two largest series [71, 130]. These results are comparable to those published for children [71, 130, 145]. In the only series which includes adequate numbers of adults with non-T, non-B ALL, T-ALL and B-ALL to make meaningful comparisons, patients with B-ALL had shorter survivals than those with T-ALL (p = 0.05) or non-T, non-B ALL (p = 0.03) (Figure 3). In two studies in children, results have been similar [71, 145, 147].

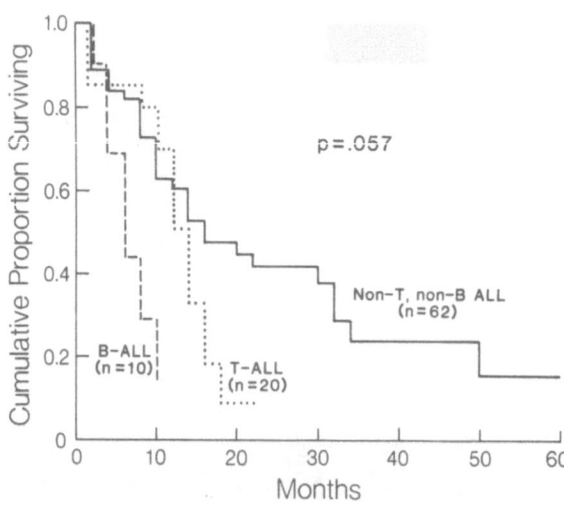

*Figure 3.* Survival according to immunologic phenotype in adult ALL. Data from the Third International Workshop on Chromosomes in Leukemia [71].

### 3.4. Immunologic Phenotype and Other Prognostic Variables

The above data suggest that immunologic classification as non-T, non-B ALL, T-ALL and B-ALL may be useful for predicting survival in adult ALL, although more large studies are needed to be certain. In the largest series reported to date [71], the p value for trend for duration of first remission was 0.12 and for survival was 0.057. Clearly these data are not as compelling as have been reported in children. In the above series, for example, among children the p value for trend for both remission duration and survival was 0.001 [71]. B-ALL clearly carries a poor prognosis. The difference in remission duration and survival is not clear between non-T, non-B ALL and T-ALL, at least in adults.

Non-T, non-B ALL encompasses a large fraction of adult ALL. It appears to include some adults who are cured and others who have short survivals. Among adults, as well as children, it has already been demonstrated that karyotype subdivides non-T, non-B ALL into groups with significantly different survivals [71]. It is quite possible that immunologic subclassification of non-T, non-B ALL may also separate the adult long-term survivors from other patients. It has been suggested by some preliminary studies in children that such will be the case.

Even if further study demonstrates that immunologic classification has prognostic or therapeutic significance in adult ALL, it will be necessary to demonstrate that it does so independent of other known prognostic factors. No multivariate analyses have been published evaluating immunologic class as an independent prognostic variable among adults with ALL. Even among children, the only published multivariate analyses of prognostic factors which have included immunologic class have involved no more than 100 patients, and thus cannot be considered definitive [74, 143].

Professor Anne Goldman has performed a multivariate analysis of prognostic factors on 152 patients from the Third International Workshop on Chromosomes in Leukemia; this series included a slight predominance of adult patients. Seven risk factors at diagnosis were evaluated including age, WBC, percent circulating blasts, FAB classification, the presence of a mediastinal mass, central nervous system leukemia, and immunologic class (non-T, non-B, T, B) [71]. The multiple survivorship model containing all seven risk factors effectively predicted survival (i.e., was significantly better for estimating survival than the model which assumed all patients had the same hazard). However, only age, WBC, and immunologic class contributed significantly to the model (each $p<0.05$). The model containing only these three risk factors predicted survival in a fashion similar to the model containing all seven factors. Similar results were obtained when the 121 patients who achieved a complete remission were analyzed for risk factors important in predicting duration of the first remission.

In almost all large series of ALL, multivariate analyses of prognostic factors have identified WBC at diagnosis as the major independent prognostic factor in addition to age [72, 142, 149]. Patients who present with low leukocyte counts have significantly longer initial remissions and survivals. Among childhood non-T, non-B ALL it has been shown that patients presenting with low leukocyte counts have significantly longer survivals [147]. Similar results for common-ALL in patients under 20 years of age for remission duration have been reported [3]. In this latter study, significant differences in remission duration between common-ALL and T-ALL disappeared when cases were adjusted for WBC. Thus, patients with common-ALL with high counts had remissions comparable to patients with T-ALL with similar counts. Analysis of survival according to presenting WBC in one adult series, also showed no significant difference between non-T, non-B ALL and T-ALL in each WBC group [71]. These data raise questions regarding the independent prognostic significance of immunologic class. However, in one study in children immunologic classification as T (T+) vs. non-T (Ia+) added significant prognostic information to age and WBC, although the numbers in some groups were very small [7].

These studies demonstrate the complexity of prognostic factors in ALL and reemphasize the need for a large prospective clinicopathologic study of adults with ALL. Such a study should include careful pretreatment evaluation of clinical features, detailed characterization of the leukemic blasts relative to immunologic markers, cytogenetics and morphology, and standardized treatment and follow-up evaluation.


4. PROSPECTS

This review suggests that the various immunologic classes of adult ALL have characteristic biologic and clinical features. This review also clearly indicates that little information is published, even relative to the broadest immunologic categories. Current studies that are on-going in cooperative cancer clinical trial groups and the larger single institutions will hopefully in the next five to ten years better define the biology and clinical course of both the general immunologic groups and their subclasses. These studies will also determine if immunologic phenotype has prognostic significance and whether this is independent of other clearly associated clinical features such as age, WBC, labelling index, and karyotype.

There is no obvious explanation for why immunologic markers should relate to response to treatment or survival. These gene products presumably have important cellular functions but there is no evidence that they in any way influence susceptibility to chemotherapy. If phenotype is related to prognosis it is presumably due to a non-random property of the cell type. Even so, several different uses of immunologic phenotype for selecting therapy have been proposed. None of these approaches have been adequately tested in patients with ALL, either adults or children, but they are interesting to consider.

It has been suggested that leukemic lymphoblasts with different immunologic phenotypes may have different sensitivities to specific drugs. Supporting data come from *in vivo* animal and *in vitro* cell culture studies. Thus the thymus derived AKR leukemia shows great sensitivity to cyclophosphamide and cytarabine and less sensitivity to methotrexate and 6MP [150]. The results are reversed in conventional non-T cell mouse lymphoid leukemia systems [7]. Similarly, differential chemosensitivity [151, 152] and radiosensitivity [153] of cultured T, B and non-T, non-B leukemic lymphocytes has been demonstrated. L-asparaginase, for example, was more active in T than in B or non-T, non-B ALL cell lines [151]. Similarly, thymidine was more active against T cells than B cells [152]. Confirmation of differential sensitivity in patients has not been done in a rigorous fashion. L-asparaginase and cytarabine have been reported to be effective in refractory T-ALL [154, 155]. However, in both reports, there were not significant differences between response rates in T-ALL and non-T, non-B ALL. Similarly, thymidine has been tried in T-ALL with peripheral clearing of blasts in one patient [156]. It is of interest that since regimens that include drugs such as L-asparaginase, adriamycin, and high dose cyclophosphamide, which may be particularly effective in T-ALL, have been used for therapy, studies have reported less difference in remission duration between T and non-T, non-B ALL.

A similar therapeutic approach has been to exploit differences in enzyme levels among immunologic phenotypes. For example, ADA levels have been highest in most series in T-ALL (see Table 5). Thus, the adenosine deaminase inhibitor 2′ deoxycoformycin has been used in refractory T-ALL, and has been reported to induce striking responses, including complete remissions [157, 158]. The specificity of these results for T-ALL however is unclear; insufficient numbers of cases of various immunologic types of ALL have been tested, but responses in B-CLL have been reported to low dose deoxycoformycin [159].

A second approach to using immunologic phenotype for selecting therapy is derived from the differences in clinical course of the various immunologic classes. Thus, since extramedullary relapses appear to be more frequent in T-ALL, it has been suggested that more intensive CNS therapy may be required for these patients, and that as a minimum they be monitored more carefully. Similarly, since patients with B- and T-ALL have been suggested to have poor survivals, especially following relapse, some investigators have performed marrow transplantation early in the course of these patients [160–162]. Preliminary results in children and young adults with relapsed T-ALL and newly diagnosed B-ALL have been promising, with long-term survivors reported. Further exploration of such approaches is required.

A final approach to the use of immunologic phenotype for therapy relates to the cell surface antigens themselves. Antisera have been raised to specific antigens, such as the common-ALL antigen. Such antibodies have been used in at least three ways. They have been used for serotherapy, for the removal of leukemic blasts from autologous marrow prior to reinfusion, and for the development of immunofluorescent assays that can detect leukemic cells not visable by light microscopy.

With the development of monoclonal hybridoma antibodies it is now possible to generate unlimited quantities of specific antibodies, thereby markedly increasing the feasibility of serotherapy. Serotherapy has been attempted in patients with refractory common-ALL with infusions of J5 monoclonal antibody [163, 164] and in a patient with T-ALL with infusion of L17512 antibody [165]. In all patients, decreases in circulating tumor cells were noted but antigenic modulation occurred and clinical benefit was limited. However these preliminary experiments demonstrate that serotherapy is feasible and further study is indicated. In mouse leukemia, therapy with monoclonal antibodies against a thymus differentiation antigen has been curative [166].

Antibodies prepared against the common-ALL antigen have also been used to treat marrow from patients with common-ALL collected during remission, with the aim of ridding the marrow of any residual leukemic cells. These marrows have then been reinfused following intensive treatment for relapse [167, 168]. Although only a few patients have been studied, it is clear that such autotransplantation is feasible. Further study is required to determine its efficacy.

A final potential use of immunologic markers for therapy relates to the use of the leukemic cell surface antigens for identifying malignant cells when they are present in such small quantities that they can not be detected morphologically. Thus, an immunofluorescent technique has been used to demonstrate common-ALL antigen on normal appearing lymphocytes in patients with common-ALL [169]. The potential of such an approach for early identification of relapse or detection of leukemic cells in extramedullary sites is obvious. Whether such monitoring will detect occult disease can, of course, only be determined by prospective study.

While these potential therapeutic approaches based on immunologic phenotype are of interest, even if none of them prove useful, lymphocyte surface markers should contribute to our understanding of the biology of the lymphoproliferative malignancies and leukemogenesis. For example, the fact that the antineuroblastoma monoclonal p1153/3 reacts with all common-ALL, most null-ALL, mature B-cell leukemias and normal B cells, but not T cells, suggests that most cases of non-T ALL are of B cell lineage [3, 26].

In addition, it is possible that immunologic phenotype will eventually allow us to understand one of the major clinical puzzles relative to ALL, i.e., why children have such a different response to treatment than adults. Current data suggest that for patients with T- and B-ALL, survival is similar in children and adults; the difference in survival by age appears to relate primarily to non-T, non-B ALL ($p = 0.001$) (Figure 2). Immunologic subclasses of non-T, non-B ALL appear to differ in frequency between children and adults (Table 2). At least one study suggests that when adults and children have the same immunologic phenotype (e.g., common-ALL) disease-free survival is similar [50]. The frequency of various karyotypes also differs between children and adults with non-T, non-B ALL; when identical karyotypes are present, survival is identical [71]. Further immunologic study (presumably with monoclonals) of non-T, non-B ALL is necessary to determine if patients with identical immunologic phenotypes will also have similar survivals independent of age. With more precise immunologic phenotyping highly selective therapy for adult ALL may finally be possible.

ACKNOWLEDGEMENT

The author is indebted to Ellis G. Levine, M. D. for critical review of the manuscript.

REFERENCES

1. Bloomfield CD, Gajl-Peczalska KJ: The clinical relevance of lymphocyte surface markers in leukemia and lymphoma. Curr Top Hematol 3:175-240, 1980.
2. Humphrey GB, Blackstock R, Filler J: Cell surface markers in acute lymphoblastic leukemia. Ann Clin Lab Sci 10:169-180, 1980.
3. Greaves MF: Analysis of the clinical and biological significance of lymphoid phenotypes in acute leukemia. Cancer Res 41:4752-4766, 1981.
4. Greaves M, Paxton A, Janossy G, Pain C, Johnson S, Lister TA: Acute lymphoblastic leukaemia associated antigen. III. Alterations in expression during treatment and in relapse. Leukemia Res 4:1-14, 1980.
5. LeBien TW, Hurwitz RL, Kersey JH: Characterization of a xenoantiserum produced against three molar KCl-solubilized antigens obtained from a non-T, non-B (pre-B) acute lymphoblastic leukemia cell line. J Immunol 122:82-88, 1979.
6. Pesando JM, Ritz J, Levine H, Terhorst C, Lazarus H, Schlossman SF: Human leukemia-associated antigen: relation to a family of surface glycoproteins. J Immunol 124:2794-2799, 1980.

7. Sallan SE, Ritz J, Pesando J, Gelber R, O'Brien C, Hitchcock S, Coral F, Schlossman, SF: Cell surface antigens: prognostic implications in childhood acute lymphoblastic leukemia. Blood 55:395–402, 1980.

8. Pesando JM, Ritz J, Lazarus H, Costello SB, Sallan S, Schlossman SF: Leukemia-associated antigens in ALL. Blood 54:1240–1248, 1979.

9. Thiel E, Rodt H, Huhn D, Netzel B, Grosse-Wilde H, Ganeshaguru K, Thierfelder S: Multimarker classification of acute lymphoblastic leukemia: evidence for further T subgroups and evaluation of their clinical significance. Blood 56:759–772, 1980.

10. Foon KA, Billing RJ, Terasaki PI, Cline MJ: Immunologic classification of acute lymphoblastic leukemia. Implications for normal lymphoid differentiation. Blood 56:1120–1126, 1980.

11. Morgan E, Hsu CCS: Prognostic significance of the acute lymphoblastic leukemia (ALL) cell-associated antigen in children with null-cell ALL. Am J Pediatr Hematol Oncol 2:99–102, 1980.

12. Veit BC, Melvin SL, Bowman WP: Identification of a leukemia-associated antigen of human acute lymphocytic leukemia. J Natl Cancer Inst 64:1321–1328, 1980.

13. Pullen DJ, Falletta JM, Crist WM, Vogler LB, Dowell B, Humphrey GB, Blackstock R, van Eys J, Cooper MD, Metzgar RS, Meydrech EF: Southwest Oncology Group experience with immunologic phenotyping in acute lymphocytic leukemia of childhood. Cancer Res 41:4802-4809, 1981.

14. Anderson JK, Moore JO, Falletta JM, Terry WF, Metzgar RS: Acute lymphoblastic leukemia: classification and characterization with antisera to human T-cell and Ia antigens. J Natl Cancer Inst 62:293–298, 1979.

15. Foon KA, Billing RJ, Terasaki PI: Dual B and T markers in acute and chronic lymphocytic leukemia. Blood 55:16–20, 1980.

16. Davey FR, Dock NL, Wolos JA, Terzian JA, Gottlieb AJ: Studies of mixed lymphocyte reactions, surface B cell antigens, and intracytoplasmic immunoglobulins in 'null cell' acute lymphocytic leukemia. Cancer 44:1622–1628, 1979.

17. Nadler LM, Reinherz EL, Weinstein HJ, D'Orsi CJ, Schlossman SF: Heterogeneity of T-cell lymphoblastic malignancies. Blood 55:806–810, 1980.

18. Reinherz EL, Nadler LM, Sallan SE, Schlossman SF: Subset derivation of T-cell acute lymphoblastic leukemia in man. J Clin Invest 64: 392–397, 1979.

19. Janossy G, Bollum FJ, Bradstock KF, Ashley J: Cellular phenotypes of normal and leukemic hemopoietic cells determined by analysis with selected antibody combinations. Blood 56:430–441, 1980.

20. Vogler LB, Crist WM, Bockman DE, Pearl ER, Lawton AR, Cooper MD: Pre-B-cell leukemia. A new phenotype of childhood lymphoblastic leukemia. N Engl J Med 298:872–878, 1978.

21. LeBien TW, Hozier J, Minowada J, Kersey JH: Origin of chronic myelocytic leukemia in a precursor of pre-B lymphocytes. N Engl J Med 301:144–147, 1979.

22. Brouet JC, Preud'Homme JL, Penit C, Valensi F, Rouget P, Seligmann M: Acute lymphoblastic leukemia with pre-B-cell characteristics. Blood 54:269–273, 1979.

23. Greaves M, Verbi W, Vogler L, Cooper M, Ellis R, Ganeshaguru K, Hoffbrand V, Janossy G, Bollum FJ: Antigenic and enzymatic phenotypes of the pre-B subclass of acute lymphoblastic leukaemia. Leukemia Res 3:353–362, 1979.

24. Greaves MF, Verbi W, Reeves BR, Hoffbrand AV, Drysdale HC, Jones L, Sacker LS, Samaratunga I: 'Pre-B' phenotypes in blast crisis of Ph[1] positive CML: evidence for a pluripotential stem cell 'target.' Leukemia Res 3:181–191, 1979.

25. Abramson CS, Kersey JH, LeBien TW: A monoclonal antibody (BA-1) reactive with cells of human B lymphocyte lineage. J Immunol 126:83–88, 1981.

26. Kennett RH, Gilbert F: Hybrid myelomas producing antibodies against a human neuro-blastoma antigen present on fetal brain. Science 203:1120–1121, 1979.

27. Greaves MF: Analysis of human leukaemic cell populations using monoclonal antibodies and the fluorescence activated cell sorter. In: Proc IX Int Conf on Comparative Research on Leukaemia and Related Diseases, Yohn D (ed). Elsevier/North Holland (in press).

28. Brooks DA, Beckman I, Bradley J, McNamara PJ, Thomas ME, Zola H: Human lympho-cyte markers defined by antibodies derived from somatic cell hydrids. I. A hybridoma secreting antibody against a marker specific for human B lymphocytes. Clin Exp Immunol 39:477–485, 1980.

29. Stashenko P, Nadler LM, Hardy R, Schlossman SF: Characterization of a human B lym-phocyte-specific antigen . J Immunol 125:1678–1685, 1980.

30. Nadler LM, Stashenko P, Hardy R, Schlossman SF: A monoclonal antibody defining a lymphoma-associated antigen in man. J Immunol 125:570–577, 1980.

31. Brooks DA, Beckman IGR, Gradley J, Zola H: A hybridoma antibody directed against a B cell subpopulation marker. Proc 4th Internatl Congr. Immunol: 6:603, 1980 (Abstr).

32. Brodsky FM, Parham P, Barnstable CJ, Crumpton MJ, Bodmer WF: Monoclonal antibod-ies for analysis of the HLA system. Immunol Rev 47:3–61, 1979.

33. Hansen JA, Martin PJ, Nowinski RC: Monoclonal antibodies identifying a novel T-cell antigen and Ia antigens of human lymphocytes. Immunogenetics 10:247–260, 1980.

34. Reinherz EL, Kung PC, Pesando JM, Ritz J, Goldstein G, Schlossman SF: Ia determinants on human T-cell subsets defined by monoclonal antibody. J Exp Med 150:1472–1482, 1979.

35. Kamoun M, Martin PJ, Hansen JA, Brown MA, Siadak AW, Nowinski RC: Identification of a human T lymphocyte surface protein associated with the E-rosette receptor. J Exp Med (in press).

36. Kung PC, Talle MA, DeMaria ME, Butler MS, Lifter J, Goldstein G: Strategies for gen-erating monoclonal antibodies defining human T-lymphocyte differentiation antigens. Transplant Proc Vol XII, No 3, Suppl 1 (Sept), 141–146, 1980.

37. Royston I, Majda JA, Baird SM, Meserve BL, Griffiths JC: Human T cell antigens defined by monoclonal antibodies: The 65,000-Dalton antigen of T cells (T65) is also found on chronic lymphocytic leukemia cells bearing surface immunoglobulin. J Immunol 125:725–731, 1980.

38. Zipf TF, Fox RI, Dilley J, Levy R: Definition of the high risk acute lymphoblastic leu-kemia patient by immunologic phenotyping with monoclonal antibodies. Cancer Res 41:4786–4789, 1981.

39. Wang CY, Good RA, Ammirati P, Dymbort G, Evans RL: Identification of a p69,71 complex expressed on human T cells sharing determinants with B-type chronic lymphatic leukemic cells. J Exp Med 151:1539–1544, 1980.

40. Reinherz EL, Kung PC, Goldstein G, Levey RH, Schlossman SF: Discrete stages of human intrathymic differentiation: analysis of normal thymocytes and leukemic lymphoblasts of T-cell lineage. Proc Natl Acad Sci 77:1588–1592, 1980.

41. Reinherz EL, Schlossman SF: Derivation of human T-cell leukemias Cancer Res 41:4767–4770, 1981.

42. Kung PC, Goldstein G, Reinherz EL, Schlossman SF: Monoclonal antibodies defining distinctive human T cell surface antigens. Science 206:347–349, 1979.

43. McMichael AJ, Pilch JR, Galfré G, Mason DY, Fabre JW, Milstein C: A human thymo-cyte antigen defined by a hybrid myeloma monoclonal antibody. Eur J Immunol 9:205–210, 1979.

44. Bradstock KF, Janossy G, Pizzolo G, Hoffbrand AV, McMichael A, Pilch JR, Milstein C, Beverley P, Bollum FJ: Subpopulations of normal and leukemic human thymocytes: an analysis with the use of monoclonal antibodies. J Natl Cancer Inst 65:33–42, 1980.

45. Bradstock KF, Janossy G, Bollum FJ, Milstein C: Anomalous phenotype in thymic acute lymphoblastic leukaemia. Nature 284:455–457, 1980.

46. Levy R, Dilley J, Fox RI, Warnke R: A human thymus-leukemia antigen defined by hybridoma monoclonal antibodies. Proc Natl Acad Sci 76:6552–6556, 1979.

47. Ritz J, Pesando JM, Notis-McConarty J, Lazarus H, Schlossman SF: A monoclonal antibody to human acute lymphoblastic leukaemia antigen. Nature 283:583–585, 1980.

48. Kersey JH, LeBien TW, Abramson CS, Newman R, Sutherland DR, Greaves M: p24: A human leukemia-associated and lymphohemopoietic progenitor cell surface structure identified with monoclonal antibody. J Exp Med 153:726–731, 1981.

49. Catovsky D, Pittman S, O'Brien M, Cherchi M, Costello C, Foa R, Pearce E, Hoffbrand AV, Janossy G, Ganeshaguru K, Greaves MF: Multiparameter studies in lymphoid leukemias. Am J Clin Pathol 72:736–745, 1979.

50. Lister TA, Roberts MM, Brearley RL, Woodruff RK, Greaves MF: Prognostic significance of cell surface phenotype in adult acute lymphoblastic leukaemia. Cancer Immunol Immunother 6:227–230, 1979.

51. LeBien TW, Parkin JL, Brunning RD, Kersey JH: Immunologic and ultrastructural heterogeneity of acute lymphoblastic leukemia-associated antigen-positive human leukemias. J Natl Cancer Inst 65: 1231–1236, 1980.

52. Richie ER, Culbert SJ, Sullivan MP, van Eys J: Complement receptor-positive, sheep erythrocyte receptor-negative lymphoblasts in childhood acute lymphocytic leukemia. Cancer Res 38:3616–3620, 1978.

53. Richie ER, Sullivan MP, van Eys J: A unique surface marker profile in T-cell acute lymphocytic leukemia. Blood 55:702–705, 1980.

54. Levin S, Russell EC, Blanchard D, McWilliams NB, Maurer HM, Mohanakumar T: Receptors for peanut agglutinin (Arachus hypogea) in childhood acute lymphoblastic leukemia: possible clinical significance. Blood 55:37–39, 1980.

55. Beck JD, Haghbin M, Wollner N, Mertelsmann R, Garrett T, Koziner B, Clarkson B, Miller D, Good RA, Gupta S: Subpopulations of human T lymphocytes. VI. Analysis of cell markers in acute lymphoblastic leukemia with special reference to FC receptor expression on E-rosette-forming blasts. Cancer 46:45–49, 1980.

56. Burns GF, Cawley JC, Worman CP, Barker CR, Hayhoe FGJ: The distribution of a receptor for IgM (µFcR) on haemic cells. Am J Hematol 6:243–251, 1979.

57. Brouet JC, Seligmann M: The immunological classification of acute lymphoblastic leukemias. Cancer 42:817–827, 1978.

58. Magrath IT, Ziegler JL: Bone marrow involvement in Burkitt's lymphoma and its relationship to acute B-cell leukemia. Leukemia Res 4:33–59, 1979.

59. Nakahara K, Ohashi T, Oda T, Hirano T, Kasai M, Okumura K, Tada T: Asialo $GM_1$ as a cell-surface marker detected in acute lymphoblastic leukemia. N Engl J Med 302:674–677, 1980.

60. Balch CM, Dougherty PA, Vogler LB, Ades EW, Ferrone S: A new B-cell differentiation antigen (BDA) on normal and leukemic human B lymphocytes that is distinct from known DR (Ia-like) antigens, J Immunol 121:2322–2328, 1978.

61. Koziner B, Kempin S, Passe S, Gee T, Good RA, Clarkson BD: Characterization of B-cell leukemias: a tentative immunomorphological scheme. Blood 56: 815–823, 1980.

62. LeBien TW, McKenna RW, Abramson CS, Gajl-Peczalska KJ, Nesbit ME, Coccia PF, Bloomfield CD, Brunning RD, Kersey JH: Use of monoclonal antibodies, morphology, and cytochemistry to probe the cellular heterogeneity of acute leukemia and lymphoma. Cancer Res 41:4776-4780.

63. Heideman RL, Falletta JM, Mukhopadhyay N, Fernbach DJ: Lymphocytic leukemia in children: prognostic significance of clinical and laboratory findings at time of diagnosis. J Pediatr 92:540–545, 1978.

64. Borella L, Casper JT, Lauer SJ: Shifts in expression of cell membrane phenotypes in childhood lymphoid malignancies at relapse. Blood 54:64–71, 1979.

65. Bennett JM, Catovsky D, Daniel MT, Flandrin G, Galton DAG, Gralnick HR, Sultan C: Proposals for the classification of the acute leukaemias. Br J Haematol 33:451–458, 1976.

66. Bennett JM, Catovsky D, Daniel MT, Flandrin G, Galton DAG, Gralnick HR, Sultan C: The morphological classification of acute lymphoblastic leukaemia: concordance among observers and clinical correlations. Br J Haematol 47:553–561, 1981.

67. Miller DR, Leikin S, Albo V, Hammond D: Prognostic significance of lymphoblast morphology (FAB classification) in childhood leukemia (ALL). Proc Am Soc Clin Oncol 20:345, 1979. (Abstr)

68. Brearley RL, Johnson SAN, Lister TA: Acute lymphoblastic leukaemia in adults: clinico-pathological correlations with the French-American-British (FAB) co-operative group classification. Eur J Cancer 15:909–914, 1979.

69. Leimert JT, Burns CP, Wiltse CG, Armitage JO, Clarke WR: Prognostic influence of pretreatment characteristics in adult acute lymphoblastic leukemia. Blood 56:510–515, 1980.

70. Ruggero D, Baccarani M, Gobbi M, Tura S: Adult acute lymphoblastic leukaemia: study of 32 patients and analysis of prognostic factors. Scand J Haematol 22:154–164, 1979.

71. Third International Workshop on Chromosomes in Leukemia: Clinical significance of chromosomal abnormalities in acute lymphoblastic leukemia. Cancer Genet Cytogenet 4:111-137, 1981.

72. McKenna RW, Brynes RK, Nesbit ME, Bloomfield CD, Kersey JH, Spanjers E, Brunning RD: Cytochemical profiles in acute lymphoblastic leukemia. Am J Pediatr Hematol Oncol 3:263-275, 1979.

73. Coccia PF, Miller DR, Kersey JH, Bleyer WA, Gross S, Siegel SE, Sather HN, Hammond GD: Relationship of blast cell surface markers and morphology (FAB classification) in childhood acute lymphocytic leukemia (ALL). Blood 54(Suppl 1):182a, 1979. (Abstr)

74. Palmer MK, Hann IM, Jones PM, Evans DIK: A score at diagnosis for predicting length of remission in childhood acute lymphoblastic leukemia. Br J Cancer 42:841–849, 1980.

75. Bloomfield CD: Classification and prognosis of acute lymphoblastic leukemia. Progress in Clinical and Biological Research 58 (The Lymphocyte):167–183, 1981.

76. Hurd DD, LeBien TW, Peterson BA, Kersey J, Gajt Pectalska K, Bloomfield CD: Clinical relevance of immunologic classification in adult acute lymphoblastic leukemia (in preparation).

77. Koziner B, Mertelsmann R, Andreeff M, Arlin Z, Hansen H, De Harven E, McKenzie S, Gee T, Good RA, Clarkson B: Heterogeneity of cell lineages in L3 leukemias. Blood 55:694–698, 1980.

78. Ganick DJ, Finlay JL: Acute lymphoblastic leukemia with Burkitt cell morphology and cytoplasmic immunoglobulin. Blood 56:311–314, 1980.

79. McKenna RW, Parkin J, Brunning RD: Morphologic and ultrastructural characteristics of T-cell acute lymphoblastic leukemia. Cancer 44:1290–1297, 1979.

80. Hann IM, Evans DIK, Palmer MK, Jones PJM, Haworth C: The prognostic significance of morphological features in childhood acute lymphoblastic leukaemia. Clin Lab Haemat 1:215–226, 1979.

81. Raney RB, Jr., Festa RS, Waldman MTG, Manson D, Hann HWL: The periodic acid–Schiff reaction and prognosis in children with acute lymphoblastic leukemia. Am J Hematol 6:27–34, 1979.

82. Brouet JC, Valensi F, Daniel MT, Flandrin G, Preud'homme JL, Seligmann M: Immunological classification of acute lymphoblastic leukaemias: evaluation of its clinical significance in a hundred patients. Br J Haematol 33:319–328, 1976.

83. Goldberg AF, Barka T: Acid phosphatase activity in human blood cells. Nature 195:297, 1962.
84. Li C-Y, Yam LT, Lam KW: Acid phosphatase isoenzyme in human leukocytes in normal and pathologic conditions. J Histochem Cytochem 18:473–481, 1970.
85. Lilleyman JS, Britton JA, Laycock BJ, Sugden PJ: Sex and acid phosphatase in childhood non-T lymphoblastic leukaemia. J Clin Pathol 33:151–154, 1980.
86. Berger R, Bernheim A, Brouet JC, Daniel MT, Flandrin G: t(8;14) translocation in a Burkitt's type of lymphoblastic leukaemia (L3). Br J Haematol 43:87–90, 1979.
87. Kulenkampff J, Janossy G, Greaves MF: Acid esterase in human lymphoid cells and leukaemic blasts: a marker for T lymphocytes. Br J Haematol 36:231–240, 1977.
88. Knowles DM, Halper JP, Machin GA, Sherman W: Acid §-naphthyl acetate esterase activity in human neoplastic lymphoid cells. Am J Pathol 96:257–277, 1979.
89. Yam LT, Li CY, Crosby WH: Cytochemical identification of monocytes and granulocytes. Am J Clin Pathol 55:283–290, 1971.
90. Barr RD, Perry S: Lysosomal acid hydrolases in human lymphocyte subpopulations. Br J Haematol 32:565–572, 1976.
91. Machin GA, Halper JP, Knowles DM: Cytochemically demonstrable β-glucuronidase activity in normal and neoplastic human lymphoid cells. Blood 56:1111–1119, 1980.
92. Bollum FJ: Terminal deoxynucleotidyl transferase as a hematopoietic cell marker. Blood 54:1203–1215, 1979.
93. Janossy G, Bollum FJ, Bradstock KF, McMichael A, Rapson NT, Greaves MF: Terminal transferase-positive human bone marrow cells exhibit the antigenic phenotype of common acute lymphoblastic leukemia. J Immunol 123:1525–1529, 1979.
94. Bradstock KF, Janossy G, Hoffbrand AV, Ganeshaguru K, Llewellin P, Prentice HG, Bollum FJ: Immunofluorescent and biochemical studies of terminal deoxynucleotidyl transferase in treated acute leukaemia. Br J Haematol 47:121–131, 1981.
95. Janossy G, Hoffbrand AV, Greaves MF, Ganeshaguru K, Pain C, Bradstock KF, Prentice HG, Kay HEM, Lister TA: Terminal transferase enzyme assay and immunological membrane markers in the diagnosis of leukaemia: a multiparameter analysis of 300 cases. Br J Haematol 44:221–234, 1980.
96. Srivastava BIS, Khan SA, Minowada J, Henderson ES, Rakowski I: Terminal deoxynucleotidyl transferase activity and blast cell characteristics in adult acute leukemias. Leukemia Res 4:209–215, 1980.
97. Shaw MT, Dwyer JM, Allaudeen HS, Weitzman HA: Terminal deoxyribonucleotidyl transferase activity in B-cell acute lymphocytic leukemia. Blood 51:181–187, 1978.
98. Gordon DS, Hutton JJ, Smalley RV, Meyer LM, Vogler WR: Terminal deoxynucleotidyl transferase (TdT), cytochemistry, and membrane receptors in adult acute leukemia. Blood 52:1079–1088, 1978.
99. Smyth JF, Poplack DG, Holiman BJ, Leventhal BG, Yarbro G: Correlation of adenosine deaminase activity with cell surface markers in acute lymphoblastic leukemia. J Clin Invest 62:710–712, 1978.
100. Liso V, Tursi A, Specchia G, Troccoli G, Loria MP, Bonomo L: Adenosine deaminase activity in acute lymphoblastic leukaemia: Cytochemical, immunological and clinical correlations. Scand J Haematol 21:167–175, 1978.
101. Ben-Bassat I, Simoni F, Holtzman F, Ramot B: Adenosine deaminase activity of normal lymphocytes and leukemic cells. Isr J Med Sci 15:925–927, 1979.
102. Chechik BE, Rao J, Greaves MF, Hoffbrand AV: Human thymus/leukaemia-associated antigen (a low-molecular weight form of adenosine deaminase) and the phenotype of leukaemic cells. Leukemia Res 4:343–349, 1980.
103. Ellis RB, Rapson NT, Patrick AD, Greaves M: Expression of hexosaminidase isoenzymes in childhood leukemia. N Engl J Med 298:476–480, 1978.

104. Dewji N, Rapson N, Greaves M, Ellis R: Isoenzyme profiles of lysosomal hydrolases in leukaemic cells. Leukemia Res 5:19–27, 1981.

105. Besley GTN, Broadhead DM, Bain AD, Dewar AE, Eden OB: Enzyme markers in acute lymphoblastic leukaemia. Lancet ii:1311, 1978.

106. Broadhead DM, Besley GTN, Moss SE, Bain AD, Eden OB, Sainsbury CPQ: Recognition of abnormal lysosomal enzyme patterns in childhood leukaemia by isoelectric focusing, with special reference to some properties of abnormally expressed components. Leukemia Res 5:29–40, 1981.

107. Reaman GH, Levin N, Muchmore A, Holiman BJ, Poplack DG: Diminished lymphoblast 5'-nucleotidase activity in acute lymphoblastic leukemia with T-cell characteristics. N Engl J Med 300:1374–1377, 1979.

108. Blatt J, Reaman GH, Levin N, Poplack DG: Purine nucleoside phosphorylase activity in acute lymphoblastic leukemia. Blood 56:380–382, 1980.

109. Blatt J, Reaman G, Poplack DG: Biochemical markers in lymphoid malignancy: N Engl J Med 303:918–922, 1980.

110. Bloomfield CD, Lindquist LL, Arthur D, McKenna RW, LeBien TW, Peterson BA, Nesbit ME: Chromosomal abnormalities in acute lymphoblastic leukemia. Cancer Res 41:4838–4843, 1981.

111. Arthur DC, Bloomfield CD, Lindquist LL, Peterson BA, Nesbit ME: Chromosome abnormalities in acute lymphoblastic leukemia (ALL): frequency and clinical implications. Proc Amer Soc Clin Oncol 22:345, 1981. (Abstr)

112. Borgström GH, Teerenhovi, Vuopio P, Andersson LC, Knuutila S, Elonen E, de la Chapelle A: Chromosome studies in acute lymphoblastic leukaemia (ALL). Scand J Haematol 26:241–251, 1981.

113. Kaneko Y, Rowley JD: Correlation of karyotype with prognosis in acute lymphocytic leukemia (ALL). Proc Amer Soc Clin Oncol 22:338, 1981. (Abstr)

114. Brodeur GM, Williams DL, Bowman WP, Look AT, Kalwinsky DK, Aur RJA, Rivera G, Dahl GV: Cytogenetic features of acute lymphoblastic leukemia (ALL) in children. Proc Amer Assoc Cancer Res 22:45, 1981. (Abstr)

115. Oshimura M, Freeman AI, Sandberg AA: Chromosomes and causation of human cancer and leukemia. Cancer 40:1161–1172, 1977.

116. Bloomfield CD, Brunning R, Kersey J, Gajl-Peczalska KJ: Adult acute lymphocytic leukemia (ALL): the therapeutic significance of surface markers (SM) and the Philadelphia chromosome (Ph). Proc Amer Assoc Cancer Res 17:166, 1976. (Abstr)

117. Vogler LB, Crist WM, Vinson PC, Brattain MG, Sarrif AM, Coleman MS: Philadelphia chromosome-positive pre-B cell leukemia presenting as blastic myelogenous leukemia. Blood 52:279, 1978. (Abstr)

118. Kaneko Y, Rowley JD, Check I, Variakojis D, Moohr JW: The 14q+ chromosome in pre-B-ALL. Blood 56:782–785, 1980.

119. Roozendaal KJ, van der Reijden HJ, Geraedts JPM: Philadelphia chromosome positive acute lymphoblastic leukaemia with T-cell characteristics. Br J Haematol 47:145–147, 1981.

120. Mastrangelo R, Malandrino R, Riccardi R, Longo P, Ranelletti FO, Iacobelli S: Clinical implications of glucocorticoid receptor studies in childhood acute lymphoblastic leukemia. Blood 56:1036–1040, 1980.

121. Bloomfield CD, Peterson BA, Zaleskas J, Frizzera G, Smith KA, Hildebrandt L, Gajl-Peczalska KJ, Munck A: In-vitro glucocorticoid studies for predicting response to glucocorticoid therapy in adults with malignant lymphoma. Lancet i:952–956, 1980.

122. Bloomfield CD, Smith KA, Peterson BA, Munck A: Glucocorticoid receptors in adult acute lymphoblastic leukemia. Cancer Res 41:4857–4860, 1981.

123. Lippman ME, Yarbro GK, Leventhal BG: Clinical implications of glucocorticoid receptors in human leukemia. Cancer Res 38:4251–4256, 1978.

124. Nakao Y, Tsuboi S, Fujita T, Masaoka T, Morikawa S, Watanabe S: Glucocorticoid receptors and terminal deoxynucleotidyl transferase activities in leukemic cells. Cancer 47:1812–1817, 1981.

125. Bell PA: Glucocorticoids and leukaemia. Clinics in Oncology (in press).

126. Ho AD, Brandeis WE, Hunstein W, Denk B: Terminal deoxynucleotidyl transferase activity, glucocorticoid receptors and sensitivity in acute lymphoblastic leukaemia (in press).

127. Yarbro GSK, Lippman ME, Johnson GE, Leventhal BG: Glucocorticoid receptors in subpopulations of childhood acute lymphocytic leukemia. Cancer Res 37:2688–2695, 1977.

128. Konior G, Johnson G, Lippman M, Ziegler J, Leventhal BG: Glucocorticoid receptors in Burkitt's lymphoma (BL) and poorly differentiated lymphocytic lymphoma (PDLL). Blood 48:995, 1976. (Abstr).

129. Crist W, Vogler L, Sarrif A, Pullen J, Bartolucci A, Falletta J, Humphrey B, van Eys J, Cooper M: Clinical and laboratory characterization of pre-B cell leukemia in children. Blood 54 (Suppl 1):183a, 1979. (Abstr).

130. Preud'Homme JL, Brouet JC, Danon F, Flandrin G, Schaison G: Acute lymphoblastic leukemia with Burkitt's lymphoma cells: membrane markers and serum immunoglobulin. J Natl Cancer Inst 66:261–264, 1981.

131. Bloomfield CD, Peterson LC, Yunis JJ, Brunning RD: The Philadelphia chromosome (Ph[1]) in adults presenting with acute leukaemia: a comparison of Ph[1]+ and Ph[1]– patients. Br J Haematol 36:347–358, 1977.

132. Arthur DC, Bloomfield CD, Lindquist LL, Nesbit ME: Translocation 4;11 in acute lymphoblastic leukemia: Clinical characteristics and prognostic significance. Blood 59:96-99, 1982.

133. Burns CP, Armitage JO, Aunan SB, Gingrich RD, Dick FR, Maguire LC, Leimert JT: Therapy of adult acute lymphoblastic leukemia: superior results of null vs. T-cell disease. Proc Am Soc Clin Oncol 22:485, 1981. (Abstr).

134. Bitran JD: Prognostic value of immunologic markers in adults with acute lymphoblastic leukemia. N Engl J Med 299:1317, 1978.

135. Baccarani M, Gobbi M, Tura S: Prognostic value of immunologic markers in adults with acute lymphoblastic leukemia. N Engl J Med 302:123, 1980.

136. French AJ, Lilleyman JS: Bleeding tendency of T-cell lymphoblastic leukaemia. Lancet ii:469–470, 1979.

137. Hutchins MR, Hussein KK, Bottomley RH: Burkitt cell variant of acute lymphoblastic leukemia (ALL). Proc Am Soc Clin Oncol 21:444, 1980. (Abstr).

138. Cohen LF, Balow JE, Magrath IT, Poplack DG, Ziegler JL: Acute tumor lysis syndrome . A review of 37 patients with Burkitt's lymphoma. Am J Med 68:486–491, 1980.

139. Tsokos GC, Balow JE, Spiegel RJ, Magrath IT: Renal and metabolic complications of undifferentiated and lymphoblastic lymphomas. Medicine 60:218–229, 1981.

140. Champion LAA, Luddy RE, Schwartz AD: Disseminated intravascular coagulation in childhood acute lymphocytic leukemia with poor prognostic features. Cancer 41:1642–1646, 1978.

141. Greaves MF, Lister TA: Prognostic importance of immunologic markers in adult acute lymphoblastic leukemia. N Engl J Med 304:119–120, 1981.

142. Grossi M, Minowada J, Jung O, Sagawa K, Morita M, Freeman AI: Prognostic factors and surface markers in children and adolescents with acute lymphoblastic leukemia (ALL). Proc Am Assoc Clin Res 22:152, 1981. (Abstr).

143. Hann HWL, Listbader ED, Evans AE, Toledano SR, Lillie PD, Jasko LB: Lack of influence of T-cell marker and importance of mediastinal mass on the prognosis of acute lymphocytic leukemias of childhood. J Natl Cancer Inst 66:285–290, 1981.

144. Lilleyman JS, Sugden PJ: T lymphoblastic leukaemia and the central nervous system. Br J Cancer 43:320–323, 1981.

145. Kersey J, Coccia P, Bloomfield C, Nesbit M, McKenna R, Brunning R, Hallgren H, Gajl-Peczalska K: Surface markers define human lymphoid malignancies with differing prognoses. Haematol and Blood Transfusion 20:17–24, 1977.

146. Frei E, Sallan SE: Acute lymphoblastic leukemia: treatment. Cancer 42:828–838, 1978.

147. Coccia PF, Kersey JH, Gajl-Peczalska KJ, Krivit W, Nesbit ME: Prognostic significance of surface marker analysis in childhood non-Hodgkin's lymphoproliferative malignancies. Am J Hematol 1:405–417, 1976.

148. Pasino M, Rosanda-Vadala C, Astaldi A, Tonini GP, Astaldi GCB, Perutelli P, Comelli A, De Bernardi B, Giovanelli A, Mori PG, Massimo L: Scand J Haematol 20:147–152, 1978.

149. Robison LL, Nesbit ME, Sather HN, Hammond GD, Coccia PF: Assessment of the inter-relationship of prognostic factors in childhood acute lymphoblastic leukemia. A report from Childrens Cancer Study Group. Am J Pediatr Hematol Oncol 2:5–13, 1980.

150. Frei E, Schabel FM, Goldin A: Comparative chemotherapy of AKR lymphoma and human hematological neoplasia. Cancer Res 34:184–193, 1974.

151. Beranek JT, Takahashi I, Ohnuma T, Holland JF, Minowada J: Differential chemosensitivity of T, B, and non T-non B leukemic cells in culture. Proc Am Soc Clin Oncol 21:443, 1980. (Abstr).

152. Fox RM, Piddington SK, Tripp EH, Dudman NP, Tattersall MHN: Thymidine sensitivity of cultured leukaemic lymphocytes. Lancet i:391–393, 1979.

153. Nakazawa S, Minowada J, Tsubota T, Sinks LF: Profound radiosensitivity in 'leukemic' T-cell lines and T-cell-type acute lymphoblastic leukemia demonstrated by sodium {$^{51}$Cr} chromate labeling. Cancer Res 38:1661–1666, 1978.

154. Steuber CP, Levy GJ, Nix WL, Shepherd DA, Starling KA, Fernbach DJ: Use of L-asparaginase and cytosine arabinoside for refractory acute lymphocytic leukemia with particular reference to T-cell leukemia. Med Pediatr Oncol 5:33–38, 1978.

155. Rivera G, Dahl GV, Bowman WP, Avery TL, Wood A, Aur RJ: VM-26 and cytosine arabinoside combination chemotherapy for initial induction failures in childhood lymphocytic leukemia. Cancer 46:1727–1730, 1980.

156. Howell SB, Chu B, Mendelsohn J, Carson DA, Kung FH, Seegmiller JE: Thymidine as a chemotherapeutic agent: pharmacologic, cytokinetic, and biochemical studies in a patient with T-cell acute lymphocytic leukemia. J Natl Cancer Inst 65:277–284, 1980.

157. Prentice HG, Smyth JF, Ganeshaguru K, Wonke B, Bradstock KF, Janossy G, Goldstone AH, Hoffbrand AV: Remission induction with adenosine-deaminase inhibitor 2'-deoxycoformycin in thy-lymphoblastic leukaemia. Lancet ii:170–172, 1980.

158. Mitchell BS, Koller CA, Heyn R: Inhibition of adenosine deaminase activity results in cytotoxicity to T lymphoblasts in vivo. Blood 56:556–559, 1980.

159. Grever MR, Siaw MFE, Jacob WF, Neidhart JA, Miser JS, Coleman MS, Hutton JJ, Balcerzak SP: The biochemical and clinical consequences of 2'-deoxycoformycin in refractory lymphoproliferative malignancy. Blood 57:406–417, 1981.

160. O'Leary M, Ramsay NKC, Nesbit ME, Krivit W, Coccia PF, Kim TH, Kersey JH: Bone marrow transplantation (BMT) for childhood non-Hodgkin's lymphoma (NHL). Proc Am Assoc Cancer Res 21:173, 1980. (Abstr)

161. Garrett TJ, Grossbard E, Hopfan S, Koziner B, Clarkson BD, Good RA, O'Reilly R: Bone marrow transplantation for the therapy of refractory adult T cell acute lymphoblastic leukemia. Cancer 45:2006–2008, 1980.

162. Vellekoop L, Dicke KA, Zander AR, Spitzer G, Verma DS: Repeated autologous bone marrow transplantation in adult ALL in first remission. Proc Am Soc Clin Oncol 22:490, 1981. (Abstr).

163. Nadler LM, Ritz J, Griffin JD, Todd RF, Reinherz EL, Schlossman SF: Diagnosis and treatment of human leukemias and lymphomas utilizing monoclonal antibodies. In: Progress in Hematology XII (in press).

164. Ritz J, Pesando JM, Notis-McConarty J, Schlossman SF: Modulation of human acute lymphoblastic leukemia antigen induced by monoclonal antibody *in vitro*. J Immunol 125:1506-1514, 1980.

165. Miller RA, Levy R: Treatment of human T cell neoplasms with murine hybridoma monoclonal antibody. Proc Am Soc Clin Oncol 22:376, 1981. (Abstr).

166. Bernstein ID, Tam MR, Nowinski RC: Mouse leukemia: Therapy with monoclonal antibodies against a thymus differentiation antigen. Science 207:68-71, 1980.

167. Netzel B, Haas RJ, Rodt H, Kolb HJ, Thierfelder S: Immunological conditioning of bone marrow for autotransplantation in childhood acute lymphoblastic leukaemia. Lancet i:1330-1332, 1980.

168. Wells JR, Billing R, Herzog P, Feig SA, Gale RP, Terasaki P, Cline MJ: Autotransplantation after *in vitro* immunotherapy of lymphoblastic leukemia. Exp Hematol 7 (Suppl 5):164-169, 1979.

169. Morgan E, Hsu CCS: Relationship of a leukemia-associated antigen to the presence of lymphoblasts in the peripheral blood in children with acute lymphocytic leukemia. Blood 57:879-882, 1981.

170. Galili U, Galili N, Or R, Polliack A: Analysis of the peanut agglutin binding site as a differentiation marker of normal and malignant human lymphoid cells. Clin Exp Immunol 43:311-318, 1981.

171. Coleman MS, Greenwood MF, Hutton JJ, Holland P, Lampkin B, Krill C, Kastelic JE: Adenosine deaminase, terminal deoxynucleotidyl transferase (TdT), and cell surface markers in childhood acute leukemia. Blood 52:1125-1131, 1978.

172. Muchi H, Wang YM, Frankel LS, van Eys J: Hexosaminidase isoenzymes in leukemia. Proc Am Assoc Cancer Res 22:184, 1981 (Abstr).

173. Koziner B, Evans R, Gebhard D, Clarkson BD, Good RA: Analysis of monoclonal hybridoma antibodies to T-cell antigens in acute lymphatic leukemia (ALL). Proc Am Soc Clin Oncol 22:337, 1981 (Abstr).

174. Lu AY, Leung KL, Kung FH, Sobol RE, Royston I: Utility of monoclonal antibodies in the immunologic phenotyping of acute lymphoblastic leukemia (ALL). Proc Am Soc Clin Oncol 22:409, 1981 (Abstr).

175. Gordon DS, Vogler WR, Brynes RK, Meyer LM, Dowell BL, Metzgar RS: Immunological characterization of adult acute undifferentiated leukemia. Proc Am Soc Clin Oncol 22:390, 1981 (Abstr).

176. Roper M, Crist W, Metzgar R, Nix W, Smith S, Pullen J, Ragab A, Cooper MD: Immune phenotypes in childhood T cell lymphoid malignancies. Proc Am Soc Clin Oncol 22:374, 1981 (Abstr).

# 10. The Therapy of Adult Acute Lymphoblastic Leukemia

ROBERT J. ESTERHAY, JR. and PETER H. WIERNIK

CONTENTS

## 1. INTRODUCTION

Although acute lymphoblastic leukemia (ALL) is predominantly a childhood disease, adult ALL accounts for approximately 15% of all cases of adult acute leukemia [1]. In children, major progress has been achieved in the past 5–10 years in the treatment of this disease with an increase in frequency of remission, reduction in the incidence of central nervous system (CNS) leukemia, and an increase in survival. At the present time, 50–60% of patients with childhood ALL can be expected to experience long-term disease-free survival [2]. In contrast, improvement in the management of adult ALL has not advanced as rapidly. Currently, it is the rare patient with adult ALL that survives disease-free for longer than five years, and the best reported median duration of continuous complete remission is only 25 months [3]. However, progress has been achieved in the therapy of adult ALL. The purpose of this paper is to review that progress with respect to remission induction, prophylactic CNS, remission continuation, and relapse reinduction therapy and to propose new ideas and areas for future clinical therapeutic research in this disease. The topic of bone marrow transplantation for adult ALL will not be discussed in any detail here since it is reviewed elsewhere in this volume by Kay.

## 2. CLASSIFICATION

In analyzing the results of published studies of adult ALL and in proposing new ideas for future clinical therapeutic research, one must now consider ALL as a biologically heterogeneous disease. Classically ALL was thought to be a homogeneous disease. However, certain pretreatment disease characteristics which have important clinical implications with respect to therapeutic response and survival are now recognized. For instance, several subgroups of ALL have been identified which have different prognoses [4-6]. These subgroups of ALL have been identified by classifying lymphoblasts according to certain morphological, cytochemical, immunologic, biochemical, and cytogenetic characteristics (see chapter by Bloomfield). The clinical classification and lymphoblast subclassification will be briefly reviewed to provide further understanding of the biology of this disease so that different therapeutic results can be more effectively compared.

Some of the clinical features at diagnosis of childhood ALL that have been associated with poor prognosis are black race, male sex, age less than two or greater than ten years, a high white blood cell count, a mediastinal mass and CNS leukemia at presentation [4-6]. Not all of these features are equally important and combinations of them such as a high white blood cell count, mediastinal mass, and CNS leukemia at diagnosis, are often found in the same patient. Similar clinical features in untreated adult ALL have been assigned prognostic significance; however the importance of these various clinical features has been less well studied. One recent study demonstrated that many of the important prognostic indicators as mentioned for childhood ALL do not necessarily apply to the disease in adults [7]. For example, age was not related to the attainment of complete remission. Other studies have shown a decreasing complete remission rate and survival with increasing age. A high white blood cell count and mediastinal mass, indices of disease extent, were not prognostically significant. Other studies have shown a worse prognosis for those patients with extreme leukocytosis or extensive tissue infiltration. In adult ALL it appears that with increasingly aggressive treatment, the response rate, duration of remission and survival have been slowly improving, thereby minimizing the importance of what were thought to be important clinical prognostic indicators. To what extent these clinical prognostic indicators for childhood ALL will be useful in assigning good or poor risk prognosis to more aggressively treated adult ALL is yet to be clearly defined.

Factors of reported prognostic value based on leukemic cell characteristics include morphological features, cytochemical reactions, immunologic cell surface and biochemical markers, and cytogenetic findings. A system of morphological classification proposed for ALL by Mathé *et al.* has attempted to correlate nuclear chromatin pattern and cell size with prognosis [8, 9]. Bennett *et al.* (the French-American-British Cooperative Group) were not able to duplicate Mathé's findings and instead proposed their own (FAB) classification scheme (Table 1): acute prolymphocytic (L1) leukemia, acute prolymphoblastic (L2) leukemia, and acute Burkitt's cell (L3) leukemia [10]. The clinical correlation of prognosis with these subgroups for either childhood or adult ALL is yet to be clearly defined. Other morphologic subclassifications have been proposed based on cell size, amount of cytoplasm, number of nucleoli, nuclear chromatin pattern, and overall lymphoid differentiation [11–16]. That there is little or no agreement between the various systems of morphologic classification should not be surprising and several authors have even suggested that these various proposed schemes have no prognostic significance [17–19]. Despite the lack of agreement among the various proposed morphologic classification schemes, patients with more

*Table 1.* Morphologic classification of ALL : French-American-British (FAB) criteria.

| Cytological features | Prolymphocytic (L1) | Prolymphoblastic (L2) | Burkitt's cell (L3) |
|---|---|---|---|
| Cell size | Small cells | Large cells, heterogeneous | Large cells, homogeneous |
| Nuclear chromatin | Homogeneous | Variable, heterogeneous | Finely stippled, homogeneous |
| Nuclear shape | Regular, occasional clefting/identation | Irregular, clefting/identation common | Regular, oval to round |
| Nucleoli | Not visible or small and inconspicious | One or more present, often large | Prominent, one or more vesicular |
| Amount of cytoplasm | Scanty | Variable, often moderately abundant | Moderately abundant |
| Basophilia of cytoplasm | Slight or moderate, rarely intense | Variable, deep in some | Very deep |
| Cytoplasmic vacuolation | Variable | Variable | Often prominent |

Adapted from Bennett *et al.*, Br J Haematol 33:451–458, 1976. See Bennett *et al.*, Br J Haematol 47:553–561, 1981 for recent modifications.

*Table 2.* Cytochemical reactions in acute lymphoblastic leukemia.

| Cytochemical stain | Reaction |
|---|---|
| Sudan black or peroxidase | Negative |
| Specific esterase (chloroacetate esterase) | Negative |
| Nonspecific esterase (alpha-naphythyl-butyrate) | Negative |
| Periodic acid–Schiff (PAS) | Block to granular positivity |
| Acid phosphatase | Block positivity for T-cell ALL, otherwise granular positivity |

immature lymphoblasts (larger cell size with more cytoplasm, more nucleoli, and with a more primitive chromatin pattern, the L2 type of the FAB classification) have a less favorable prognosis compared to patients in whom the lymphoblasts have a more mature appearance (the L1 type of the FAB classification). In fact, most children with ALL appear to have the L1 type of morphology and adults usually have the L2 type [20]. The third type of ALL, acute Burkitt's cell leukemia (L3 in the FAB classification), has a well-defined morphologic appearance. Most of these patients are thought to have B-cell leukemia; however, not all patients with B-cell leukemia have acute Burkitt's cell leukemia. Patients with the L3 type of ALL have a poorer prognosis than patients with either L1 or L2 type of ALL [21–25]. The L3 type is associated with the lowest complete remission rate, shortest duration of complete remission, and the highest incidence of early CNS leukemia [20].

Lymphoblasts from some patients with ALL have a characteristic reaction to periodic acid–Schiff (PAS) stain (Table 2). The periodic acid oxidizes glycols and related compounds to aldehydes. Glycogen and certain mucopolysaccharides are primarily responsible for positive staining with PAS. The stain in conjunction with sudan black or peroxidase stain can be helpful in discriminating acute lymphoblastic from acute non-lymphoblastic leukemia. Lymphoblasts may contain multiple PAS granules of varying size. The very large 'coarse-looking' granules appear to be 'blocks' and patients with ALL whose lymphoblasts demonstrate PAS block positivity have been reported to have an improved prognosis [12, 16, 26, 27]. Lymphoblasts from other patients with ALL may demonstrate a characteristic reaction for acid phosphatase stain. The enzyme hydrolyzes the substrate releasing a naphthol which couples with a diazonium salt to form a colored insoluble product. The stain may be of value in discriminating T-cell ALL from non-T, non-B (common and null) ALL (see chapter by Bloomfield). Patients with acid phosphatase positive ALL have T-cell ALL about 75 % of the time and have been reported to have a shorter duration of response to therapy and survival [27, 28]. Other cytochemical stains such as beta glucuronidase and acid alpha naphthyl esterase have been reported to be positive (60–80%) for T-cell ALL and therefore may have utility [26]. Other cytochemical stains have also been described but either they have not been useful in establishing the diagnosis of ALL or they have not been helpful in determining prognosis.

Immunologic cell surface markers on lymphoblasts have been found to be very important determinants of prognosis in childhood ALL [4, 29, 30]. There appears to be a correlation between immunologic classification and clinical response. However, in adult ALL there has been some conflicting data on the relationship of prognosis to cell surface markers [32, 33]. Adult ALL, like childhood ALL, can be immunologically classified into four major subgroups [28]: common ALL, null (or unclassified) ALL, T-cell ALL, and B-cell ALL (see detailed discussion in chapter by Bloomfield). T-cell (sheep erythrocyte-rosette positive or E+) ALL accounts for approximately 15% of childhood and adult ALL; B-cell (presence of surface immunoglobulin or sIg+) ALL constitutes approximately 5% of adult ALL; and, non-T, non-B (E− and sIg−) ALL accounts for about 80% of childhood and adult ALL. Non-T, non-B ALL can be further separated into common (cALL+) and null (cALL−) ALL. The cALL antigen is found in approximately 60% of the non-T, non-B ALL cases. The presence of E+ lymphoblasts (T-cell ALL) in both children and adults correlates strongly with clinical high-risk features such as a high white blood cell count, mediastinal mass, and early CNS involvement. T-cell ALL forms a distinct clinical subgroup with a poor prognosis and more aggressive treatment needs to be studied in this ALL variant. On the other hand, patients with common ALL have a prognosis that is better than that of children and adults with null, T-cell, or B-cell ALL [28–35]. A very recent study suggests that the prognosis of adults with common ALL approaches that of children with common ALL [35]. Null ALL is thought to have a somewhat variable prognosis between that of common and T-cell ALL, while the prognosis of B-cell ALL (non-Burkitt's) is unknown because it is rarely encountered. The prognosis for acute Burkitt's leukemia (also a B-cell ALL) is worse than T-cell ALL. Other immunologic subgroups such as pre-B-cell ALL (cALL+, cytoplasmic IgM+, sIg−) have been reported in adults and, as more data accumulates, may come to be associated with a characteristic prognosis [28, 36, 37].

Terminal deoxynucleotidyl transferase (TdT), a biochemical enzyme marker, may also have prognostic significance in patients with ALL. Elèvated levels of TdT have been detected in cases of non-T, non-B ALL and T-cell ALL [38]. It appears that there is no direct correlation between the presence of E+ lymphoblasts and TdT+ cells because TdT is present in immature or undifferentiated cells which are the precursors of mature T cells [39–42]. Although in most cases classification based on morphologic features, cytochemical stains, and cell surface markers is sufficient, there are a number of cases in which it is difficult to classify the type of leukemia. With the availability of biochemical assays and immunological techniques for the detection of TdT, it should be possible to classify leukemias based on the presence or absence of TdT in the leukemic cells, and design clinical therapeutic research studies based on this classification. Future prospects include development of TdT as a biologic marker for following patients during treatment and remission, further subclassification of ALL, and correlation with the immunologic subgroups of ALL. Other biochemical enzymes studied to date include adenosine deaminase and hexosaminidase isoenzymes. Only a few studies have been reported and confirmation of the results is needed [28].

Cytogenetic analyses with nonbanding procedures for more than 400 ALL patients have been reported and have demonstrated no correlation with either clinical features or prognosis [43, 44]. Banding studies have been more recently applied to chromosomal analysis in patients with ALL [45–47] (see chapters by Golomb and Bloomfield). Approximately two-thirds of patients with ALL show abnormal karyotypes [47]. A number of specific chromosomal abnormalities have been associated with ALL. In particular, the presence of the Philadelphia (Ph$^1$) chromosome has been found in up to 30% of patients with non-T, non-B ALL, usually those who are subclassified as common ALL (E−, sIg−, cALL+, Ia+) [48, 49]. Cytogenetic analysis with banding techniques should be done on all adults presenting with ALL who are being considered for clinical therapeutic research studies at least to identify Ph$^1$+ cases for more aggressive therapy and/or separate therapeutic analysis since these patients do not respond as well to 'standard' ALL chemotherapy [50, 51]. Future banding studies of chromosomal abnormalities in patients with adult ALL should be correlated with the various immunologic subgroups of the disease.

The correlation between morphologic classification, cytochemical reactions, immunologic cell surface and biochemical markers, and cytogenetic findings with respect to response frequency, remission duration, and survival is only beginning to be studied. As discussed there appears to be a correlation between a positive acid-phosphatase reaction, T-cell ALL, and a poor prognosis. Moreover, it seems quite clear that the subclassification of ALL based on methods of characterizing lymphoblasts described above will have important treatment implications in the design of future clinical therapeutic research studies.

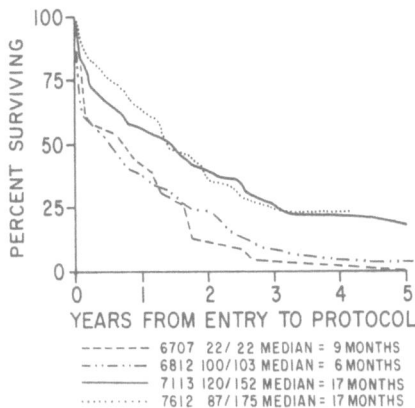

*Figure 1.* Survival in adult acute lymphoblastic leukemia for the years 1967–1980 as reported by Cancer and Leukemia Group B (CALGB) (Reproduced with permission of Oliver Glidewell and CALGB).

## 3. THERAPY

The therapy of adult ALL has recently resulted in significant improvement in the remission induction rate as well as in remission duration and survival. There are now adults with ALL, in some reported studies, surviving disease-free for longer than three years. The changes in survival in adult ALL from 1967 to 1980 by one large cooperative study group, Cancer and Leukemia Group B (CALGB), are shown in Figure 1. In this section, the current status of remission induction, prophylactic CNS, remission continuation, and relapse reinduction therapy will be discussed.

### 3.1. Remission Induction Therapy

The most effective chemotherapeutic agents used alone for remission induction therapy in both childhood and adult ALL are vincristine, prednisone, daunorubicin, and asparaginase [2, 52]. Combinations of these individually active agents have increased remission induction rates. Vincristine and prednisone have been employed in virtually all remission induction therapy programs in both childhood and adult ALL with complete remissions of 85–95% in childhood ALL and 50–60% in adult ALL [2, 52]. The addition of an anthracycline antibiotic such as daunorubicin and doxorubicin, and asparaginase has increased the complete remission rate for adults with ALL to 70–80% as shown in Table 3 [3, 25, 53–71]. Other agents, when combined with prednisone and vincristine, have also resulted in improved initial remission induction rates in both childhood and adult ALL. Such drugs include methotrexate and mercaptopurine as in the POMP

*Table 3.* Combination chemotherapy for previously untreated adult ALL.

| Author (reference) | Remission induction regimen | Number of patients | Percent complete remission | Prophylactic CNS regimen | CNS Leukemia (percent) | Remission continuation regimen | Median duration CR in mos. | Median survival in mos. |
|---|---|---|---|---|---|---|---|---|
| Whitecar [53] | V+P+ARA+C | 21 | 43 | None | NA | Maintenance V+P+ARA+C | 14.5 | 5.5 |
| Smyth [54] | V+D+PYR+TG | 17 | 53 | PYR & CCNU | 6/17 (35.3) | Consolidation V+D+PYR+TG Maintenance V+D+PYR+TG & CCNU | 6.0 | 13.5 |
| Gahrton [55] | P+ARA+C+ASP | 12 | 58 | None | NA | Maintenance MTX, MP, C | 4.1 | 6.6 |
| Armitage [56] | V+P±ARA | 13 | 67 | IT–MTX+CI | 0/13 (0) | Maintenance MTX+MP+C | 11.0 | 26.0 |
| Gingrich [57] | V+P+ARA | 13 | 69 | IT–MTX+CI | NA | Maintenance MTX+MP | 9.5 | 14.0 (CR pts.) |
| Lister [25] | V+P+DOX+ASP | 51 | 71 | IT–MTX+CI | 3/51 (5.9) | Maintenance MTX+MP+C | 18.5 | 21.0 |
| Shaw [58] | V+P+DOX | 25 | 72 | None* or IT–MTX+CI | 4/25 (16.0) | Maintenance MTX+MP Reinforcement V+P | 10.2 | NA |
| Willemze [59] | V+P+DNR | 21 | 72 | IT-MTX+CI | 1/21 (4.8) | Maintenance MTX+MP Reinforcement V+P | 15.0 | 16.0+ |
| Henderson [60] | V+P+ASP±DNR | 149 | 72 | IT–MTX+CI | 12/149 (8.0) | Maintenance MTX+MP Reinforcement V+P | 15.0 | 17.0 |

*Table 3.* (Continued).

| Author (reference) | Remission induction regimen | Number of patients | Percent complete remission | Prophylactic CNS regimen | CNS Leukemia (percent) | Remission continuation regimen | Median duration CR in mos. | Median survival in mos. |
|---|---|---|---|---|---|---|---|---|
| Jacquillat [61] | V+P+DNR | 30 | 73 | IT–MTX | 4/30 (13.3) | Maintenance MTX+MP | 11.0 | 15.0 |
| Muriel [62] | V+P+(DNR or DOX) | 20 | 75 | None* or IT–MTX+CI | NA | Consolidation ASP Maintenance MTX+MP Reinforcement V+P | NA | NA |
| Esterhay [63] | V+D+MTX+ASP | 24 | 75 | IV-HDMTX | 2/24 (8.3) | Consolidation MTX+ASP Cytoreduction HDMTX+CL Maintenance MTX+MP Reinforcement V+D | 11.1 | 17.0 |
| Gottlieb [64] | V+P+DNR+ASP | 89 | 77 | IT–MTX+CI | NA | Maintenance MTX+MP Reinforcement V+P | NA | NA |
| Gee [3] | V+P+DNR | 23 | 78 | IT–MTX * or OM–MTX | 4/23 (17.4) | Consolidation ARA+TG, ASP+V+BCNU Maintenance TG+V, H+DNR, MTX+BCNU, H+C | 25.0 | 33.0 |

Table 3. (Continued).

| Author (reference) | Remission induction regimen | Number of patients | Percent complete remission | Prophylactic CNS regimen | CNS Leukemia (percent) | Remission continuation regimen | Median duration CR in mos. | Median survival in mos. |
|---|---|---|---|---|---|---|---|---|
| Rodriguez [65] | V+P+MTX+MP | 14 | 79 | None | NA | Maintenance V+P+MTX+MP | 8.0 | 13.0 (CR pts.) |
| Omura [66] | V+P+MTX | 99 | 80 | None or IT−MTX+CI | 14/99 (14.1) | Consolidation ARA+TG, ASP+V+P Maintenance MTX+MP+C Reinforcement V+P | 16.9 (CR pts.) | 24.2 |
| Curtis [68] | V+P | 17 | 82 | None* or IT−MTX+CI | NA | Consolidation MTX Maintenance MTX+MP | NA | 15.7+ (CR pts.) |
| Schauer [67] | V+P+DOX | 61 | 85 | IT−MTX* or OM−MTX | 5/61 (8.2) | Consolidation MTX+ARA+TG, ASP+C Maintenance DOX, MTX+MP, DAC, BCNU, C Reinforcement V+P | NA | NA |
| Spiers [69] | V+P | 9 | 89 | IT−MTX+CI | 0/9 (0) | Consolidation V+P+C+ARA Maintenance V+P+MTX+MP, ARA+ASP+DNR+TG, V+P+C+ARA | NA | NA |

*Table 3.* (Continued).

| Author (reference) | Remission induction regimen | Number of patients | Percent complete remission | Prophylactic CNS regimen | CNS Leukemia (percent) | Remission continuation regimen | Median duration CR in mos. | Median survival in mos. |
|---|---|---|---|---|---|---|---|---|
| Scavino [70] | V+P | 14 | 93 | IT–MTX+CI | 1/14 (7.1) | Maintenance MTX+MP+C Reinforcement V+P | 10.0 | 11.0+ |
| Einhorn [71] | V+P+DNR | 9 | 100 | None,* CSI, IT–MTX+CI | 1/9 (11.1) | Maintenance MTX+MP Reinforcement V+P+DNR | 14.0+ | 19.0+ |

NA = data not available, * = non-randomized study, CR = complete remission.
ARA = cytarabine, ASP = asparaginase, BCNU = carmustine, C = cyclophosphamide, CCNU = lomustine, CI = cranial irradiation, CL = calcium leucovorin, CSI = craniospinal irradiation, D = dexamethasone, DAC = dactinomycin, DNR = daunorubicin, DOX = doxorubicin, H = hydroxyurea, IT–MTX = intrathecal methotrexate, IV–HDMTX = intravenous high-dose methotrexate, MP = mercaptopurine, MTX = methotrexate, OM–MTX = methotrexate via Ommaya reservoir, P = prednisone, PYR = pyrimethamine, TG = thioguanine, V = vincristine.

*Table 4.* Drugs used in the currently most effective remission induction regimens for adult ALL.

| Drug | Dose | Route | Schedule |
|------|------|-------|----------|
| Vincristine | 1.0–2.0 mg/m² * | IV | Weekly |
| Prednisone | 40–100 mg/m² † | PO | Daily |
| Daunorubicin | 45–80 mg/m² ‡ | | Daily × 2–3 |
| or | or | IV | or |
| doxorubicin | 30–75 mg/m² | | weekly |
| Asparaginase | 500–1000 IU/kg | | Daily × 5–10 |
| | or | IV | or |
| | 10 000 IU/m² | | weekly |

\* Most studies have a maximum of 2.0 mg.

† Most studies use 40 mg/m²/day.

‡ The lower dose is used for a daily × 2–3 schedule, the higher dose for a weekly schedule.

regimen [65, 72]. In addition, thioguanine (instead of mercaptopurine) has been shown to be effective in the treatment of adult ALL and dexamethasone has been demonstrated to have antileukemic activity equal to prednisone in both childhood and adult ALL [54, 73].

Although a multitude of remission induction regimens have been studied in adult ALL, the most effective regimen appears to be a combination of weekly injections of vincristine (usually a maximum of 2.0 mg), daily oral prednisone (usually 40 mg/m²/day), daily × 2–3 or weekly injections of daunorubicin and daily × 5–10 or weekly infusions of asparaginase (Table 4). Using the doses and schedules shown in Table 4, close to 80% of adults can be expected to achieve a complete remission. The most effective scheduling of daunorubicin is unknown. Whether daunorubicin should be given in a daily × 2–3 or weekly schedule has not been tested in a comparative study. In CALGB study #7612, the highest remission frequency is produced with vincristine, prednisone, and daunorubicin given only on days 1–3 of induction [64]. In sequential CALGB studies, the data suggest but do not prove that daily rather than weekly daunorubicin is more effective [60, 64]. There has been only one study comparing daunorubicin and doxorubicin in adult ALL, but the number of patients in the study was too small to provide a definite conclusion [62]. The most effective scheduling of asparaginase appears to be daily rather than weekly, as determined by sequential CALGB studies [60, 64].

Sequentially administered methotrexate and asparaginase, with scheduling based on *in vitro* pharmacologic studies, has significant activity in refractory childhood and adult ALL [74–78]. It appears that asparaginase not only increases the sensitivity of leukemic cells to methotrexate by producing a rapid regrowth phase nine to ten days after asparaginase administration, but also mutes the toxicity of methotrexate when given 24 hours after methotrexate [74–76]. The primary toxicity observed in these studies was an allergic reaction to asparaginase after several months of intermittent treatment [76–78]. When such reactions occurred it was possible to continue asparaginase treatment utilizing enzyme prepared from *Erwinia* species [79]. This sequentially administered regimen has been used not only for remission induction therapy, but indefinitely as remission continuation therapy with reported remission durations of greater than one year [76–78].

The remission induction therapy protocol used at the Baltimore Cancer Research Center incorporates this sequential cycling of methotrexate and asparaginase in combination with vincristine and dexamethasone. A course of MOAD remission induction therapy is shown in Table 5. Each remission induction course consists of a 10 day period. Courses are continuous with the second course beginning on day 11, the third on day 21, etc. Each course consists of: methotrexate, 100 mg/m$^2$ IV push on day 1, increasing subsequent doses by 50% each course to 225 mg/m$^2$, thereafter by 25% each course to minimal toxicity; vincristine, 2 mg regardless of body surface, IV push on day 2; asparaginase (*E. coli*), 500 IU/kg by a 30 minute infusion on day 2, 24 hours after methotrexate is given (if asparaginase allergy develops *Erwinia* asparaginase is used); and dexamethasone, 6 mg/m$^2$/day, PO for

*Table 5.* MOAD for adult ALL: induction therapy.

| | | | | | Each course | | | | | |
|---|---|---|---|---|---|---|---|---|---|---|
| Day | 1 | 2 | 3 | 4 | 5 | 6 | 7 | 8 | 9 | 10 |
| | MTX | | | | | | | | | |
| | D | D | D | D | D | D | D | D | D | D |
| | | V | | | | | | | | |
| | | ASP | | | | | | | | |

| | Drug | Dose | Route | Schedule |
|---|---|---|---|---|
| MTX | Methotrexate | 100 mg/m$^2$ * | IV push | Day 1 |
| D | Dexamethasone | 6 mg/m$^2$ | PO | Days 1–10 |
| V | Vincristine | 2 mg | IV push | Day 2 |
| ASP | Asparaginase | 500 IU/kg | IV infusion | Day 2 |

* Increase dose by 50% to 225 mg/m$^2$ then by 25% until minimal toxicity.
A minimum of 5 remission induction courses is given every 10 days before starting remission continuation therapy (see text).

days 1–10. Patients who do not have bone marrow improvement after three induction courses or who have not obtained a complete remission after five induction courses (without continuing marrow improvement after each course) are considered remission induction therapy failures. Patients who achieve a complete remission receive two additional induction therapy courses. A minimum of five remission induction courses is required before beginning remission continuation therapy. This remission induction regimen resulted in a 75% complete remission rate for previously untreated adult ALL patients and a 79% complete remission rate for previously treated (relapsed/refractory) adult ALL patients at the Baltimore Cancer Research Center [63].

The rationale behind the design of this study and in particular this remission induction therapy regimen was based on a number of considerations. The remission induction rate of adult ALL can be improved by adding other active agents to the combination of vincristine and prednisone (or dexamethasone). In childhood ALL, the addition of asparaginase or an anthracycline antibiotic contributes little to an improved remission rate because 85–95% of the patients achieve a complete remission with vincristine and prednisone alone. Additional induction agents cause additional toxicity and even early drug-related deaths [80, 81]. Although the addition of either asparaginase or an anthracycline antibiotic contributes little to an improved remission rate, a third induction agent provides an advantage because more patients will continue in complete remission who have had more intensive or aggressive initial remission induction therapy [82]. Whether more intensive remission induction therapy will have an effect on the duration of complete remission for adult ALL is not known because of the variety of remission continuation therapies utilized (see Table 3). However, the remission induction rate for adult ALL is improved when a third and fourth drug such as an anthracycline antibiotic and asparaginase are used in addition to vincristine and prednisone. As mentioned, as other active agents are added to vincristine and prednisone toxicity obviously increases also. For example, CALGB studied the use of a remission induction regimen for adult ALL (Protocol #7612) including vincristine and prednisone followed by asparaginase, with and without daunorubicin [64]. With daunorubicin the complete remission rate was 80% and 75% of the patients had severe (3+) or life-threatening (4+) leukopenia and 50% had 3+ or 4+ thrombocytopenia. Without daunorubicin the CR rate was 50% and only 41% had 3+ leukopenia and only 38% had 3+ thrombocytopenia. However, it should be noted that there was no difference in the incidence of severe infection or hemorrhage related to the use of daunorubicin [64], which is a tribute to the quality and quantity of supportive care available to patients on that study. Thus, the remission induction rate improves with the

*Table 6.* MOAD for adult ALL: consolidation therapy.

| | Each course | | | | | | | | | |
|---|---|---|---|---|---|---|---|---|---|---|
| Day | 1 | 2 | 3 | 4 | 5 | 6 | 7 | 8 | 9 | 10 |
| | MTX | | | | | | | | | |
| | | ASP | | | | | | | | |

| | Drug | Dose | Route | Schedule |
|---|---|---|---|---|
| MTX | Methotrexate | Established dose * | IV push | Day 1 |
| ASP | Asparaginase | 5000 IU/kg | IV infusion | Day 2 |

* Or continue to increase dose by 25% until minimal toxicity.
After complete remission is obtained and remission induction therapy is completed consolidation therapy is repeated every 10 days for 6 courses.

addition of daunorubicin to vincristine, prednisone and asparaginase, but at the expense of potentially serious increased hematologic toxicity.

Increasing the doses of remission induction agents without adding additional agents may also increase the response rate, and may or may not increase hematologic toxicity. In the MOAD study, the methotrexate dose was increased on subsequent courses of remission induction and consolidation therapy (Tables 5 and 6). However, the myelosuppressive effect of MOAD decreased with bone marrow improvement for the previously untreated patients, even with escalation of the methotrexate dose from 100 to 550 mg/m$^2$ (Table 7). Hematologic toxicity observed with the first three courses of MOAD for the previously untreated patients was not observed for previously treated patients because they were treated earlier and had fewer blasts in the peripheral blood and bone marrow at the time of treatment.

*Table 7.* MOAD for adult ALL: hematologic toxicity during induction and consolidation previously untreated patients.

| Methotrexate dose (mg/m$^2$) | Number of evaluable courses | WBC count ($\times 10^3$) median nadir (range) | Platelet count ($\times 10^3$) median nadir (range) |
|---|---|---|---|
| 100 | 35 | 0.7 (0.1–13.9) | 23 (5–348) |
| 150 | 30 | 1.1 (0.3–13.4) | 65 (17–150) |
| 225 | 32 | 2.2 (0.4–6.0) | 114 (3–270) |
| 280 | 16 | 2.6 (1.9–5.0) | 120 (60–245) |
| 350–550 | 12 | 3.1 (2.2–6.4) | 230 (106–306) |

Although the majority of adult ALL patients do not have severe or life-threatening infections during remission induction therapy, the number of severe infections increases as more myelosuppressive therapy is attempted. In CALGB study #7113, life-threatening infections occurred in 13 of 27 (48%) patients who were given asparaginase simultaneously with vincristine and prednisone [60]. When doxorubicin was added to vincristine and prednisone in a Southwest Oncology Group study, 14 (56%) of 25 patients developed an infection during remission induction therapy [58]. When cytarbine was added to vincristine and prednisone, six of 13 (46%) patients developed bacteremias and despite appropriate antibiotic therapy, three (23%) of these patients died [56]. Even with vincristine and prednisone alone, eight of 14 (57%) patients had infections or fever without proven infection during remission induction therapy [70]. Therefore, more intensively treated adult ALL patients are at an increased risk of infection and require infection prevention measures, especially during remission induction therapy.

Patients on the MOAD study were given oral prophylactic antibiotics during periods of prolonged, severe granulocytopenia [83, 84]. None of the patients were placed in reverse isolation. They were empirically given intravenous broad-spectrum antibiotics for granulocytopenia and fever [83, 84]. Prophylactic platelet transfusions and therapeutic granulocyte transfusions were used when indicated. Although myelosuppression was tolerable there were ten severe or life-threatening infections in 24 (41.7%) of the previously untreated patients (Table 8). Four patients died of infection, two while in

*Table 8.* MOAD for adult ALL: response to therapy.

|  | Previously untreated | Previously treated |
|---|---|---|
| No. of patients | 24 | 14 |
| Complete remissions (CR) (%) | 18 (75%) | 11 (79%) |
| Median treatment days (range) to CR | 48 (27–85) | 39 (9–109) |
| Patients (%) with severe infections during induction | 10 (41.7%) | 3 (21.4%) |
| Median duration (range) of CR in months | 11.1 (0.7+ to 55.9+) | 7.5 (1.9+ to 55.3+) |
| CNS leukemia (%) | 2 (8.3%) | 0 |
| Median survival (range) of CR patients in months | 17.8 (0.7+ to 55.9+)* | 17.2 (2.6+ to 55.3+) |
| Median survival (range) of all patients in months | 17.0 (0.4 to 55.9+) | 11.2 (1.1 to 55.3+) |

* The median survival of previously untreated CR patients has not been reached. However, the median cannot be less than 17.8 months.

CR. There were three severe infections in 14 (21.4%) of the previously treated patients. Most of the severe infections for the previously untreated patients occurred early in induction when myelosuppression was maximal (Table 7). The incidence of severe infections for the previously untreated patients is less than that reported in our previous study in which ten of 17 patients (59%) had severe infections during induction [54]. In that study patients were not given oral prophylactic antibiotics. In addition, the number of severe infections is less that that reported for adults with acute non-lymphoblastic leukemia undergoing initial induction with the protection of oral prophylactic antibiotics without reverse isolation [83, 84]. Most of the infections for the previously untreated and treated ALL patients during induction were due to hospital acquired pathogens. The organisms causing the bacteremias had been shown by surveillance cultures to be colonizing the alimentary canal, the mucosa of which may have been damaged by methotrexate during induction therapy. Although the frequency of infections was less than in our previous study when no prophylactic antibiotics were used, it is clear from other studies and the MOAD study that intensively treated adult ALL patients are at high risk of infection and require increased effort at infection prevention.

In summary, remission induction therapy studies for adult ALL have resulted in increased frequency of remission from 50–60% to 70–80%. This has been accomplished by adding asparaginase and an anthracycline antibiotic to the combination of vincristine and prednisone. Sequentially administered methotrexate and asparaginase also has significant activity in adult ALL and when added to vincristine and dexamethasone as in the MOAD combination, results in an effective regimen for inducing complete remission in previously untreated patients. MOAD is also highly effective as a reinduction regimen for refractory adult ALL patients who have not previously received asparaginase. This schedule-dependent therapeutic synergism between methotrexate and asparaginase suggests that this regimen in combination with vincristine and dexamethasone be further explored for remission induction therapy in larger cooperative group studies.

More intensive remission induction therapy causes more toxicity, in particular myelosuppression with an increased risk of severe or life-threatening granulocytopenia and thrombocytopenia. Patients with adult ALL, in particular poor prognostic subgroups such as T-cell ALL, are likely to receive more intensive remission induction therapy and therefore will clearly be at an increased risk of fatal infection. Therefore, all patients with adult ALL should be treated with full supportive care. Infection prophylaxis should include, during intensive remission induction therapy when prolonged granulocytopenia can be expected, careful personal hygiene (hand washing, bathing and shampooing with an antiseptic soap such as chlorhexidine), slippers when out of bed, and scrupulous attention to dental hygiene with brushing and flossing. A low microbial diet (the so-called cooked food diet) should be prescribed and oral trimethoprim/sulfamethoxazole (one double strength tablet every 8 hours) and nystatin suspension (1 million units every 6 hours) should be given to suppress alimentary canal microbial organisms [85]. This combination of techniques will reduce new organism acquisition and suppress colonizing microorganisms. Prophylactic platelet transfusions and therapeutic granulocyte transfusions (see chapter by Strauss and Connett) should be used when indicated.

### 3.2. Prophylactic CNS Therapy

The addition of prophylactic CNS therapy with intrathecal methotrexate combined with cranial irradiation immediately following completion of remission induction therapy delays the onset of CNS leukemia, and thus prolongs complete remission and survival in childhood ALL [2]. It was assumed that the benefit of CNS prophylaxis in childhood ALL would translate directly to adult ALL. However, this has not yet happened. Since the effect of CNS prophylaxis on remission duration in childhood ALL is not observed during the first 24 months of remission, it is reasonable to expect that the effect of CNS prophylaxis on adult ALL will not become evident until improved remission duration and survival is achieved [66]. The reported incidence of CNS leukemia in adult ALL has ranged from 7% to 75% [86, 87].

A Southeastern Cancer Group study tested the effect of CNS prophylaxis in adult ALL, using cranial irradiation (2400 rads in 12 fractions over 2.5 weeks through opposing lateral ports to the head with each field treated each day) and intrathecal methotrexate ($10 \, mg/m^2$, given twice weekly for 5 doses) [66]. A significant prolongation of the CNS relapse-free survival was demonstrated in those adult ALL patients who received CNS prophylaxis. Only three of 28 (10.7%) evaluable patients in the prophylactic group developed CNS relapse by 24 months compared with 11 of 34 (32.3%) evaluable patients in the untreated group. The difference between the two groups was significant ($p = 0.03$). If one takes into account the time at risk for CNS relapse (i.e., that interval of time from the completion of CNS prophylaxis to the date of last follow-up), the difference is also significantly different ($p = 0.008$) in favor of CNS prophylaxis. However, there was no significant difference in either remission duration or survival between the no-prophylaxis and the CNS prophylaxis groups. The median remission duration was 16.9 months for complete remission patients. The median survival for all patients on this study was 24.2 months (see Table 3).

Table 9 lists different methods that have been used for either prophylaxis or therapy of CNS leukemia for both childhood and adult ALL. Although

*Table 9.* Prophylaxis and therapy of CNS leukemia.

| Therapeutic modalities | Comments and risks |
| --- | --- |
| Cranial irradiation + intrathecal methotrexate | Current standard CNS prophylaxis<br>Risk of acute, subacute, delayed neurotoxicity |
| Craniospinal irradiation | Severe prolonged myelosuppression<br>Risk of life-threatening infection<br>Risk of relapse during myelosuppression |
| Intrathecal methotrexate | Therapeutic concentration achieved only around lumbar space<br>Risk of acute, subacute neurotoxitiy |
| Intraventricular methotrexate | Invasive procedure (Ommaya reservoir)<br>Risk related to insertion and use of reservoir, e.g., infection, bleeding, neurologic deficits |
| Intravenous, high-dose methotrexate + calcium leucovorin | Therapeutic (greater than $10^{-7}$M) CSF methotrexate levels can be achieved<br>Full evaluation of this modality incomplete |
| Oral pyrimethamine (Daraprim) | Does not prevent or delay CNS leukemia |
| Intrathecal cytarabine | Usually employed when intrathecal methotrexate becomes refactory |
| Intrathecal triethylenethio-phosphoramide (Thiotepa) | Neurotoxicity too great for routine use |
| Intrathecal (methotrexate + cytarabine + hydrocortisone) | Intrathecal triple drug therapy as good as intrathecal methotrexate alone or combined with intrathecal cytarabine |
| Prophylactic CNS therapy for selected patients | Identify patients who need CNS prophylaxis<br>Risk of CNS leukemia, e.g., extreme leukocytosis, L3 morphology |

craniospinal irradiation (2400 rads) is as effective as cranial irradiation (2400 rads) combined with intrathecal methotrexate (5 doses) in preventing CNS leukemia, it results in increased myelosuppression because the entire spine is irradiated [2, 52, 88, 89]. Consequently, many patients who have received craniospinal irradiation for CNS prophylaxis have had remission continuation therapy interrupted for long periods of time because of severe myelosuppression. This places them at increased risk for bone marrow relapse. Therefore, craniospinal irradiation is no longer considered standard prophylactic CNS therapy for either childhood or adult ALL. This treatment is presently reserved for children and adults with CNS relapse. Other toxicities from cranial irradiation occur and include a somnolence syndrome seen in about 10% of childhood ALL. The syndrome presents with fever, anorexia and nausea, sometimes associated with dizziness and CSF pleocytosis, occurring five to eight weeks after irradiation and lasting for three to 15 days. This probably represents a transient radiation encephalo-pathy and has no apparent long-term manifestations [88, 89]. With intensive remission induction and remission continuation regimens, intrathecal methotrexate alone has been shown to be statistically equivalent to standard CNS prophylaxis (intrathecal methotrexate plus cranial irradiation) for childhood and adult ALL [2, 52]. However, studies have reported that the concentration of methotrexate in ventricular CSF after intrathecal injection of the drug into the lumbar subarachnoid space is not adequate for a significant antitumor effect [90, 92]. In addition, as many as 11–24% of the intrathecal methotrexate administrations may be injected inadvertently into the epidural or subdural space rather than into the subarachnoid space [90, 92, 93]. Also, the lumbar puncture may create a leak in the meninges and thereby alter the flow, pressure and volume of the CSF, as well as result in a lumbar puncture syndrome [90, 94]. The most distressing complication of intrathecal methotrexate therapy is an acute, subacute or delayed neurotoxicity.

Chemical arachnoiditis is the most common form of neurotoxicity [90]. It presents as an acute syndrome usually starting within hours after injection and resolving within 1–5 days. The symptoms and physical findings are due to meningeal irritation and increased intracranial pressure: headache, backache, vomiting, fever, and leg pain. The CSF reveals a granulocytic pleocytosis and the findings can mimic bacterial meningitis [95]. The severity of this acute syndrome is related to the dose of methotrexate and to the peak methotrexate concentration in the CSF [96]. Five symptomatic patients of 25 (20%) (age range from 2 to 37 years) in one reported study had CSF methotrexate concentrations averaging 13.8 times higher than the mean and these concentrations were consistently higher than the range of methotrexate values in the 20 asymptomatic patients [96]. This study suggested that the chemical arachnoiditis was related to a prolonged exposure of an elevated concentration of methotrexate in the CSF, which in turn might be a result of impaired elimination of methotrexate from the CSF or increased dosage in relation to CSF volume (particularly in adolescents). The investigators suggested that frequent monitoring of CSF methotrexate concentration and appropriate adjustment of drug dosage or treatment interval might be helpful in decreasing or preventing this syndrome. Intrathecal cytarabine can also cause acute chemical arachnoiditis but it occurs less commonly than with methotrexate [97].

The subacute form of intrathecal methotrexate neurotoxicity occurs a few weeks after therapy is started. This form of neurotoxicity is rare and usually presents as brain or spinal cord motor dysfunction. The symptoms and physical findings are due to paraparesis, cerebellar dysfunction and cranial nerve palsies. Paraplegia, quadriplegia, seizures and obtundation also have been reported [98]. This form of neurotoxicity is more likely to occur in patients receiving more than two intrathecal injections on a weekly basis and is apparently related to a continuously elevated concentration of methotrexate ‘in the CSF [96]. This complication may be transient or permanent [99, 101].

In childhood ALL, the delayed (or chronic) form of neurotoxicity, a demyelinating leukoencephalopathy, occurs months to years after the administration of intrathecal methotrexate. It presents insidiously and progresses to severe dementia, dysarthria, dysphagia, ataxia, spasticity, seizures and coma [102–104]. The risk of leukoencephalopathy depends not only on the combination of the CNS therapeutic modalities, but also on the dose of drug given. In every case, the patients who developed leukoencephalopathy had received greater than 2 000 rads of cranial irradiation, greater than 50 mg/m$^2$ of intrathecal methotrexate and/or greater than 40 mg/m$^2$/week of intravenous methotrexate [103–107]. The higher the dose of cranial irradiation, the greater the cummulative dose of intrathecal methotrexate, or the higher the dose of intravenous methotrexate, the greater the risk of leukoencephalopathy [103, 104]. The incidence with all three modalities combined (at the stated doses) is approximately 45%. The estimated risk of leukoencephalopathy with any of the modalities alone is reported to be less than 1%. Whether the risk of developing leukoencephalopathy is less at lower dose levels is unknown [90].

Methotrexate administered intraventricularly via an Ommaya reservoir for either prophylaxis or therapy of CNS leukemia has been shown to be a significant therapeutic improvement over intrathecally administered methotrexate. In one reported study the number of episodes of CNS leukemia per month in the ventricular treatment period was one-fourth that in the lumbar treatment period (p<0.01) [108]. At one institution, those children and adults presenting with a white blood cell count greater than 20 000 are given CNS prophylaxis with intraventricular methotrexate via an Ommaya reservoir because it was noted on a previous study that the rate of CNS relapse was greater with those children and adults who presented with an elevated white blood cell count [3, 67]. In another study, a direct comparison of intraventricular versus intralumbar methotrexate for treatment of CNS leukemia showed a significantly greater therapeutic effect (p<0.07) for the group having Ommaya reservoirs [109].

The major limitations and toxicities of intraventricular methotrexate are due to complications related to the insertion and use of the Ommaya reservoir [110]. Misplacement and occlusion of the cannula tip, transient or persistent focal neurologic deficits, bleeding and infection have been reported. In one study, complications occurred with 20 (18%) of 110 reservoirs [108].

In another study, two of 23 (8.7%) reservoirs had clinically significant complications related to the reservoir [109]. The complication rate can be reduced by strict adherence to sterile technique, by the use of small-gauge, scalpvein ('butterfly') needles for injections in the reservoir, by insertion of the reservoir transfrontally instead of transoccipitally and by the use of fluoroscopy during insertion [108].

Neurotoxicity of intrathecal methotrexate can be reduced by simultaneous administration of intrathecal hydrocortisone. This has been reported to reduce the severity but not the incidence of acute chemical arachnoiditis [111]. Elliott's B solution, an investigational artificial CSF, has also been used to decrease the acute toxicity of intrathecal methotrexate [112, 113]. Another approach which has been used is to adjust each patient's dosage relative to the concentration of the drug in his or her CSF. The use of the methotrexate concentration in the CSF as a therapeutic guide has been reported to reduce the incidence and severity of the acute and subacute neurotoxicities of intrathecal methotrexate [90, 96].

The combination of intrathecal methotrexate and intrathecal cytarabine has been used with intrathecal hydrocortisone for prophylactic CNS therapy and has been reported to be as good as intrathecal methotrexate alone [111, 114]. The rationale for this approach is to increase the therapeutic effect of methotrexate by adding cytarabine and to decrease the severity of acute chemical arachnoiditis by using hydrocortisone. Thiotepa, an alkylating agent, has been evaluated as an alternative to either intrathecal methotrexate or intrathecal cytarabine. However, in clinical phase I trials, the drug was found to be too toxic for routine use [115]. Other approaches to CNS prophylaxis have been the combined use of methotrexate intrathecally and intravenously [116] or intravenously alone in high doses without cranial irradiation and without intrathecal methotrexate [63]. When methotrexate is given intravenously in large enough doses over a sufficient period of time, effective levels of methotrexate can be achieved in the CSF. Intraventricular CSF methotrexate levels as discussed are variable after intrathecal injections and are more consistently achieved after high-dose intravenous infusions [91]. Therapeutic (greater than $10^{-7}$ M) CSF methotrexate levels can be obtained 24 hours after bolus injections of 400–600 mg/m$^2$ of methotrexate [75]. Other pharmacologic studies using higher doses of intravenous bolus and prolonged infusions of methotrexate have also demonstrated that therapeutic CSF methotrexate levels can be achieved [117, 118].

At the Baltimore Cancer Research Center, once patients with adult ALL are in complete remission they are given remission continuation therapy which includes as the second phase intravenous, high-dose methotrexate that is used without prophylactic cranial irradiation and without prophylac-

*Table 10.* MOAD for adult ALL: cytotredution therapy for remission continuation.

| | | | | Each course | | | | |
|---|---|---|---|---|---|---|---|---|
| Day | 1 | 2 | 3 | 4 | 5 | 6 | No treatment | 30 |
| | V | | | | | | | |
| | | D | D | D | D | D | | |
| | HDMTX | | | | | | | |
| | CL | CL | CL | | | | | |

| | Drug | Dose | Route | Schedule |
|---|---|---|---|---|
| V | Vincristine | 2 mg | IV push | Day 1 |
| D | Dexamethasone | 6 mg/m$^2$ | PO | Days 2–6 |
| HDMTX | High Dose Methotrexate | 100 mg/kg * | IV infusion [†] | Day 1 |
| CL | Calcium Leucovorin | 5% of HDMTX dose [‡] | IV infusion-PO [§] | Days 1–3 ** |

\* Increase by 25% until minimal toxicity develops.
[†] Over 6 hours.
[‡] Total dose of 5% of HDMTX dose given in 12 equally divided doses over 3 days.
[§] Short IV infusion every 6 hours for first 8 doses (days 1–2), and then last 4 doses given orally (day 3).
\** Start calcium leucovorin exactly 2 hours after the end of the methotrexate infusion.
After the completion of consolidation therapy, monthly cytoreduction therapy is given for 12 courses.

tic intrathecal methotrexate because of its activity alone as prophylaxis against CNS leukemia. See Table 10 for the cytoreduction regimen which is used both as prophylactic CNS and remission continuation therapy (see discussion below).

Only two of 24 (8.3%) previously untreated patients on the MOAD study developed CNS leukemia as the initial site of relapse. Before CNS prophylaxis was given with the cytoreduction regimen, one patient relapsed simultaneously in the CNS and bone marrow during consolidation therapy at 3.3 months from the start of MOAD induction therapy. After CNS prophylaxis was given, another patient relapsed in the CNS alone during maintenance therapy at 42.7 months from the start of MOAD. Figure 2 shows that therapeutic (greater than $10^{-7}$ M) CSF methotrexate levels were achieved during cytoreduction with high-dose methotrexate starting at 100 mg/kg. It appears that increasing the dose of methotrexate did not increase the CSF methotrexate concentration. Therapeutic CSF methotrexate levels were not achieved during induction and consolidation when lower doses of drug were used starting at 100 mg/m$^2$. It appears that intravenous, high-dose metho-

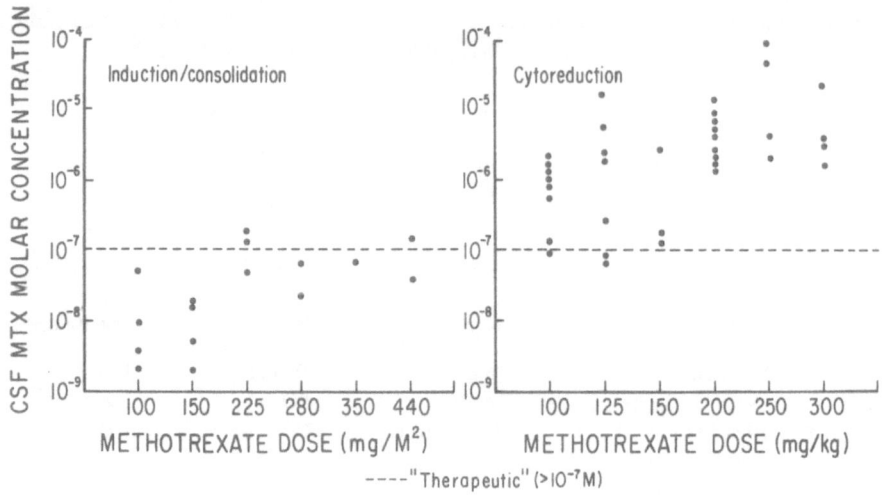

*Figure 2.* Methotrexate CSF levels 24 hours after IV administration during induction/consolidation and during cytoreduction.

trexate alone without cranial irradiation and without intrathecal methotrexate delays the onset or reduces the incidence of CNS leukemia compared to our historical experience with either no CNS prophylaxis (42.5%) or with oral pyrimethamine (Daraprim) prophylaxis (33.3%) [54, 63]. Full evaluation of this therapeutic modality for CNS prophylaxis must await for a longer period of follow-up.

In summary, results for adult ALL indicate that CNS prophylaxis is of value in decreasing the occurrence of CNS relapse. The combination of cranial irradiation plus intrathecal methotrexate has proven effective as CNS prophylaxis for both childhood and adult ALL. However, prophylactic CNS therapy for adult ALL has not resulted in improved remission duration or survival to date. Although there are both acute and delayed side effects for both cranial irradiation and intrathecal methotrexate the overall incidence is low. In the future, CNS irradiation and/or intrathecal chemotherapy may be replaced by systemic administration of antineoplastic agents that result in therapeutic CSF levels. Intravenous, high-dose methotrexate appears promising in this regard. Finally, it should be obvious that new methods are needed to better identify those patients who are clearly at an increased risk for CNS relapse as well as those patients who may not need CNS prophylaxis. In the future, it may be possible to not only reliably select prophylactic CNS therapy for certain patients according to certain prognostic factors, but also to individualize that therapy based on pharmacologic monitoring and individual dosage modification.

## 3.3. Remission Continuation Therapy

Remission continuation therapy following the attainment of a hematologic complete remission attempts to prevent or delay bone marrow relapse. In childhood ALL it has been clearly shown that remission continuation therapy prolongs the duration of complete remission [2]. Withholding remission continuation therapy after the induction of complete remission results in a median time to relapse of two months [119]. Remission continuation therapy with single agents such as methotrexate and mercaptopurine, extends median remission duration to 5-9 months, but long-term remission durations are few [72]. Various remission continuation therapy combinations of low-dose, oral methotrexate and mercaptopurine or other drug combinations with vincristine and prednisone given as periodic reinduction or 'reinforcement pulses' have significantly extended remission duration in some earlier childhood ALL studies [120, 121]. The addition of a third or fourth drug (cyclophosphamide and cytarabine, respectively) to the methotrexate and mercaptopurine combination did not improve remission duration and survival and was associated with an increased risk of infection secondary to increased myelosuppression [89, 122]. However, in comparative childhood studies that use an adequate remission induction regimen (vincristine, prednisone and either an anthracycline or asparaginase) and effective remission continuation therapy (weekly methotrexate and daily mercaptopurine), 'pulses' of vincristine and prednisone or other drug combinations do not make a significant contribution to the overall results [2].

The role of remission continuation therapy in adult ALL is unknown, primarily because few comparative studies have been done and many different remission continuation regimens have been reported (see Table 3). In the MOAD program, for example, remission continuation therapy consists of three phases, a consolidation phase, a cytoreduction phase and a maintenance phase (see Tables 6, 10, 12). The general approach to prolong the duration of complete remission in adult ALL has been to adapt the successful remission continuation therapy programs for childhood ALL. However, since neither remission duration nor survival is as good for adult ALL as it is for childhood ALL, several different approaches have been attempted to prolong the duration of complete remission in adult ALL. Some studies have used an early intensification or consolidation phase following remission induction therapy as the first phase of remission continuation therapy in adult ALL with excellent results [3, 67, 69]. The best reported median duration of continuous complete remission (25 months) and median survival (33 months) in adult ALL is a study that used an intensive consolidation phase with cytarabine and thioguanine (see Table 3).

However, there are no reported comparative studies that have been done in a prospective randomized fashion to answer the question whether early intensification or consolidation therapy (as the first phase of remission continuation therapy) is of value in prolonging the duration of complete remission and survival in adults with ALL. One such study is underway in CALGB. That study (protocol #8011) tests whether consolidation with two courses of cytarabine and daunorubicin after remission induction therapy with vincristine, prednisone, daunorubicin, asparaginase, and intrathecal methotrexate will increase the duration of remission and survival. Following the consolidation phase, remission continuation therapy will be identical for both treatment groups and will consist of a maintenance phase with oral methotrexate and mercaptopurine plus periodic reinforcement with vincristine and prednisone. This approach has merit because all adults with ALL are in the high-risk or poor prognostic group of patients with this disease.

Other studies have employed a cytoreduction treatment phase as part of the remission continuation therapy program. The problem that is encountered with this approach is that the initiation of systemic combination chemotherapy for cytoreduction during cranial irradiation for prophylactic CNS therapy is usually associated with significant bone marrow suppression resulting in either an increase in the risk of infection or a decrease in the planned chemotherapy dose for many patients, placing them at risk for relapse. In childhood ALL, aggressive cytoreductive therapy given simultaneously with prophylactic CNS therapy did not prolong remission duration and was associated with significant morbidity [2]. The MOAD study in adult ALL has attempted to give aggressive cytoreductive therapy with simultaneous CNS prophylaxis [63]. This therapy was essentially non-toxic. Hematologic toxicity was minimal and there were no significant infections. Usually what has been attempted in other studies is to give either oral methotrexate or mercaptopurine until cranial irradiation and intrathecal methotrexate are finished. The contribution of a cytoreduction phase to remission continuation therapy will not be known until a comparative study is done in a prospective randomized fashion to answer the question whether this therapy (which includes systemic chemotherapy and CNS prophylaxis) is of value in prolonging the duration of complete remission and survival in adults with ALL. Currently there is no such known study underway.

The next phase of remission continuation therapy is maintenance. The most commonly used maintenance regimen for adult ALL is directly adapted from the successful regimen for childhood ALL (see Table 11). Weekly oral, low-dose methotrexate and daily oral mercaptopurine have been employed in more than half of the reported studies for the maintenance phase of remission continuation therapy for adult ALL (see Table 3). Although the addition of a third or fourth drug such as cyclophophamide and cytarabine to methotrexate and mercaptopurine did not extend remission duration in childhood ALL, the addition of cyclophosphamide to

*Table 11.* Drugs most commonly used in remission continuation regimens for adult ALL.

| Therapy | Drug | Dose | Route | Schedule |
|---------|------|------|-------|----------|
| Consolidation 1 or 2 courses after CR, before CNS prophylaxis | Cytarabine + Thioguanine Asparaginase | $100-150 \, \text{mg/m}^2$ $100-125 \, \text{mg/m}^2$ $500-35\,000 \, \text{IU/m}^2$ | IV PO IV | q 12 h × 10–20 doses q 12 h × 10–20 doses Daily × 5–28 |
| Maintenance after CR, consolidation, and CNS prophylaxis | Mercaptopurine + Methotrexate +/− Cyclophosphamide | $50-100 \, \text{mg/m}^2$ $15-30 \, \text{mg/m}^2$ $200-300 \, \text{mg/m}^2$ | PO PO PO | Daily Weekly Weekly |
| Reinforcement every 1 to 6 months after CR | Vincristine + Prednisone | $1.0-2.0 \, \text{mg/m}^2$ $40-100 \, \text{mg/m}^2$ | IV PO | Weekly × 1–3 Daily × 5–15 |

CR = complete remission.
CNS = central nervous system.

methotrexate and mercaptopurine has been utilized in approximately one of every five reported studies for adult ALL. Whether cyclophosphamide improves remission duration and survival in adult ALL cannot be evaluated because of the differences in prophylactic CNS, maintenance, and reinforcement therapies. However, a standard maintenance phase, consisting of weekly oral, low-dose methotrexate and daily oral, low-dose mercaptopurine with periodic reinforcement with vincristine and prednisone appears to prolong the duration of complete remission and survival for adult ALL, but not to the extent that it does for childhood ALL.

The median duration of complete remission with remission continuation therapy on the MOAD study with consolidation, cytoreduction and maintenance therapy (see Tables 6, 10, and 12) was 11.1 months for the previously untreated patients (see Figure 3) and is comparable to many reported studies (see Table 3). The median duration of complete remission of 7.5 months for the previously treated patients (see Figure 3) is superior to most reported studies [63, 65, 123–127] (see Table 13). The median survival of previously untreated complete remission patients has not been reached (17.8 months). The median survival of previously treated complete remission patients was 17.2 months. The median survival of all previously untreated patients was 17.0 months and of all previously treated patients was 11.2 months (see Figure 4). The median survival of 17.0+ months for all the previously untreated patients is comparable to many reported studies (see Table 3). The median survival of 11.2 months for the previously treated patients is superior to most reported studies (see Table 13). Hematologic

*Table 12.* MOAD for adult ALL: maintenance therapy.

| | | | | | Each course | | | | |
|---|---|---|---|---|---|---|---|---|---|
| Day | 1 | 2 | 3 | 4 | 5 | 6 | 7 | 8 | 28 |
| | V | | | | | | | | |
| | D | D | D | D | D | | | | |
| | MTX | | | | | | | MTX | Weekly |
| | MP | MP | MP | MP | MP | MP | MP | MP | Daily |

| | Drug | Dose | Route | Schedule |
|---|---|---|---|---|
| V | Vincristine | 2 mg | IV push | Day 1 |
| D | Dexamethasone | 6 mg/m$^2$ | PO | Days 1–5 |
| MTX | Methotrexate | 15 mg/m$^2$ | PO | Weekly |
| MP | Mercaptopurine | 100 mg/m$^2$ | PO | Daily |

Following the completion of cytoreduction therapy, maintenance therapy is given until relapse.

toxicity from remission continuation therapy was minimal and no significant infections developed. As previously discussed (under prophylactic CNS therapy) only two of 24 (8.3%) previously untreated patients developed CNS leukemia. Remission continuation therapy resulted in an increase in

*Table 13.* Combination chemotherapy for previously treated adults.

| Author (reference) | Relapse reinduction regimen | Number of patients | Percent complete remission | Median duration CR in mos. | Median survival in mos. |
|---|---|---|---|---|---|
| Bloomfield [123] | P+DNR | 11 | 18 | 1.0 | 2.0 |
| Bodey [24] | DNR+ASP | 34 | 38 | 3.0 (includes AML pts.) | 7.5 (CR pts.) |
| Elias [125] | V+P+DOX | 10 | 50 | 3.8 | 3.3 |
| Amadori [126] | MTX+ASP | 17 | 59 | 2.5 (includes AML pts.) | 4.8 |
| Rodriguez [65] | V+P+MTX+MP | 21 | 62 | 3.3 (includes AML pts.) | 7.0 |
| Yap [78] | MTX+ASP | 21 | 62 | 5.0 (includes AML pts.) | 11.3 (CR pts.) |
| Woodruff [127] | V+P+DOX+ASP | 23 | 69 | 2.0 | 7.0 |
| Esterhay [63] | V+D+MTX+ASP | 14 | 79 | 7.5+ | 11.2+ |

ASP = cytarabine,  D = dexamethasone,  DNR = daunorubicin,  DOX = doxorubicin,
MP = mercaptopurine, MTX = methotrexate, P = prednisone, V = vincristine.

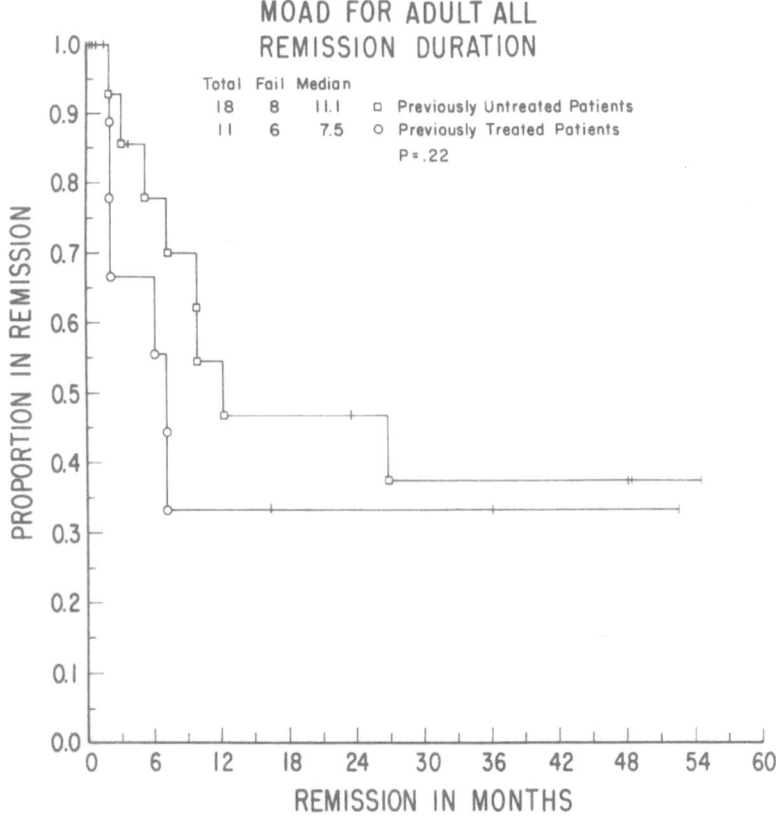

*Figure 3.* Remission duration from date of CR or reinduced CR to relapse for previously untreated and previously treated patients.

the median survival for previously untreated patients at our institution (see Table 14 and Figure 5).

The question of when remission continuation therapy should be stopped has not yet clearly been resolved for adult ALL. The usual practice for childhood ALL is to discontinue treatment after 2.5–5 years of continuous complete remission following institution of effective treatment regimens [2]. However, even if a continuous complete remission has been maintained for 2.5–3 years in childhood ALL, the overall frequency of relapse following cessation of treatment is about 25 % [2]. The current policy of some programs or studies for adult ALL is not to stop the maintenance phase of remission continuation therapy after three years of continuous complete remission, but to continue therapy indefinitely until relapse occurs.

In summary, remission continuation therapy results for previously untreated adult ALL indicate that therapy during remission is of value in

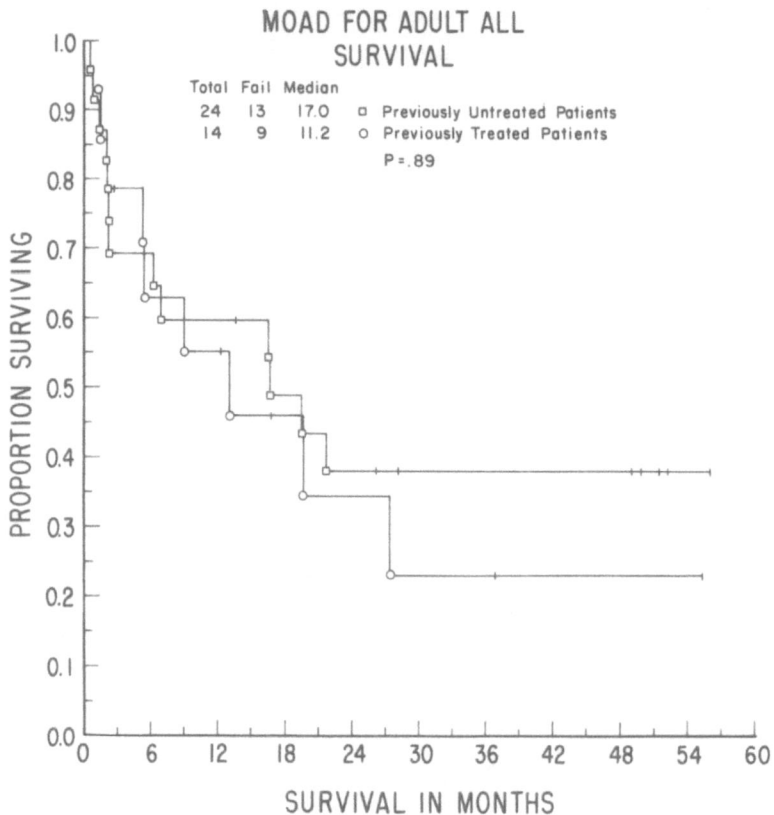

*Figure 4.* Survival for all patients from date of MOAD therapy for previously untreated and previously treated patients.

prolonging the duration of complete remission and survival. Whether an intermittent, intensive consolidation phase following remission induction therapy adds to the benefits of remission continuation therapy for adult ALL is yet to be established. Comparative studies are underway to answer this question. In addition, the role of a cytoreduction phase prior to the maintenance phase to simultaneously deliver both systemic remission continuation and prophylactic CNS therapy is not established, although intravenous, high-dose methotrexate appears promising. It has been shown that standard CNS prophylaxis (with cranial irradiation plus intrathecal methotrexate) superimposed on systemic remission continuation therapy is associated with sufficient marrow suppression to require a significant decrease in the planned therapy doses for many patients placing them at risk for relapse. A standard maintenance phase, consisting of weekly oral, low-dose methotrexate and daily oral mercaptopurine given along with periodic rein-

*Table 14.* Baltimore Cancer Research Center: therapy of previously untreated adult ALL 1965-1980.

| | VCR + PRED or POMP (1965–71) | TODD (1972–74) | MOAD (1975–80) |
|---|---|---|---|
| Patients | 40 | 18 | 24 |
| Median age | 24 | 26 | 31 |
| Complete remission (CR) | 42% | 53% | 75% |
| Partial remission | 7% | 30% | — |
| Median duration CR | 7.0 months | 6.0 months | 11.1 months |
| CNS leukemia | 42.5% | 33.3% | 8.3% |
| Median survival, all treated | 7.0 months | 13.5 months | 17.0 months |

VCR = vincristine; PRED = prednisone; POMP = prednisone, vincristine, methotrexate, mercaptopurine; TODD = thioguanine, vincristine, dexamethasone, pyrimethamine; MOAD = methotrexate, vincristine, asparaginase, dexamethasone.

forcement with vincristine and steroid has been shown to be effective remission continuation therapy for adults with ALL. However, periodic reinforcement with vincristine and steroid (for patients who have received intensive remission induction and standard prophylactic CNS therapy) has not been tested in a comparative study to see how it contributes to the benefits of standard maintenance with mercaptopurine and methotrexate.

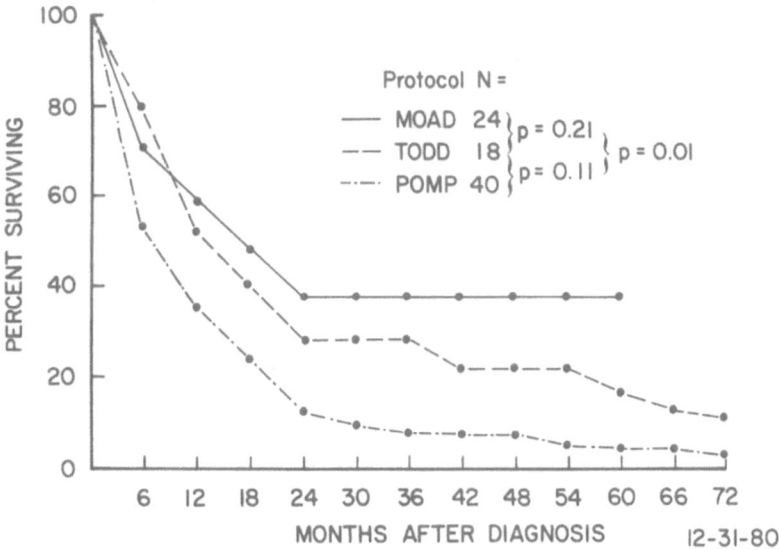

*Figure 5.* Therapy of previously untreated adult ALL patients at the Baltimore Cancer Research Center 1965–1980.

## 3.4. Relapse Reinduction Therapy

In childhood ALL, remission reinduction therapy with vincristine, prednisone, and an anthracycline or asparaginase is usually employed and a high proportion (about 80%) of patients achieve a second complete remission [2]. In adult ALL, a lower proportion (about 60%) of patients achieve a second complete remission (see Table 13). However with both childhood and adult ALL the duration of a second complete remission is usually short. The reported median duration of subsequent complete remission for previously treated/relapsed adult ALL patients is three months (range 1.0–7.5) and survival is seven months (range 2.0–11.0) (see Table 13). Obviously, the problem that has to be addressed is the lack of effective remission continuation therapy once the second complete remission is obtained.

Another problem that must be dealt with is the risk of CNS leukemia following the bone marrow relapse. Usually, survival is so short once a bone marrow relapse occurs during remission continuation therapy that CNS leukemia is not a major problem in disease control. The different therapeutic modalities for CNS leukemia therapy are outlined in Table 9. The approach at the Baltimore Cancer Research Center is to give intrathecal chemotherapy with methotrexate for CNS leukemia. Others, as previously discussed, have advocated using intrathecal triple drug (methotrexate, cytarabine, and hydrocortisone) therapy. Whether single or combination intrathecal chemotherapy is more effective is unknown [111]. After CSF remission has been obtained, periodic intrathecal chemotherapy is required to maintain that remission. Intrathecal cytarabine is usually employed after the patient becomes refractory to methotrexate and craniospinal irradiation. As previously discussed under the prophylactic CNS therapy section, some patients with CNS leukemia will benefit from intraventricular methotrexate or cytarabine via an Ommaya reservoir. With CNS leukemia, subsequent systemic chemotherapy should be given as relapse reinduction therapy with at least vincristine and steroid as part of the reinduction regimen. The reason for this is that there has probably been seeding of lymphoblasts to the bone marrow and other sites and the goal of reinduction therapy is to prevent subsequent relapses. The major site of relapse in addition to the bone marrow and CNS is for males, the testes [2, 52]. Testicular relapse should be treated with bilateral testicular irradiation and should be followed with relapse reinduction therapy.

## 4. FUTURE TREATMENT RESEARCH

Future research in adult ALL will obviously be centered about the classification of ALL in an attempt to improve our understanding of the biologic heterogeneity of this disease. Ongoing and future studies will attempt to correlate morphologic classification, cytochemical reactions, immunologic cell surface and biochemical markers and cytogenetic findings with respect to response frequency, remission duration, and survival. In addition, studies that monitor the levels of terminal deoxynucleotidyl transferase during remission induction and continuation therapy are underway. More intensive remission induction regimens for adult ALL using comparative trials to evaluate aggressive consolidation regimens are either planned or underway by cooperative cancer study groups such as CALGB. Studies also need to be done to determine optimal CNS prophylaxis. It is not clear what the best CNS therapeutic modality will ultimately be for adult ALL. There are dose-schedule pharmacokinetic interactions between methotrexate and vincristine and methotrexate and asparaginase that need to be further explored for both CNS prophylaxis and systemic therapy [74–78, 128]. More effective remission continuation and reinduction regimens need to be found which result in prolonged second remissions.

New agents such as AMSA, AZQ, and deoxycoformycin need to be further evaluated. AMSA (acridinylamino-methanesulfon-m-anisidide), a non-cardiotoxic acridine derivative, possesses antileukemic activity against ALL [129–131]. There are phase I–II studies underway to determine the efficacy of this new agent in refractory adult acute leukemia [132, 133]. Preliminary data indicate that the activity in refractory acute non-lymphoblastic leukemia is greater than the activity in ALL [132, 133]. AZQ (aziridinylbenzoquinone), which is undergoing phase I–II studies in refractory adult acute leukemia, appears attractive because preliminary results suggest that this new agent penetrates into the brain and brain tumors readily with a tendency to persist [134]. This agent may be useful as an alternative to methotrexate and cytarabine for CNS prophylaxis and therapy. Deoxycoformycin, a selectively lymphocytotoxic compound that acts by inhibition of the enzyme adenosine deaminase, has been reported to induce complete remissions in patients with refractory T-cell ALL [135]. In ALL, very rapid reductions of lymphoblasts in both the peripheral blood and bone marrow have been reported [136, 137]. A dose of 0.25 mg/kg/day for five days produces a response with acceptable toxicity [135, 136, 138]. This antilymphocytic agent will be studied further and new clinical trials in adult ALL are anticipated.

New modalities of therapy need to be investigated. Bone marrow transplantation, biological response modifiers such as immunotherapeutic agents, interferon, interferon inducers (e.g., poly I: poly C) and differentiating inducing proteins are new modalities that will be investigated further in the 1980s.

## 5. SUMMARY

The next decade should prove to be very interesting as our understanding of ALL evolves and our application of therapeutic modalities becomes tailored to this new understanding. The prognosis in adult ALL is improving dramatically and although the end results are not as good as those in childhood ALL, steady progress has been made. Because adult ALL occurs infrequently the approach to therapy will continue to be largely taken from the experience in children. More effective systemic therapy for both induction and continuation therapy and the application of optimal CNS prophylaxis will lead to continued improvements in the therapy of adult ALL in the 1980s.

## REFERENCES

1. Hayhoe FGJ: Clinical and cytological recognition and differentiation of the leukemias. In: Proceedings of the International Conference on Leukemia-Lymphoma. Zarafonetis CJE (ed). Philadelphia: Lea and Febiger, 1968, p. 307.
2. Mauer AM: Therapy of acute lymphoblastic leukemia in childhood. Blood 56:1-10, 1980.
3. Gee TS, Haghbin M, Dowling MD, Cunningham I, Middleman MP, Clarkson BD: Acute lymphoblastic leukemia in adults and children. Differences in response with similar therapeutic regimens. Cancer 37:1256-1264, 1976.
4. Chessels JM, Hardisty RM, Rapson NT, Greaves MF: Acute lymphoblstic leukaemia in children: classification and prognosis. Lancet ii:1307-1309, 1977.
5. Miller DR:Prognostic factors in childhood leukemia. J Pediatr 87:672-676, 1975.
6. Dow LW, Borella L, Sen L, Aur RJA, George SL, Mauer AM, Simone JV: Initial prognostic factors and lymphoblast-erythrocyte rosette formation in 109 children with acute lymphoblastic leukemia. Blood 50:671-682, 1977.
7. Leimert JT, Burns CP, Wiltse CG, Armitage JO, Clarke WR: Prognostic influence of pretreatment characteristics in adult acute lymphoblastic leukemia. Blood 56:510-515, 1980.
8. Mathé G, Pouillart P, Sterescu M, Amiel JL: Subdivision of classical varieties of acute leukemia. Correlation with prognosis and cure expectancy. Eur J Clin Biol Res 16:554-563, 1971.
9. Mathé G, Belpomme D, Dantchev D, Pouillart P, Navares L, Hauss G, Schlumberger JR, Lafleur M: Search for correlations between cytological types and therapeutic sensitivity of acute leukemias. Blood Cells 1:37-52, 1975.
10. Bennett JM, Catovsky D, Daniel M-T, Flandrin G, Galton DAG, Gralnik HR, Sultan C: Proposals for the classification of the acute leukemias. Br J Haematol 33:451-458, 1976.
11. Flandrin G, Daniel MT, Couderc O: Classification cytologiques des leucémies aiguës lympholbastiques: incidences cliniques et prognostiques. Actualités Hemat 7:25-32, 1973.
12. Pantazopoulos N, Sinks LF: Morphological criteria for prognostication of acute lymphoblastic leukemia. Br J Haematol 27:25-29, 1974.
13. Bloomfield CD, Brunning RD: Prognostic implications of cytology in acute leukemia in the adult. Hum Pathol 5:641-659, 1974.

14. Galton DAG, Dacie JV: Classification of the acute leukemias. Blood Cells 1:17–24, 1975.

15. Brouet JC, Valensi F, Daniel M, Flaudrin G, Prend'Homme J, Seligmann M: Immunological classification of acute lymphoblastic leukemias: evaluation of its clinical significance in a hundred patients. Br J Haematol 33:319–328, 1976.

16. Lee SL, Kopel S, Glidewell O: Cytomorphological determinants of prognosis in acute lymphoblastic leukemia in children. Semin Oncol 3:209–217, 1976.

17. Murphy SB, Borella L, Sen L: Lack of correlation of lymphoblast cell size with presence of T-cell markers or with outcome in childhood acute lymphoblastic leukemia. Br J Haematol 31:95–102, 1975.

18. Masera P, Matera L, Gavosto F: Lymphoblast size and prognosis of acute lymphoblastic leukaemia (ALL). Haematologica 61:250–251, 1976.

19. Wagner VM, Baehner RL: Lack of correlation between blast cell size and length of first remission in acute lymphocytic leukemia in childhood. Med Pediatr Oncol 3:373–377, 1977.

20. Brearley RL, Johson SAN, Lister TA: Acute lymphoblastic leukaemia in adults: clinicopathological correlations with the French-American-British (FAB) cooperative group classification. Eur J Cancer 15:909–914, 1979.

21. Flandrin G, Brouet JC, Daniel MT, Preud'Homme JL: Acute leukemia with Burkitt's tumor cells: a study of six cases with special reference to lymphocyte surface markers. Blood 45:183–188, 1975.

22. Arsenean JC, Canellos GP, Banks PM, Berard CW, Gralnick HR, DeVita VT: American Burkitt's lymphoma: a clinicopathologic study of 30 cases. I. Clinical factors relating to prolonged survival. Am J Med 58:314–321, 1975.

23. Brearley RL, Lister TA, Whitehouse JMA, Stansfeld AG: Burkitt's lymphoma in British adults: clinical features and response to chemotherapy. Br J Cancer 35:484–487, 1977.

24. Ziegler JL: Treatment results of 54 American patients with Burkitt's lymphoma are similar to the African experience. N Engl J Med 297:75–80, 1977.

25. Lister TA, Whitehouse JMA, Beard MEJ, Brearley RL, Wrigley PFM, Oliver RTD, Freeman JE, Woodruff RK, Malpas JS, Paxton AM, Crowther D: Combination chemotherapy for acute lymphoblastic leukemia in adults. Br Med J 1:199–203, 1978.

26. Raney RB, Festa RS, Waldman MTG, Manson D, Hann HWL: The periodic acid-Schiff reaction and prognosis in children with acute lymphoblastic leukemia. Am J Hematol 6:27–34, 1979.

27. McKenna RW, Brynes RK, Nesbit ME, Bloomfield CD, Kersey JH, Spanjers E, Brunning RD: Cytochemical profiles in acute lymphoblastic leukemia. Am J Pediatr Hematol Oncol 1:263–275, 1979.

28. Bloomfield CD, Gajl-Peczalska KJ: The clinical relevance of lymphocyte surface markers in leukemia and lymphoma. Curr Topics Hematol 3:175–240, 1980.

29. Sen L, Borella L: Clinical importance of lymphoblasts with T markers in childhood acute leukemia. N Engl J med 292:828–832, 1975.

30. Tsukimoto I, Wong KY, Lampkin BC: Surface markers and prognostic factors in acute lymphoblastic leukemia. N Engl J Med 294:245–248, 1976.

31. Sallan SE, Ritz J, Pesando J: Cell surface antigens: prognostic implications in childhood acute lymphoblastic leukemia. Blood 55:395–402, 1980.

32. Bitran JD: Prognostic value of immunologic markers in adults with acute lymphoblastic leukemia. N Engl J Med 299:1317, 1978.

33. Baccarani M, Gobbi M, Tura S: Prognostic value of immunologic markers in adults with acute lymphoblastic leukemia. N Engl J Med 302:123, 1980.

34. Lister TA, Roberts MM, Brearley RL: Prognostic significance of cell surface phenotype in adult acute lymphoblastic leukemia. Cancer Immunol Immunotherap 6:227–230, 1979.

35. Greaves MF, Lister TA: Prognostic importance of immunologic markers in adult acute lymphoblastic leukemia. N Engl J Med 304:119-120, 1981.

36. Brouet JC, Preud'Homme JL, Penit C, Valensi F, Rouget P, Seligmann M: Acute lymphoblastic leukemia with pre-B-cell characteristics. Blood 54:269-273, 1979.

37. Volger LB, Crist WM, Bockman DE, Pearl ER, Lawton AR, Cooper MD: Pre-B-cell leukemia. A new phenotype of childhood lymphoblastic leukemia. N Engl J Med 298:872-878, 1978.

38. Coleman MS, Greenwood MF, Hutton JJ, Holland P, Lampkin B, Krill C, Kastelic JE: Adenosine deaminase, terminal deoxynucleotidyl transferase (TdT), and cell surface markers in childhood acute leukemia. Blood 52:1125-1130, 1978.

39. Sarin PS, Anderson PN, Gallo RC: Terminal deoxynucleotidyl transferase activities in human blood leukocytes and lymphoblast cell lines. Blood 47:11-20, 1976.

40. Coleman MS, Greenwood MF, Hutton JJ, Bollum FJ, Lampkin B, Holland P: Serial observations on terminal deoxynucleotidyl transferase activity and lymphoblast surface marker in acute lymphoblastic leukemia. Cancer Res 36:120-127, 1976.

41. Hoffbrand AV, Ganeshaguru K, Kanossy G, Greaves MF, Catovsky D, Woodruff RK: Terminal deoxynucleotidyl-transferase levels and membrane phenotypes in diagnosis of acute leukemia. Lancet ii:520-523, 1977.

42. Brouet JC, Seligmann M: The immunological classification of acute lymphoblastic leukemias. Cancer 42:817-827, 1978.

43. Reismann LE, Mitani M, Zuelzer WW: Chromosome studies in leukemia. I. Evidence for the origin of leukemia stem lines from aneuploid mutants. N Engl J Med 270:591-597, 1964.

44. Whang-Peng J, Knutsen MT, Ziegler J, Leventhal B: Cytogenetic studies in acute lymphocytic leukemia: Special emphasis on long-term survival. Med Pediatr Oncol 2:333-351, 1976.

45. Oshimura M, Freeman AI, Sandberg AA: Chromosomes and causation of human cancer and leukemia. XXXI. Banding studies in acute lymphoblastic leukemia (ALL). Cancer 40:1161-1172, 1977.

46. Cimino MC, Rowley JD, Kinnealey A, Variakojis D, Golomb HM: Banding studies of chromosomal abnormalities in patients with acute lymphocytic leukemia. Cancer Res 39:227-238, 1979.

47. Third International Workshop on Chromosomes in Leukemia: Clinical significance of chromosomal abnormalities in acute lymphoblastic leukemia. Cancer Genet Cytogenet ( in press).

48. Bloomfield CD, Brunning R, Kersey J, Gajl-Peczalska KJ: Adult acute lymphocytic leukemia (ALL): The therapeutic significance of surface markers (SM) and the Philadelphia chromosome (Ph) (abstr). Proc Am Assoc Cancer Res 17:166, 1976.

49. Janossy G, Greaves MF, Sutherland R, Durrant J, Lewis C: Comparative analysis of membrane phenotypes in acute lymphoid leukemia and in lymphoid blast crisis of chronic myeloid leukemia. Leukemia Res 1:289-300, 1977.

50. Bloomfield CD, Peterson LC, Yunis JJ, Brunning RD: The Philadelphia chromosome (Ph$^1$) in adults presenting with acute leukaemia: a comparison of Ph$^1$+ and Ph$^1$- patients. Br J Haematol 36:347-358, 1977.

51. Rosenthal S, Cannellos GP, Whang-Peng J, Gralnick HR: Blast crisis of chronic granulocytic leukemia. Morphologic variants and therapeutic implications. Am J Med 63:542-547, 1977.

52. Woodruff R: The management of adult lymphoblastic leukemia. Cancer Treat Rev 5:95-113, 1978.

53. Whitecar JP, Bodey GP, Freireich EJ, McCredie KB, Hart JS: Cyclophosphamide (NSC-26271), vinvristine (NSC-67574), cytosine arabinoside (NSC-63878), and prednisone

(NSC-10023) (COAP) combination chemotherapy for acute leukemia in adults. Cancer Chemother Rep 56:543–550, 1972.

54. Smyth AC, Wiernik PH: Combination chemotherapy of adult acute lymphocytic leukemia. Clin Pharmacol Ther 19:240–245, 1976.

55. Gahrton G, Engstedt L, Franzen S, Gullbring B, Holm G, Hoglund S, Killander A, Killander D, Lockner D, Mellstedt H, Palmbald J, Reizenstein P, Skarberg K-O, Swedberg B, Uden A-M: Induction of remission with l-asparaginase, cyclophosphamide, cytosine arabinoside and prednisone in adult patients with acute leukemia. Cancer 34:472–479, 1974.

56. Armitage JO, Burns CP: Remission maintenance of adult acute lymphoblastic leukemia. Med Pediatr Oncol 3:53–58, 1977.

57. Gingrich RD, Armitage JO, Burns CP: Treatment of adult acute lymphoblastic leukemia with cytosine arabinoside, vincristine, and prednisone. Cancer Treat Rep 62:1389–1391, 1978.

58. Shaw MT, Raab SO: Adriamycin in combination chemotherapy of adult acute lymphoblastic leukemia. A Southwest Oncology Group Study. Med Pediatr Oncol 3:261–266, 1977.

59. Willemze R, Hillen H, Hartgrink-Groeneveld CA, Haanen C: Treatment of acute lymphoblastic leukemia in adolescents and adults: a retrospective study of 41 patients (1970–1973). Blood 46:823–834, 1975.

60. Henderson ES, Scharlau C, Cooper MR, Haurani FI, Silver RT, Brunner K, Carey RW, Falkson G, Blom J, Nawab I, Levine AS, Bank A, Cuttner J, Cornwell GG Ill, Henry P, Nissen NI, Wiernik PH, Leone L, Whol H, Rai K, James GW, Weinberg V, Glidewell O, Holland JF: Combination chemotherapy and radiotherapy for acute lymphocytic leukemia in adults: results of CALGB protocol 7113. Leukemia Res 3:395–407, 1979.

61. Jacquillat C, Weil M, Gemon MF, Auclerc G, Loisel J, Delobel G, Flaudrin G, Schaison G, Izrael V, Brussel A, Dresch C, Weisgerber C, Rain D, Tanzer J, Najean Y, Seligmann M, Boiron M, Bernard J: Combination therapy in 130 patients with acute lymphoblastic leukemia (protocol 66 LA 66-Paris). Cancer Res 33:3278–3284, 1973.

62. Muriel FS, Pavlovsky S, Penalver JA, Hidalgo G, Bonesana AC, Eppinger-Helft M, de Macchi GH, Pavlovsky A: Evaluation of induction of remission, intensification, and central nervous system prophylactic treatment in acute lymphoblastic leukemia. Cancer 34:418–426, 1974.

63. Esterhay RJ Jr, Wiernik PH, Grove WR, Markus SD, Wesley MN: Moderate dose methotrexate, vincristine, asparaginase and dexamethasone for treatment of adult acute lymphocytic leukemia. Blood 59 (2):1982 (in press).

64. Gottlieb AJ, Weinberg V: Efficacy of daunorubicin in induction therapy of adult acute lymphocytic leukemia (ALL): a controlled phase III study (CALGB #7612). Blood 54:Suppl 1, 188a, 1979.

65. Rodriquez V, Hart JS, Freireich EJ, Bodey GP, McCredie KB, Whitecar JP, Goltman CA: POMP combination chemotherapy of adult leukemia. Cancer 32:69–75, 1973.

66. Omura GA, Moffitt S, Vogler WR, Salter MM: Combination chemotherapy of adult acute lymphoblastic leukemia with randomized central nervous system prophylaxis. Blood 55:199–204, 1980.

67. Schauer P, Arlin Z, Dowling M, Gee T, Mertelsmann R, Burchenal J, Dufour P, Cirrincione C, Clarkson B: The treatment of acute lymphoblastic leukemia (ALL) in adults: results of the L-10/L-10M protocol (Abstract and Personal Communication). Proc Am Assoc Cancer Res 21:180, 1980.

68. Curtis JE, Cowan DH, Bergsagel DE, Hasselback R, McCulloch EA: Acute leukemia in adults: assessment of remission induction with combination chemotherapy by clinical and cell-culture criteria. Can Med Assoc J 113:289–294, 1975.

69. Spiers ASD, Roberts PD, Marsh GW, Parekh SJ, Franklin AJ, Galton DAG, Szur ZL, Paul EA, Husband P, Wilsthaw E: Acute lymphoblastic leukaemia: cyclical chemotherapy with

three combinations of four drugs (COAP-POMP-CART regimen). Br Med J 4:614–617, 1975.

70. Scavino HF, George JN, Sears DA: Remission induction in adult acute lymphocytic leukemia. Cancer 38:672–677, 1976.

71. Einhorn LH, Bond WH: Remission induction with daunomycin, vincristine, and prednisone in adult acute lymphocytic leukemia. Oncology 34:25–28, 1977.

72. Aur RJA, Simone JV, Verzosa MS, Hustu HO, Barker LF, Pinkel DP, Rivera G, Dahl GV, Wood A, Stagner S, Mason C: Childhood acute lymphocytic leukemia. Study VIII. Cancer 42:2123–2134, 1978.

73. Jones B, Holland J, Glidewell O: Lower incidence of central nervous system leukemia using dexamethasone instead of prednisone for induction in acute lymphocytic leukemia (Abstr). Proc Am Cancer Res 16:730, 1975.

74. Capizzi RL: Biochemical interaction between asparaginase (A'se) and methotrexate (MTX) in leukemic cells (Abstr). Proc Am Assoc Cancer Res 15:77, 1974.

75. Capizzi RL: Schedule-dependent synergism and antagonism between methotrexate and asparaginase. Biochem Pharmacol (Suppl 2)23:151–161, 1974.

76. Capizzi RL, Castro O, Aspnes G, Bobrow S, Bertino J, Finch S, Pearson HA: Treatment of acute lymphocytic leukemia (ALL) with intermittent high-dose methotrexate and asparaginase (A'ase) (Abstr). Proc Am Soc Clin Oncol 15:182, 1974.

77. Lobel JS, O'Brien RT, McIntosh S, Aspnes GT, Capizzi RL: Methotrexate and asparaginase combination chemotherapy in refractory acute lymphoblastic leukemia of childhood. Cancer 43:1089–1094, 1979.

78. Yap B-S, McCredie KB, Benjamin RS, Bodey GP, Freireich EJ: Refractory acute leukaemia in adults treated with sequential colaspase and high-dose methotrexate. Br Med J 2:791–793, 1978.

79. King OY, Sutow WW: Therapy with Erwinia 1-asparaginase in children with acute leukemia after anaphylaxis to E. Coli l-asparaginase. Cancer 33:611–614, 1974.

80. Komp DM, George SL, Falletta J, Land VJ, Starling KA, Humphrey GB, Lowman J: Cyclophosphamide – asparaginase – vincristine – prednisone induction therapy in childhood acute lymphocytic and nonlymphocytic leukemia. Cancer 37:1243–1247, 1976.

81. Sallan SE, Camitta BM, Frei E III, Furman L, Leavitt P, Bishop Y, Jaffe N: Clinical and cytokinetic aspects of remission induction of childhood acute lymphoblastic leukemia (ALL): addition of an anthracycline to vincristine and prednisone. Med Pediatr Oncol 3:281–287, 1977.

82. Aur R, Simone J, Hustu O, Rivera G, Dahl G, Bowman P, George S: Multiple combination therapy for childhood acute lymphocytic leukemia (ALL) (Abstr). Blood 52:238, 1978.

83. Schimpff SC, Greene WH, Young VM, Fortner CL, Jepsen L, Cusack N, Block JB, Wiernik PH: Infection prevention in acute nonlymphocytic leukemia. Laminar air flow room isolation with oral nonabsorbable antibiotic prophylaxis. Ann Intern Med 82:351–358, 1975.

84. Hahn DM, Schimpff SC, Fortner CL, Smyth AC, Young VM, Wiernik PH: Infection in acute leukemia patients receiving oral nonabsorbable antibiotics. Antimicrob agents Chemother 13:958–964, 1978.

85. Wade J, Schimpff S, Hargadon M, Bender J, Aisner J, Young V, Wiernik P: Trimethoprim/sulfamethoxazole: infection prophylaxis during granulocytopenia. Proc Am Soc Clin Oncol 20:350, 1979.

86. Wilkinson T, Kronenbert H, Richard K: Acute leukemia in adults. Med J Aust 1:785–788, 1972.

87. Wolk R, Masse S, Conklin R, Freireich E: The incidence of central nervous system leukemia in adults with acute leukemia. Cancer 33:863–869, 1974.

88. Hustu HO, Aur RJA, Verzosa MS, Simone JV, Pinkel D: Prevention of central nervous system leukemia by irradiation. Cancer 32:585–597, 1973.
89. Aur RJA, Hustu HO, Verzosa MS, Wood A, Simone JV: Comparison of two methods of preventing central nervous system leukemia. Blood 42:349–357, 1973.
90. Bleyer WA: Current status of intrathecal chemotherapy for human neoplasms. Natl Cancer Inst Monogr 46:171–178, 1977.
91. Shapiro WR, Young DF, Mehta BM: Methotraxate: distribution in cerebrospinal fluid after intravenous, ventricular and lumbar injections. N Engl J Med 293:161–166, 1975.
92. Bleyer WA, Savitch J, Poplack DG: Methotrexate in cerebrospinal fluid. N Engl J Med 293:1152, 1975.
93. Benson DF, LeMay M, Patten DH, Rubens AB: Diagnosis of normal pressure hydrocephalus. N Engl J Med 283:609–615, 1970.
94. DiChiro G, Hammock MK, Bleyer WA: Spinal descent of cerebrospinal fluid in man. Neurology 26:1–8, 1976.
95. Mott MG, Stevenson P, Wood CBS: Methotrexate meningitis. Lancet ii:656, 1972.
96. Bleyer WA, Drake JC, Chabner BA: Neurotoxicity and elevated cerebrospinal fluid methotrexate concentration in meningeal leukemia. N Engl J Med 289:770–773, 1973.
97. Wang JJ, Pratt CB: Intrathecal arabinosyl cytosine in meningeal leukemia. Cancer 25:531–534, 1970.
98. Weis HD, Walker MD, Wiernik PH: Neurotoxicity of commonly used antineoplastic agents. N Engl J Med 291:75–81, 127–133, 1974.
99. Duttera MJ, Bleyer WA, Pomeroy TC, Leventhal CM, Leventhal BG: Irradiation, methotrexate toxicity and the treatment of menigeal leukemia. Lancet ii:703–707, 1973.
100. Gagliano RG, Costanz JJ: Paraplegia following intrathecal methotrexate. Cancer 37:1663–1668, 1976.
101. Pochedly C: Neurotoxicity due to CNS therapy for leukemia. Med Pediatr Oncol 3:101–115, 1977.
102. Kay HEM, Knapton PJ, O'Sullivan JP, Wells DG, Harris RF, Innes EM, Stuart J, Schwartz FCM, Thompson EN: Encephalopathy in acute leukemia associated with methotrexate therapy. Arch Dis Child 47:344–354, 1972.
103. Price RA, Jamieson PA: The central nervous system in childhood leukemia. II. Subacute leukoencephalopathy. Cancer 35:306–318, 1975.
104. Rubinstein LJ, Herman MM, Long TF, Wilbur JR: Disseminated necrotizing leukoencephalopathy: a complication of treated central nervous system leukemia and lymphoma. Cancer 35:291–305, 1975.
105. Aur R, Veroza M, Hutsu O, Simone J, Barker L: Leukoencephalopathy during initial complete remission in children with acute lymphocytic leukemia receiving methotrexate (Abstr). Proc Am Assoc Cancer Res 16:92, 1975.
106. Smith B: Brain damage after intrathecal methotrexate. J Neurol Neurosurg Psychiatry 38:810–815, 1975.
107. Meadows AT, Evans AE: Effects of chemotherapy on the central nervous system. A study of parenteral methotrexate in long-term survivors of leukemia and lymphoma in childhood. Cancer 37:1079–1085, 1976.
108. Shapiro WR, Posner JB, Ushio Y, Chernik NL, Young DF: Treatment of meningeal neoplasms. Cancer Treat Rep 66:733–743, 1977.
109. Bleyer WA, Poplack DG, Ziegler JL, Leventhal BG, Ommaya AK, Chabner BA: 'Concentration × time' (c × t) methotrexate (MTX) therapy of meningeal leukemia via a subcutaneous reservoir: a controlled clinical trial (Abstr). Am Soc Clin Oncol 17:253, 1976.
110. Diamond RD, Bennett JE: A subcutaneous reservoir for intrathecal therapy of fungal meningitis. N Engl J Med 288:186–188, 1973.
111. Sullivan MP, Moon TE, Trueworthy R, Vietti TJ, Humphrey GB, Komp D: Combination

intrathecal therapy for central nervous system leukemia: two versus three drugs. Blood 50:471–479, 1977.

112. Geiser CF, Bishop Y, Jaffe N, Furman L, Traggis D, Frei E: Adverse effects of intrathecal methotrexate in children with acute leukemia in remission. Blood 45:189–195, 1975.

113. Duttera MJ, Galleli JF, Kleinman LM, Tangrea JA, Wittgrove AC: Intrathecal methotrexate. Lancet i:540, 1972.

114. Haghbin M: Antimetabolites in the prophylaxis and treatment of central nervous system leukemia. Cancer Treat Rep 61:661–666, 1977.

115. Gutin PH, Weiss HD, Wiernik PH, Walker MD: Intrathecal N, N', N" - triethylenethiophosphoramide thio-TEPA (NSC 6396) in the treatment of malignant meningeal disease. Phase I–II study. Cancer 38:1471–1475, 1976.

116. Freeman AI, Wang JJ, Sinks LF: High-dose methotrexate in acute lymphocytic leukemia. Cancer Treat Rep 61:727–731, 1977.

117. Tattersal MHN, Parker LM, Pitman SW, Frei E Ill: Clinical pharmacology of highdose methotrexate (NSC-740). Cancer Chemother Rep 6:25–29, 1975.

118. Wang JJ, Freeman AI, Sinks LF: Pharmokinetic study in patients receiving highdose methotrexate for preventing meningeal leukemia (Abstr). Proc Am Soc Clin Oncol 16:231, 1975.

119. Frei E Ill, Freireich EJ: Progress and perspectives in chemotherapy of acute leukemia. Adv Chemotherapy 2:269–298, 1965.

120. Fernbach DJ, George SL, Stuow WW, Ragab AH, Lane DM, Haggard ME, Lonsdale D: Long-term results of reinforcement therapy in children with acute leukemia. Cancer 36:1552–1559, 1975.

121. Miller DR, Sonley M, Karon M, Breslow N, Hammond D: Additive therapy in the maintenance of remission in acute lymphoblastic leukemia of childhood: the effect of the initial leukocyte count. Cancer 34:508–517, 1974.

122. Simone JV: Factors that influence haematological remission duration in acute lymphocytic leukaemia. Br J Haematol 32:465–472, 1976.

123. Bloomfield CD, Brunning RD, Kennedy BJ: Daunorubicin therapy in adult acute lymphatic leukemia. Cancer 30:47–55, 1972.

124. Bodey GP, Hewlett JS, Coltman CA, Rodriquez V, Freireich EJ: Therapy of adult acute leukemia with daunorubicin and l-asparaginase. Cancer 33:626–630, 1974.

125. Elias L, Shaw MT, Raab SO: Reinduction therapy for adult acute leukemia with adriamycin, vincristine, and prednisone: a Southwest Oncology Group study. Cancer Treat Rep 63:1413-1415, 1979.

126. Amadori S, Tribalto M, Pacilli L, DeLaurentis C, Papa G, Mandelli F: Sequential combination of methotrexate and l-asparaginase in the treatment of refractory acute leukemia. Cancer Treat Rep 64:939-942, 1980.

127. Woodruff RK, Lister TA, Paxton AM, Whitehouse JMA, Malpas JS: Combination chemotherapy for haematological relapse in adult acute lymphoblastic leukaemia (ALL). Am J Hematol 4:173-177, 1978.

128. Tejada F, Zubrod CG: Vincristine effect on methotrexate cerebrospinal fluid concentration. Cancer Treat Rep 63:143-145, 1979.

129. Legha SS, Gutterman JU, Hall SW, Benjamin RS, Burgess MA, Valdivieso M, Bodey GP: Phase I clinical investigation of 4'-(9-acridinylamino) methanesulfon-m-anisidide (NSC 249992), a new acridine derivative. Cancer Res 38:3712-3722, 1978.

130. Van Hoff DD, Howser D, Gormley P, Bender RA, Glaubiger D, Levine AS, Young RC: Phase I study of methanesulfonamide, N- 4-(9-acridinylamino)-3-methoxybenyl (m-AMSA) using a single-dose schedule. Cancer Treat Rep 62:1421-1426, 1978.

131. Van Echo DA, Chiuten DF, Gormley PE, Lichtenfeld JL, Scoltock M, Wiernik PH: Phase I

clinical and pharmacological study of 4'-(9-acridinylamino) methanesulfon-*m*-anisidide using an intermittent biweekly schedule. Cancer Res 39:3881-3884, 1979.

132. Legha SS, Keating MJ, Zander AR, McCredie KB, Bodey GP, Freireich EJ: 4'-(9-acridinylamino) methanesulfon-*m*-anisidide (AMSA): a new drug effective in the treatment of adult acute leukemia. Ann Intern Med 93:17–21, 1980.

133. Arlin ZA, Sklaroff RB, Gee TS, Kempin SJ, Howard J, Clarkson BD, Young CW: Phase I and II trial of 4'-(9-acridinylamino) mathanesulfon-*m*-anisidide in patients with acute leukemia. Cancer Res 40:3304–3306, 1980.

134. Savaraj N, Lu K, Stewart D, Leavens M, Bedekian A, Feun L, Loo TL: Tissue distribution and intracerebral tumor penetration of 2,5-diaziridinyl-3, 6-biscarboethoxyamino-1, 4-benzoquinone (AZQ, NSC 182986) in man (Abstr). Proc Am Soc Clin Oncol 22:351, 1981.

135. Prentice HG, Smyth JF, Ganeshaguru K, Wonke B, Bradstock KF, Janossy G, Goldstone AH, Hoffbrand AV: Remission induction with adenosine — deaminase inhibitor 2'-deoxycoformycin in thy-lymphoblastic leukaemia. Lancet ii:170–172, 1980.

136. Koller C, Grever M, Mitchell B: Treatment of acute lymphoblastic leukemia with the adenosine deaminase inhibitor 2'-deoxycoformycin (Abstr). Proc Am Soc Clin Oncol 20:382, 1979.

137. Mitchell BS, Killer CA, Heyn R: Inhibition of adenosine deaminase activity results in cytotoxicity to T lymphoblasts in vivo. Blood 56:556–559, 1980.

138. Koller CA, Mitchell BS, Grever MR, Mejias E, Malspeis L, Metz EN: Treatment of acute lymphoblastic leukemia with 2'-deoxycoformycin: clinical and biochemical consequences of adenosine deaminase inhibition. Cancer Treat Rep 63:1949–1952, 1979.

# 11. The Role of Therapeutic and Prophylactic Granulocyte Transfusions in Adult Acute Leukemia

RONALD G. STRAUSS and JOHN E. CONNETT *

CONTENTS

1. Introduction
2. Review of Therapeutic Granulocyte Transfusion Trials
3. Analysis of Therapeutic Granulocyte Transfusion Trials
4. Review of Prophylactic Granulocyte Transfusion Trials
5. Analysis of Prophylactic Granulocyte Transfusion Trials
6. Conclusions, Current Recommendations, and Future Directions

## 1. INTRODUCTION

Great strides have been made in the induction phase of treatment for acute leukemia. Although the majority of patients will achieve an initial remission, varying periods of pancytopenia are experienced by virtually all patients as a consequence both of leukemic replacement of the bone marrow and of chemotherapy. Anemia is easily treated by transfusions because erythrocytes are accurately typed and circulate in the blood for weeks. Thrombocytopenia is more difficult to treat than anemia. Platelets exhibit a comparatively short survival in recipient blood, and many patients become refractory (unresponsive) due to donor-recipient incompatibility. Selecting donors from blood relatives with HLA-types similar to those of the recipient lessens incompatibility problems, but some patients remain refractory. However, the incidence of life-threatening hemorrhage has been markedly decreased by the use of prophylactic and therapeutic platelet transfu-

* Supported in part by contracts N01-HB6-2973 and N01-HB6-2972 from the National Heart, Lung and Blood Institute, NIH. Dr. Strauss is recipient of Research Career Development Award K04-HD00255 from the National Institute of Child Health and Human Development.

352

sions [1]. The correction of leukopenia, notably granulocytopenia, by transfusion is particularly challenging, but granulocyte transfusions (GTX) have
been clearly shown to add benefit to antibiotics in treating gram-negative
sepsis in certain patients with prolonged neutropenia [2]. Uncertainty about
GTX therapy exists because the circulating half-life of granulocytes in blood
is extremely short (under some circumstances transfused cells cannot even
be detected in recipient blood), and information is limited regarding donor-
recipient granulocyte matching. Despite these putative problems, GTX have
been employed to prevent and to treat serious infections in animals [3–5]
and man [reviewed in 2, 6–9]. Although GTX have been endorsed enthu-
siastically by many, cautionary voices raised earlier [10] have gained support [2, 11]. Concerns have been: a) the small numbers of patients studied
in controlled trials; b) the relatively small numbers of granulocytes transfused ($10^{10}$ infused per day when endogenous production during infection
may approximate $10^{12}$); c) the satisfactory, but imperfect function of neutrophils prepared for transfusion, particularly if not infused immediately [12]; d) the suspected risks of alloimmunization such as transfusion reactions, impaired granulocyte function, platelet refractoriness, and rendering
patients poor candidates for bone marrow transplantation; e) the expense in
blood resources and money (although based largely on estimates, therapeutic and prophylactic GTC were calculated to cost, respectively, $ 17.7 and
$ 57.8 million nationwide in 1978 [13]); and f) the inconveniences and
potential risks to which donors are exposed [14].

In our opinion, these problems are acceptable in certain desperate situations in which therapeutic GTX are used. They may be intolerable, however, in a prophylactic setting unless benefits of GTX are clearly shown. Thus,
it is important to critically review available information regarding the use of
therapeutic and prophylactic GTX in patients with acute leukemia and to
offer guidelines to assist physicians when they consider giving GTX.

## 2. REVIEW OF THERAPEUTIC GRANULOCYTE TRANSFUSION TRIALS

The literature published in English through August, 1980, pertaining to
the use of therapeutic GTX in neutropenic patients, will be examined. The
study populations in most papers were comprised almost entirely of patients
with acute leukemia, although a few patients with other malignancies or
aplastic anemia were included. The papers were written in styles that precluded retrieval of information applying only to the patients with leukemia,
and this minor limitation must be recognized when interpreting the data.
Data were obtained only from papers in which sufficient information was
provided to determine the types of infection for which GTX were given and

the outcome of treatment. Certain reports were excluded: a) those published in foreign languages; b) data reported in abstracts or brief reports that seemed likely to be duplicated in completed papers; c) those describing patients with qualitative neutrophil defects rather than neutropenia; d) studies employing leukocytes obtained from donors with chronic myelocytic leukemia since most pheresis centers currently use normal subjects as granulocyte donors.

Data in 17 papers were presented in sufficient detail to permit analysis [15–31]. Several features were common to all reports. Only patients with significant neutropenia (<1000 PMN/μl blood) were studied, and the count was <500/μl in all reports except two [16, 31]. All patients received antibiotics judged to be appropriate for their infections; however, in none of the papers was mention made of adjusting antibiotic dosages according to blood levels or to serum bactericidal activities. Patients in 12 of the 17 reports were eligible for study only after failing to respond to antibiotic therapy [17–19, 21–25, 27–29, 31]. Presumably, infections in these patients were unlikely to be cured by antibiotics alone. In six of the 17 studies nontransfused patients served as concurrent controls [15–20]. Controls were selected by randomization in only four of these [16, 17, 19, 20]. Granulocytes for transfusion were collected from healthy donors, but the dose of neutrophils administered was extremely variable. The dose ranges were listed in most papers, but the number of cells given to individual patients was frequently unavailable. Thus, an accurate dose-response assessment could not be made. However, most patients received $0.5-2.0 \times 10^{10}$ or $1.5-3.0 \times 10^{10}$ granulocytes per transfusion when prepared, respectively, by centrifugation and filtration techniques. Generally, post-transfusion granulocyte increments were, at best, a few hundred cells/μl. As another variable in the reports, leukapheresis and transfusion techniques were dissimilar, making comparisons difficult. Related and unrelated donors were selected on the basis of erythrocyte compatibility. Positive lymphocytotoxicity or leukoagglutinin tests excluded donors in some studies, and occasionally donors and recipients were selected to share at least one HLA haplotype. Almost never, however, were donors and recipients compatible by complete histocompatibility typing and in no instances were they matched by neutrophil specific antigens. Thus, conclusions drawn from this review of the current literature may not apply to future studies when patients will undoubtedly receive larger numbers of granulocytes that are more carefully matched, and perhaps more functionally capable.

The types of infections treated by GTX, the number of patients with each infection, and the results of therapy are listed on Table 1. Except for patients with culture-proven sepsis, the criteria for defining infection varied somewhat among investigators. Only infections which prompted GTX are listed (i.e., those for which the patients entered the studies). Infections recognized during therapy or postmortem were not tabulated. Although a list of infecting organisms was provided in most papers, it was impossible to link individual infections with causative bacteria. Thus, information about infections caused by specific microorganisms was meager. An attempt was made to define the response of each broad category of infection to GTX. Patients were called 'evaluable' (Table 1) if their course and mortality could be clearly documented. Not all patients in the treated column of Table 1 were evaluable because in many papers the characteristics of the study population, the types of infections, the microorganisms responsible, and the results of therapy were recorded in separate tables without a means of interconnecting data. Thus, it was impossible to trace the mortality of all subjects who received GTX as treatment for specific types of infections, and it was difficult to determine whether the patient died of the index infection or of a subsequent one acquired as a consequence of persistent marrow failure.

A large number of patients with gram-negative sepsis were studied, and important information has been learned. Survival was nearly identical in these patients and in those simply reported as being 'septic,' (Table 1) and it seems likely that most of this latter group had gram-negative sepsis. Survival of nontransfused, control subjects was 35% (19 of 54), although not all were evaluated concurrently. All investigators agree that patients will recover with antibiotics alone if they experience bone marrow recovery during the early days of sepsis. However, GTX will benefit those with persistent marrow failure and severe neutropenia. Originally, a minimum of four daily GTX was accepted as a therapeutic course [15, 17]. Survival of patients with gram-negative sepsis treated with ≥4 GTX was 77% (37 of 48), whereas, it was only 25% (9 of 36) in patients receiving fewer GTX (the dose was not reported in 23 patients). These data do not represent a dose-response study since patients were not prospectively assigned to treatment groups in which specific numbers of GTX were to be given as a course of therapy. Most patients were treated with fewer than four transfusions simply because they died of fulminant disease in the midst of therapy. It is likely that the septicemia was irreversible, and that they would have died regardless of further therapy. Current practice is to continue GTX until infection has completely resolved [28, 29]. The influence of the underlying disease in the response of gram-negative sepsis to GTX cannot be determined. Although 51 episodes of gram-negative sepsis were reported in patients with non-lymphocytic leukemia and 30 occurred with acute lymphoblastic leukemia, the outcome of these 81 episodes could be traced in only 19 patients. Likewise, influence of age could not be evaluated. In this regard, two uncontrolled studies of GTX in children (1–14 years) found that the majority of patients responded to only one or two transfusions [23, 24]. It is suggested by this rapid response

*Table 1.* Pooled results of 17 studies of therapeutic GTX.

| Types of infections | Patients | | Survival | |
| --- | --- | --- | --- | --- |
| | Treated | Evaluable | Number | Percent |
| Gram-negative sepsis * | 126 | 107 | 59 | 55 |
| Gram-positive sepsis | 9 | 3 | 3 | 100 |
| Polymicrobial sepsis | 8 | 8 | 3 | 38 |
| Fungemia | 1 | 0 | – | – |
| Sepsis organism unspecified | 98 | 39 | 18 | 60 |
| Total pneumonias | 53 | 18 | 13 | 72 |
| Gram-negative pneumonia | 3 | – | – | – |
| Gram-positive pneumonia | 1 | – | – | – |
| Polymicrobial pneumonia | 1 | – | – | – |
| Fungal pneumonia | 1 | – | – | – |
| Pneumonia organism unspecified | – | – | – | – |
| Localized infection, e.g., skin, genitourinary, enteric, pharynx | 68 | 31 | – | – |
| Gram-negative | 11 | – | – | – |
| Gram-positive | 7 | – | – | – |
| Polymicrobial | 2 | – | – | – |
| Fungal | 1 | – | – | – |
| Organism unspecified | 47 | – | – | – |
| Cellulitis and abscess | – | 23 | 20 | 87 |
| Genitourinary | – | 8 | 6 | 75 |
| Fever unknown origin | 86 | 16 | 14 | 87 |

* All septic patients included (patients with sepsis and pneumonia are listed here rather than under pneumonia).

to slight therapy that the needs of neutropenic children for GTX may differ from those of adults, and that the principles of GTX therapy for one age may not apply to others because of differences in underlying diseases, chemotherapy, length of marrow hypoplasia, etc.

Conclusions cannot be drawn regarding the efficacy of GTX as treatment for gram-positive sepsis because the number of evaluable patients is small (Table 1). The response to GTX of patients with pneumonia (unassociated with bacteremia) was good, as was that of other types of localized infections and fever of unknown origin (Table 1). Unfortunately, information is limited by small numbers. Of 53 patients with pneumonia treated with GTX it was possible to determine the mortality rate in 18, and the causative organism was reported in only four of these patients (three gram-negative, one gram-positive and 14 organisms unspecified).

In attempts to minimize these many variables, the response of infected neutropenic patients to treatment with GTX was compared to that of nontransfused subjects evaluated concurrently in six controlled studies (Table 2). Survival of transfused patients was significantly greater than that of controls in three of six studies [16, 17, 19] when all subjects entered were analyzed. When patients were subdivided it became clear that GTX were of benefit under only certain conditions. GTX provided an advantage to patients with severe neutropenia and persistent marrow disease who had gram-negative sepsis that failed to respond to antibiotics. To the contrary, patients with fever and no documented infection, and those who experienced even a slight increase in blood neutrophil numbers ($>200/\mu$l) as a sign of recovering marrow function did equally well whether or not GTX were added to antibiotics.

A number of criticisms have been directed at these studies previously [2, 7, 16, 31] regarding the selection of controls, the heterogeneity of the patients, the variability of transfusion and antibiotic practices, and the definitions of response. It must be emphasized that each of the four truly randomized studies [16, 17, 19, 20] has fewer than 20 patients in either the transfused or the control groups. Furthermore, the patients in these studies were selected by study design to be unusually ill so that the information provided is not applicable to many of the neutropenic patients encountered in practice [2]. For example, in three controlled studies [17–19] patients were eligible for study only after failing 48–72 hours of antibiotic therapy. Undoubtedly the intention was to avoid giving GTX to patients expected to respond simply to antibiotics, but another result was to select study subjects who were unlikely to be cured simply by continuing antibiotics alone. The numbers and fates of patients who responded favorably to antibiotics alone, and thus were ineligible for study, were rarely provided, making it impos-

*Table 2.* Controlled therapeutic granulocyte transfusion studies.

| Study | Patients entered | | Proportion septic | Percent survivors | |
|---|---|---|---|---|---|
| | Transfused | Controls | | Transfused | Controls |
| Randomized | | | | | |
| Higby et al. [17] * | 17 | 19 | ≅ 31% | 76 [†] | 26 |
| Vogler et al. [19] * | 17 | 13 | ≅ 67% | 59 [†] | 15 |
| Herzig et al. [16] | 13 | 14 | 100% | 75 [†] | 36 |
| Alavi et al. [20] | 12 | 19 | ≅ 39% | 82 | 62 |
| Not randomized | | | | | |
| Graw et al. [15] | 39 | 37 | 100% | 46 | 30 |
| Fortuny et al. [18] | 17 | 22 | ≅ 34% | 78 | 80 |

* Only patients failing 48–72 hours of antibiotic therapy.
[†] Survival of transfused > controls (p<0.05).

sible to determine the proportion of the entire population of infected-neu-tropenic patients actually studied at each institution. With modern, combination antibiotic therapy, it is likely that only a small percentage of patients would fail to respond to antibiotics [33-36].

Another factor, however, is the large number of patients in the controlled studies who were in the terminal stages of leukemia. Clearly, a fatal result is expected for patients with serious infections who have persistent marrow disease and prolonged neutropenia [16, 19, 20]. Thus, a key finding of the controlled studies is that GTX may prolong life in terminal patients. However, an advantage of GTX plus antibiotics over antibiotics alone has not been shown for patients in whom bone marrow recovery occurs during the infectious episode. This last situation is that frequently present in patients undergoing initial induction therapy. In contrast GTX may not always be considered as part of palliative therapy offered to terminal patients because of the grim long-term prognosis. Thus, patients in the early stages of therapy do not need GTX because they respond to antibiotics, whereas, the risks, costs, etc. of GTX are rarely justified for patients in terminal stages.

Several other features render information in the controlled studies difficult to apply broadly in practice. Firstly, the infections treated were heterogeneous. In only two studies did all patients in both arms have culture-proven infections [15, 16]. It is hazardous to lump the results of small groups of patients treated for several types of infection because individual infections respond differently. For example, GTX are useful for certain patients with gram-negative sepsis, but they offer nothing to those with fever of undetermined origin [20]. Secondly, GTX were initiated in different studies at varying intervals after the infection was recognized. The importance of this delay to response is unknown. It is likely that a short trial of appropriate antibiotic therapy given prior to beginning GTX carries little risk because nontransfused control subjects rarely died during the first few days of therapy [16, 17, 19, 20]. Thirdly, antibiotic therapy may not have been optimal by current standards. The antibiotics chosen and doses employed were reported, but there was no suggestion in any report that antibiotic blood levels, serum bacteriostatic/bactericidal activity, or sensitivity testing designed to detect antibiotic synergism were employed as a means to ensure adequate antibiotic therapy. Serum concentrations of antibiotics, particularly aminoglycosides, vary greatly [37], and dosage must be tailored for individual patients by determining antibiotic blood levels. The advantages of using synergistic combinations of antibiotics is supported both by clinical studies in man [38-41] and by experimental data [42-44]. The presence of synergism and the clinical response correlate well with the level of antibacterial activity in serum [44, 45]. Many subjects described in these antibiotic studies [38-45] were infected, neutropenic cancer patients, suggesting that these techniques are useful in predicting response and for monitoring antibiotic therapy in subjects with impaired body defenses. It is doubtful that modern antibiotic therapy has been given a fair chance in the GTX literature published to date, and it seems premature to conclude that GTX can always offer a therapeutic advantage over that of antibiotics that are used properly. In support of this notion are studies that demonstrate a greater than 60% response rate to antibiotic therapy even in patients whose neutrophil counts failed to increase during the infectious episode [31, 34, 35]. In addition, Singer et al. [46] found that the survival of cancer patients with sepsis was significantly better in patients receiving appropriate antibiotics than in those given therapy deemed inappropriate. Finally, Anderson et al. [47] reported that antibiotic failures in some patients were simply the consequence of inadequate blood levels of antibiotics.

## 3. ANALYSIS OF THERAPEUTIC GRANULOCYTE TRANSFUSION STUDIES

It is clear that GTX benefit patients with severe neutropenia who have gram-negative sepsis that is not responding to combination antibiotic therapy. However, published information is insufficient for the practicing physician at the bedside of an infected, neutropenic patient to decide whether GTX offer an advantage over antibiotic therapy in treating other infections. Unquestionably, the return of bone marrow function during or shortly after the onset of gram-negative sepsis is associated with a relatively good prognosis whether or not GTX are given, whereas nearly all patients with persistent marrow disease eventually die, usually of infection. In addition, GTX when added to antibiotic therapy may prolong the patient's life so that additional therapy can be given in attempts to obtain a remission. Several questions remain to be answered: 1) the importance of underlying disease and age of the patient; 2) the optimal dose and the best techniques by which GTX should be given; and 3) the role of GTX in treating conditions other than gram-negative sepsis. It must be reiterated that many patients in the controlled studies published to date seem to represent patients encountered in practice with high-risk features (late stages of leukemia, prolonged cytopenia with remission unlikely, infections unresponsive to antibiotics). Predictably, these patients would die if conventional therapy were continued. Certainly they offer an appropriate setting in which to evaluate new modes of therapy, but they fail to accurately represent most patients who still retain a hopeful prognosis (those undergoing first induction). Thus, it seems unwise to apply indiscriminately the information provided by these reports to all neutropenic patients with presumed infection.

A practical approach at present is to evaluate febrile neutropenic patients in the usual fashion (cultures, chest x-rays, urinalysis, etc.) and to begin combination antibiotic therapy with plans to alter antibiotics as dictated by the clinical course and by the results of cultures, sensitivity testing, and antibiotic drug levels. GTX should be considered for patients with documented bacterial infections and persistent neutropenia who fail to respond to antibiotics used in an optimal fashion for about 48 hours. Evidences of antibiotic failure are persistent fever *plus* either cultures that continue to be positive or clinical signs of progressive infection such as a worsening chest roentgenogram, skin lesions, and shock. GTX would not be indicated, except under investigational circumstances, for febrile patients without documented bacterial infections or for patients whose infections have resolved except for fever.

### 4. REVIEW OF PROPHYLACTIC GRANULOCYTE TRANSFUSION TRIALS

Literature published through August, 1980, pertaining to the use of prophylactic GTX in patients with acute leukemia will be reviewed. Reports of a somewhat preliminary nature will be included because of the paucity of papers published to date on this topic. Studies of prophylactic GTX in bone marrow transplantation will not be reviewed in detail. Seven trials were reviewed, and each will be discussed [9, 11, 21, 48, 50, 53, 54]. Several features of design and a brief statement of the results of these studies are presented in Table 3. One obstacle in analyzing results must be recognized. Precise information regarding rates of infection per individual patients entered was usually not available because investigators often reported total episodes of infection that occurred during the on-study period. Thus, it was frequently impossible to determine whether a given number of infections were distributed evenly through all patients entered or whether a few patients experienced many episodes of infection while others were infection-free. In addition, this style of tabulation at times resulted in the number of infections being larger than the number of patients entered. Therefore, one must often, by necessity, simply accept the conclusions reached by the investigators.

Cooper *et al.* [48] studied patients with acute myelocytic leukemia, all of whom were being treated with similar chemotherapy for remission induction. The study was not randomized. Instead, transfused patients were those with related donors who were compatible by erythrocyte testing and who shared at least one HLA haplotype with the recipient. The nontransfused control group were patients without suitable donors. Transfused patients received histocompatible blood components when the platelet count fell to

*Table 3.* Literature reports of prophylactic granulocyte transfusions in leukemia.

| Study | Design | Patients | Granulocyte transfusions | Key findings |
|---|---|---|---|---|
| Cooper et al. [48] | Controlled Not randomized | 14 transfused 26 controls | Continuous-flow centrifugation $2.6 \times 10^{10}$ twice a week 3–11 infusions (mean = 6) HLA-matched donors | Incidence of infections and hemorrhage decreased. No alloimmunization as HLA-matched donors were used. Remission rate increased. |
| Ford et al. [9] | Randomized | 10 transfused 9 controls | Intermittent-flow centrifugation $1.5 \times 10^{10}$ every other day 1–12 transfusions | No benefits detected. |
| Mannoni et al. [50] | Randomized | 22 transfused 28 controls | Intermittent-flow centrifugation $2.1 \times 10^{10}$ daily 8–15 infusions (mean = 8) | Incidence of infections decreased. Remission rate or duration not affected. Alloimmunization rate doubled in transfused patients. |
| Schiffer et al. [11] | Randomized | 10 transfused 9 controls | Intermittent-flow centrifugation $1.2 \times 10^{10}$ every other day 3–19 infusions (mean = 11) | No statistically significant benefits. Study halted due to high rates of Alloimmunization and transfusion reactions. |
| Curts et al. [21] | Controlled Not randomized | 7 transfused 20 controls | Continuous-flow centrifugation $0.07 \times 10^{10}$ schedule not given 3–5 infusions HLA-matched donors. | Incidence of clinical, but not documented, infections decreased. Remission rate not affected. |
| Hester et al. [54] | Controlled Not randomized | 18 transfused 50 controls | Centrifugation leukapheresis $1.5 \times 10^{10}$ every day or two Variable course, duration unclear HLA-matched donors | Overall infection rate not affected, but septicemia and pneumonia decreased. |
| Strauss et al. [53] | Randomized | 54 transfused 48 controls | Intermittent-flow centrifugation $0.7 \times 10^{10}$ $(0.35/m^2)$ daily 3–28 infusions (median = 18.5) | Overall infection rate not affected, but bacterial septicemia decreased. Transfusion reactions in most recipients. Pulmonary infiltrates increased. |

<30 000/μl and the granulocyte count was <1000/μl; controls received pooled platelets from unrelated donors when the platelet count was <30 000/μl. GTX were given only twice each week (Table 3). Four transfused patients had infections at the entry into the trial, and therapeutic vs. prophylactic GTX effects could not be easily distinguished. These initial infections resolved rapidly, and only one new infection occurred. In contrast, infections were more frequent (p<0.001) in controls, and eight of ten controls with severe infections died. As expected, post-transfusion platelet increments were greater in transfused patients receiving histocompatible platelets than in controls who were given pooled random donor platelets. Bleeding presented no apparent problem to transfused patients, whereas, ten of 26 controls experienced life-threatening hemorrhage. Although the time required to achieve remission was similar, the rate of complete remission was 64% in the transfused and only 27% in controls. Presumably, transfused patients had less infection and bleeding and were likely to survive long enough to receive sufficient amounts of chemotherapy to attain remission. This reasoning may prove to be fallacious, however. This study has continued to accrue patients, and with larger numbers of subjects to be analyzed, neither the rates nor the severity of infections and bleeding were significantly decreased in the transfused group. The complete remission rate of transfused patients, however, remained significantly better, particularly for patients <45 years of age (M.R. Cooper, written communication, 1980). Duration of remission and survival was not statistically different. Neither platelet nor leukocyte antibodies developed in recipients of histocompatible blood components during the study, but one-half of these patients became sensitized later after receiving random donor components.

Ford et al. [9] reported a randomized trial in which GTX were given on alternate days to adults with previously untreated nonlymphocytic leukemia. Patients were afebrile and free of infection at entry. All received prophylactic, oral, nonabsorbable antibiotics. Combined granulocyte-platelet units were started when the absolute blood neutrophil count fell to <500/μl and were continued until: a) the blood neutrophil count was spontaneously >500/μl; b) the patient was considered to be stable (three weeks after chemotherapy); or c) serious transfusion reactions developed. Granulocytes were obtained from relatives or friends irrespective of HLA types. Controls were not given prophylactic platelets, but received them at the slightest sign of clinical bleeding. GTX had no apparent effect on the rate or the course of infections. Two patients died of infection, one in each arm of the trial. Three of ten transfused subjects and five of nine controls achieved remission. The rate of transfusion reactions was similar. Only two transfused and one control patient developed anti-HLA antibodies. Thus, GTX imparted no notable effects on the clinical course of remission induction for the few patients in this study. Apparently, additional patients have entered this trial, but little data are provided in a recent letter [49]. However, the authors suggested that the duration of initial, complete bone marrow remission was longer in patients achieving remission if they had been transfused; eventual survival was similar in transfused and control patients.

The study of Mannoni et al. [50] is the largest one published to date and appears to be carefully performed. The largest number of granulocytes infused to date were used, but interpretation of results is hampered by several problems. First, it is difficult to determine the actual number of patients studied as data reported in the final paper [50] and in the preliminary reports [51, 52] seem contrary. Second, numbers recorded in the text and in the tables of the final paper do not always agree. Third, patients were heterogeneous as they were undergoing both first and later induction attempts. Fourth, only one-half of the patients in the control group truly did not receive GTX since therapeutic GTX were given to the remainder for infection or simply for fever that was unresponsive to antibiotics.

Patients with acute nonlymphocytic leukemia were eligible if they were uninfected. Patients were selected by randomization to receive or not daily GTX that began immediately after the first course of chemotherapy. GTX were continued until the blood neutrophil count increased to 1000/µl. Donors were not selected by HLA typing, but donor-recipient pairs were compatible by erythrocyte crossmatching, and recipient blood could not contain antibodies directed against donor leukocytes (microlymphocytotoxicity test). All patients received prophylactic, oral, nonabsorbable antibiotics and prophylactic platelet transfusions. The rate of infection was significantly decreased (p<0.02) in the transfused group. Although four patients died in the control group, only two were associated with progressive infection—a finding ascribed to the effectiveness of antibiotics and therapeutic GTX. No deaths were observed in the transfused group during remission induction. The mean duration of bone marrow suppression was similar, and no differences in the rate or duration of remission were observed in transfused and control patients who achieved complete remission. The rate of HLA immunization in the transfused group was 60% (9 of 15 patients studied), and 30% of the control group (7 of 23 patients studied), an apparent consequence of both prophylactic and therapeutic GTX and of platelet transfusions.

Schiffer et al. [11] randomized adults with acute nonlymphocytic leukemia who were undergoing identical first induction chemotherapy to receive either combined granulocyte-platelet or platelet transfusions. Patients were free of infection at entry into the study, but were treated with prophylactic, oral, nonabsorbable antibiotics. Transfusions were begun when the blood neutrophil count was <500/µl and the platelet count was <20 000/µl. Granulocytes were obtained from related and unrelated donors who were compatible with the recipient by erythrocyte crossmatching, but not necessarily by HLA. Infections were more numerous in the control group, but the small number of study subjects precluded meaningful statistical analysis. The days on-study spent receiving antibiotics, the fever pattern and the complete remission rate were similar in transfused and control groups. The rate of transfusion reactions was significantly higher in patients receiving prophylactic GTX (seven of ten versus one of nine controls). These reactions were characterized by fever and chills, and once by a diffuse pulmonary infiltrate. Although lymphocytotoxic antibodies were not detected in any patient at the time of entry, seven of ten patients receiving GTX and four of nine controls developed them during the on-study period. All GTX recipients who experienced transfusion reactions produced lymphocytotoxic antibodies. These antibodies were not proven to cause the reactions, but the study was terminated because of the disturbingly high rates of alloimmunization and transfusion reactions. It was concluded that prophylactic GTX should not be routine therapy, but should be employed only in investigational settings.

In the report of Curtis *et al.* [21] seven adults with acute myelocytic leukemia, undergoing initial induction therapy, were given prophylactic GTX and were compared to 20 patients treated concurrently with similar chemotherapy and supportive care. The mean ($\pm$SD) number of granulocytes collected from 50 donors at their institution was $0.7 \pm 0.8 \times 10^9$, but the actual dose of granulocytes given to the study subjects was not provided. This dose is extremely low (mean $= 0.07 \times 10^{10}$) when compared to other studies (Table 3), and only 3–5 GTX were given per patient. Granulocytes were obtained from HLA compatible siblings (degree of compatibility not defined) and were given during the later stages of induction chemotherapy. Therapeutic GTX from erythrocyte compatible donors were given to an unstated number of controls. The 20 controls had significantly more ($p = 0.043$) clinical infections than transfused patients (15 vs. 2 episodes), but bacteriologically proven infections were similar in the two groups ($p>0.10$). Transfused patients had fewer days of temperature $>38\,°C$ ($p<0.05$). The rate of achieving complete and partial remissions was similar in the two groups, but the complete remission rate was not given. Despite the small numbers of patients studied, the very small dose of granulocytes infused and the failure to demonstrate an effect on documented infections, the authors concluded that HLA-matched GTX were effective in preventing severe infections in neutropenic leukemic patients.

Hester *et al.* [54] studied 18 adults with the diagnosis of acute leukemia who were undergoing first or later attempts at remission induction. Transfused patients had donors with whom they shared at least one HLA haplotype. Prophylactic GTX were started when blood granulocytes were <500/µl and were continued until they rose to >500/µl. Fifty historical controls were selected who had been given similar chemotherapy, although 27 of the 50 who were not receiving therapeutic GTX seem to offer the best comparison. When the prophylactic GTX group was compared to the controls that did not receive therapeutic GTX (presumably not infected at entry), nearly all patients in both groups eventually experienced fever or suspected infection (17 of 18 in the prophylactic GTX and 22 of 27 in the nontransfused controls). However, pneumonia and bacteremia were decreased in prophylactic GTX patients (45%) when compared to controls (61%), and it was suggested that prophylactic GTX were of benefit. Complete remission rates and survival were not different.

A multi-institutional trial of prophylactic GTX was conducted from 1976 to 1980 [53], and a complete analysis of data will be presented herein. The primary objective of this trial was to determine if daily prophylactic GTX could reduce the rate of bacterial infections when given to patients with acute myelogenous leukemia (AML) undergoing first remission induction. In addition, the rates of other types of infections, the frequency and severity of adverse effects of GTX, and the influence of GTX on remission induction and mortality were studied. Participating institutions followed a common plan. All patients ≥12 years of age with untreated acute leukemia who were beginning first induction chemotherapy were considered for the trial when the blood neutrophil count fell to <500/µl if they were free of infection by physical examination, chest roentgenogram, urinalysis and cultures of blood and urine. Patients were randomized either to receive daily GTX collected from random donors (transfused group) or not (control group) via a telephone call to a central coordinating (statistical) center. Daily GTX were continued for a maximum of 28 days or until the occurrence of one of the following: a) marrow recovery defined as blood granulocytes persisting at >500/µl for 48 hours; b) death; c) a severe transfusion reaction; d) withdrawal of patient consent; or e) gram-negative septicemia. The primary endpoint was the occurrence of documented infection during the on-study period (usually about 28 days). Monitoring procedures and data collection were done on a daily basis and information was sent to the coordinating center for on-going analysis. As a minimum for detecting onset of infections, patients were examined daily; blood cultures were taken every three days; urine, throat and stool were cultured weekly; and a chest x-ray was taken weekly. Additional studies were performed in febrile patients or if infections were suspected clinically. General patient management was similar for transfused and control patients. Combination chemotherapy protocols were used that included cytosine arabinoside plus an anthracycline and were designed to produce severe marrow hypoplasia. Patients were assigned

*Table 4.* Reasons patients with AML were ineligible for the multi-institutional trial.

| Reason | Number of patients | Percent of all ineligible patients |
|---|---|---|
| Infection likely at randomization | 66 | 45 |
|    Documented bacterial infection | 22 | 15 |
|    Soft-tissue inflammation | 8 | 5 |
|    Abnormal chest roentgenogram | 13 | 9 |
|    Previous antibiotic therapy | 23 | 16 |
| Nonprotocol chemotherapy employed | 50 | 34 |
| Informed consent refused | 21 | 14 |
| Other | 11 | 7 |
| Total ineligible patients | 148 | 100% |

to private hospital rooms. Neither sterile environments nor antibiotics for gut sterilization were used. Systemic antibiotics were started promptly when patients became febrile (>38 °C). Minimum coverage included carbenicillin or ticarcillin plus an aminoglycoside. Aminoglycoside blood levels were determined during the first 48 hours of treatment and at least once later in the course. Dosage was adjusted to maintain a one hour postinfusion peak of $4-8$ µg/ml for gentamicin and tobramycin and $15-20$ µg/ml for amikacin. Additional antibiotics were added as indicated by culture results or by choice of the primary physician. Prophylactic platelet transfusions were given for blood platelet counts <20 000/µl. To assure comparability of platelet support, platelets were removed from granulocyte units by centrifugation prior to transfusion into patients with blood platelet counts >40 000/µl.

One hundred and two patients with AML were randomized into one of three strata depending on the presence of fever and previous antibiotic therapy, 54 to receive daily prophylactic GTX and 48 to serve as nontransfused controls. They represented only 41% of the 250 new AML patients monitored at participating institutions. Reasons for non-eligibility are shown in Table 4. The most common reason for declaring a patient ineligible was suspicion of infection as suggested by a positive culture, abnormal chest roentgenogram, physical evidence of infection, or a prolonged course of antibiotics given prior to day of randomization. Some patients were excluded because their physicians chose antileukemic chemotherapy that was considered to have insufficient myelotoxicity. Other patients refused to give consent. This illustrates the difficulty in accessing a large and homogeneous patient population for which GTX would be clearly prophylactic. Various characteristics of the patients randomized are displayed in Table 5. Randomization in this case appears to have produced good balance between the

*Table 5.* Characteristics of patients entered into the multi-institutional trial.

| Characteristic | Total | | Transfusions | | No transfusions | |
|---|---|---|---|---|---|---|
| Total patients | 102 | | 54 | | 48 | |
| Acute myelocytic leukemia | 62 | 61% | 35 | 65% | 27 | 56% |
| Acute promyelocytic leukemia | 3 | 3% | 1 | 2% | 2 | 4% |
| Acute monomyelocytic leukemia | 19 | 19% | 12 | 22% | 7 | 15% |
| Acute monocytic leukemia | 10 | 10% | 4 | 7% | 6 | 13% |
| Other acute leukemia | 8 | 8% | 2 | 4% | 6 | 13% |
| Age (mean ± SD) | 49±18 | | 49±19 | | 49±17 | |
| <60 years | 67 | 66% | 35 | 65% | 32 | 67% |
| ≤60 years | 35 | 34% | 19 | 35% | 16 | 33% |
| Males | 54 | 53% | 32 | 59% | 22 | 46% |
| Females | 48 | 47% | 22 | 41% | 26 | 54% |
| Other medical conditions | | | | | | |
| Cardiovascular | 24 | 24% | 13 | 24% | 11 | 23% |
| Overt diabetes | 5 | 5% | 1 | 2% | 4 | 8% |
| Renal | 7 | 7% | 3 | 6% | 4 | 8% |
| Hepatic | 1 | 1% | 0 | 0% | 1 | 2% |
| Pulmonary | 6 | 6% | 5 | 9% | 1 | 2% |
| Other cancer | 6 | 6% | 5 | 9% | 1 | 2% |

two treatment groups on the pre-existing factors which might be expected to influence outcome (no significant differences detected by the Yates corrected chi-square test for categorical variables or the t-test for quantitative variables).

The types of infections which were documented during the trial period, the number of patients affected and the median day after randomization for the onset of infections are presented in Table 6. Each type of infection that occurred in an individual patient was counted once. Recurrent episodes of the same type of infection in the same patient were not recounted because of the difficulty in determining whether subsequent episodes were in fact new infections. Patients with more than one type of infection were counted once under each category of infection so that the sum of the number of individual infections exceeds the total number of patients recorded as having experienced an infection.

Prophylactic GTX did not affect the overall incidence of infections (Table 6). Nearly one-half of the patients in each group experienced at least one type of infection (p = 0.96). The incidence of bacterial septicemia was significantly greater (p = 0.01) in controls (27%) than in transfused patients (9%). The occurrence of other types of infections was comparable in both groups, although the incidence of pneumonia in transfused patients was nearly double that of controls. The decreased incidence of bacterial septi-

*Table 6.* Occurrence of and median days to onset of infections in the multi-institutional trial.

| Infection | Granulocytes | | | No granulocytes | | | Significance levels | |
|---|---|---|---|---|---|---|---|---|
| | No. | Pct. | Median day onset | No. | Pct. | Median day onset | Occur-rence * | Median [†] day onset |
| Total patients | 54 | | | 48 | | | | |
| Any infections | 24 | 46% | 9 | 29 | 42% | 12 | 0.96 | NS |
| Septicemia | 8 | 15% | 12.5 | 13 | 27% | 10 | 0.047 | NS |
| Bacterial | 5 | 9% | 7 | 13 | 27% | 10 | 0.01 | NS |
| Gram-negative | 3 | 6% | 7 | 8 | 17% | 15.5 | 0.047 | NS |
| Gram-positive | 2 | 4% | 10.5 | 8 | 17% | 8.5 | 0.06 | NS |
| Fungal | 3 | 6% | 16 | 1 | 2% | 26 | 0.81 | NS |
| Pneumonia | 12 | 22% | 8.5 | 6 | 13% | 19 | 0.34 | 0.05 |
| Bacterial | 2 | 4% | 5 | 0 | 0% | – | 0.63 | – |
| Fungal | 2 | 4% | 7 | 2 | 4% | 9.5 | 0.48 | NS |
| Cause unknown | 8 | 15% | 10 | 4 | 8% | 20.5 | 0.58 | NS |
| Other infections | 11 | 20% | 10 | 7 | 15% | 20 | 0.58 | NS |
| Abscess | 3 | 6% | 5 | 4 | 8% | 18.5 | 0.85 | 0.05 |
| Cellulitis | 5 | 9% | 10 | 3 | 6% | 15 | 0.65 | NS |
| U.T.I. | 3 | 6% | 21 | 1 | 2% | 27 | 0.83 | NS |
| Bacterial | 1 | 2% | 21 | 0 | 0% | – | 0.96 | – |
| Fungal | 2 | 4% | 17 | 1 | 2% | 27 | 0.75 | NS |

* From Mantel-Haenszel corrected chi-square test, stratifying on clinical center and stratum.
[†] From Mann-Whitney test.

cemia and increased rate of pneumonia were apparent also when patients were analyzed according to age (>60 vs. <60 years of age). Prophylactic GTX did not delay the onset of infections. The median day of onset for most infections was 7–21 days after randomization, and the only significant differences (p<0.05) were for pneumonia and abscess, both of which occurred earlier in transfused patients.

Prophylactic GTX had no significant effects on the rates of bone marrow recovery, remission induction, and mortality during induction, or on the duration of first remission and survival of patients who achieved a complete remission. Bone marrow recovery, defined as a blood granulocyte count of $\geq 500/\mu l$ persisting for at least 48 hours, occurred in 49% of transfused and 52% of control patients during the 28-day on-study period. Eventually, complete remission was achieved by 57 and 60% of transfused patients and controls, respectively. Nearly twice as many transfused (12/54 = 22%) as control (6/48 = 13%) patients died during the 28-day on-study period, but this difference was not statistically significant (p = 0.28). Although many conditions including septicemia, pneumonia, fungal infections, hemorrhage, cardiovascular disease, renal failure, and drug toxicity were evident clinical-

368

Table 7. Dosage of prophylactic granulocyte transfusions given in the multi-institutional trial*.

| | All patients | No infection | Any infection | Bacterial infection[†] | Pneumonia | Any pulmonary infiltrate | Death on-study (28 days) |
|---|---|---|---|---|---|---|---|
| Number of patients | 54 | 29 | 25 | 15 | 12 | 31 | 12 |
| Median number of transfusions given | 18.5 | 20 | 17 | 15 | 18 | 20 | 14 |
| Mean dose/day | 6.9 | 6.9 | 6.9 | 7.0 | 6.6 | 6.5 | 7.0 |
| Mean dose/ m$^2$/day | 3.5 | 3.5 | 3.5 | 3.4 | 3.4 | 3.3 | 3.2 |
| Mean dose/ m$^2$/course | 69.0 | 71.0 | 68.0 | 64.0 | 69.0 | 68.0 | 48.0 |

* All dosages are × 10$^9$ cells.
[†] 'Bacterial infection' includes bacterial septicemia, bacterial pneumonia, abscess, cellulitis, and bacterial urinary tract infection.

ly or by autopsy, infections were judged to be the primary cause of death in 67% of both transfused (8 of 12) and control (4 of 6) patients. Hemorrhage was the primary cause in only one patient from each of the two groups suggesting that platelet support was adequate and comparable. The median number of days from randomization until first relapse for patients achieving complete remission, as estimated by life table analysis, was 350 for transfused and 413 for controls (p = 0.6), and the median days of survival from randomization for these patients were 561 and 586 for transfused and control subjects (p = 0.93).

Table 8. Dosages of granylocytes given prior to infections in transfused patients with or without infections.

| | No infection | Any infection | Bacterial infection* | Bacterial septicemia |
|---|---|---|---|---|
| Number of patients | 29 | 25 | 15 | 5 |
| Median days GTX given | 20 | 8 | 7 | 5 |
| Mean dose/day[†] | 6.9 | 6.6 | 6.6 | 6.0 |
| Mean dose/m$^2$/day[†] | 3.5 | 3.2 | 3.0 | 2.7 |

* 'Bacterial infection' includes bacterial septicemia, bacterial pneumonia, abscess, cellulitis, and bacterial urinary tract infection.
[†] Doses listed are granulocytes × 10$^9$ given daily prior to onset.

Table 7 presents a comparison of granulocyte dosages given to various categories of patients. There are no significant differences in dose per day or dose per $m^2$ per day between these categories. However, as shown in Table 8, the susceptibility of patients to certain infections appeared to be related to the dose of granulocytes given *prior to the onset of the infection*. In particular, the mean dose per $m^2$ per day for the five transfused patients who acquired bacterial septicemia was less than the dose given to transfused patients who never acquired an infection ($2.7 \times 10^9$ vs. $3.5 \times 10^9$, p<0.05). Differences in daily granulocyte doses given prior to onset were not significant when all types of infections were considered rather than bacterial septicemia alone.

Adverse effects of prophylactic GTX were frequent (Table 9). Nine hundred and eighty-seven prophylactic granulocyte transfusions were given to 54 patients, 39 of whom (72%) experienced at least one adverse effect. The most frequent effects were fever and chills, occurring in about one-half of patients. Dyspnea and wheezing were noted in about 20% of patients. Additional findings included cyanosis, nausea, vomiting, itching, urticaria, anxiety, and fluctuations in blood pressure, but each occurred in fewer than 10% of patients. GTX were interrupted in 15% of patients due to serious adverse effects, and 11% of patients were disqualified from further granu-

*Table 9.* Adverse reactions to granulocyte transfusions.

| Observation | Reactions in 54 patients | | Reactions with 987 transfusions | |
|---|---|---|---|---|
| | No. | Percent | No. | Percent |
| Temperature increase >2 °C | 31 | 57 | 79 | 8 |
| Shaking chills | 27 | 50 | 99 | 10 |
| Dyspnea | 10 | 19 | 21 | 2 |
| Wheezing | 9 | 17 | 13 | 1 |
| Cyanosis | 2 | 4 | 2 | 0.1 |
| Nausea | 5 | 9 | 6 | 0.6 |
| Vomiting | 1 | 2 | 2 | 0.2 |
| Itching | 2 | 4 | 4 | 0.4 |
| Urticaria | 4 | 7 | 6 | 0.6 |
| Anxiety | 4 | 7 | 6 | 0.6 |
| Hypertension | 4 | 7 | 4 | 0.4 |
| Hypotension | 2 | 4 | 2 | 0.2 |
| Transfusion interrupted | 8 | 14 | 38 | 4 |
| Transfusion discontinued | 2 | 4 | 2 | 0.2 |
| Disqualified from further transfusions | 6 | 11 | 6 | 0.6 |

locyte transfusions because of severe reactions. An adverse reaction accompanied 16% (158/987) of individual prophylactic granulocyte transfusions.

Fever was a greater problem in transfused than in control patients and could not be clearly related to infection (Table 10). Temperatures measured within four hours after starting a transfusion of any blood product were excluded from analysis as an attempt to discount fever caused by transfusions. Still, temperatures were higher and fever more frequent in patients receiving prophylactic GTX (p<0.01 by Yates corrected chi-square test).

The incidence of pulmonary infiltrates was strikingly increased (p = 0.002) in transfused (31/54 = 57%) patients when compared to controls (13/48 = 27%). The mechanisms responsible could not always be identified but fluid overload occurred more frequently (p = 0.03) in transfused patients (24%) than in controls (8%). A direct quantitative relationship between the numbers of granulocytes transfused and the presence of pulmonary infiltrates was not found, as might be expected if pulmonary infiltrates were directly related to the dose of granulocytes given. Transfused patients received similar numbers of granulocytes during the on-study period whether or not they developed pulmonary infiltrates. The median number of daily GTX given to patients who developed infiltrates was 20 with median granulocyte doses of $3.2 \times 10^9/m^2$/day and $70 \times 10^9/m^2$/course. Corresponding values for patients without infiltrates were 17 daily transfusions and granulocyte doses of $3.7 \times 10^9/m^2$/day and $67 \times 10^9/m^2$/course. (Median and mean values were nearly identical.) The average daily dose of granulocytes given on the days preceding the development of pulmonary infiltrates was actually less (p<0.01) for 31 patients with ($2.95 \times 10^9/m^2$/day) than for 23 patients without ($3.85 \times 10^9/m^2$/day) infiltrates.

Conclusions of the multi-institutional trial were: 1) prophylactic GTX reduced the incidence of bacterial septicemia in patients with AML undergoing initial remission induction chemotherapy; 2) the incidence of other types of infections was not affected; 3) prophylactic GTX did not influence bone marrow recovery, remission rate, mortality during induction, duration

Table 10. High temperatures and days febrile for patients in the multi-institutional trial.

|  | Granulocytes | No granulocytes |
|---|---|---|
| Number of patients | 54 | 48 |
| Days monitored | 1104 | 1130 |
| Patient-days with temperature ≥38.0°C | 707 (64%) | 543 (48%) |
| Patient-days with temperature ≥38.5°C | 566 (51%) | 359 (32%) |
| Patient-days Acetaminophen given | 618 (56%) | 401 (36%) |
| Mean high temperature (°C) ±SE | 38.54 ±0.03 | 38.04 ±0.03 |

of remission, or survival of patients who achieve remission; 4) the majority of patients receiving prophylactic GTX experienced one or more adverse reactions. Thus, prophylactic GTX as studied cannot be recommended as standard therapy for initial remission induction therapy for AML.


5. ANALYSIS OF PROPHYLACTIC GRANULOCYTE TRANSFUSION STUDIES

Several features of our study and others from the literature are summarized on Table 3 and will be briefly reviewed. Information is limited due to several factors, and comparison is difficult due to differences in study design. Patients in four studies were randomized, but two of them enrolled no more than ten subjects into either arm [9, 11]. In only one study were fairly large doses of granulocytes given daily [50]. GTX were given daily in three studies and 2–4 times/week in three; the schedule was not reported in one. Granulocytes for all studies were collected by centrifugation leukapheresis, and the number of granulocytes per transfusion in six of the studies ranged from 0.7 to $2.6 \times 10^{10}$. The study of Curtis et al. [21] was a notable exception. A seemingly insignificant quantity of granulocytes $(0.07 \times 10^{10})$ was infused per GTX, with the total number given to each patient during the entire course of 3–5 GTX computed to be only $0.21-0.35 \times 10^{10}$ granulocytes [21]. It seems hazardous to conclude that granulocytes contained in the GTX accounted for any differences between transfused and control subjects since $0.35 \times 10^{10}$ is the number of granulocytes that could be infused in a single unit (450 ml) of fresh CPD whole blood [55]. The lack of success in preventing infections in some studies is probably related to inadequate doses of granulocytes since it seems almost undeniable that infections could be prevented if circulating granulocyte counts were restored to normal, as might be accomplished by the infusion of massive numbers of perfectly matched granulocytes. Donors were selected on the basis of HLA matching in three studies [21, 48, 51], although the degree of compatibility was not reported. At least two studies [50, 54] included patients in later attempts at remission induction. It is likely that success in achieving prompt remission would be increased in studies enrolling only first remission patients. Finally, the studies do not agree regarding benefits and risks of prophylactic granulocyte transfusions.

Despite these difficulties it is possible to arrive at the following conclusions by review of all current information. Most importantly, data reported to date do not support the use of prophylactic granulocyte transfusions as part of standard therapy for patients with ANLL undergoing first induction chemotherapy for three major reasons. First, controversy exists as to whether prophylactic granulocyte transfusions prevent infections. The overall rate of infections was not decreased or was only marginally affected in five reports [9, 11, 21, 53, 54]. On the other hand, the overall rate was decreased in two studies [48, 50], although it appears that this conclusion will be reversed in one study [48] when it is completed. In two reports bacterial septicemia [53] and septicemia and pneumonia [54] were decreased when these infections were analyzed separately. The study with the most striking infection prevention benefit transfused the largest number of granulocytes daily [50]. However, the importance of daily dose as an independent factor is unclear since the incidence of bacterial septicemia was decreased by only modest doses of granulocytes per day in our study [53].

Second, little influence of prophylactic granulocyte transfusions has been demonstrated on remission rates, duration of remission or on mortality (i.e., on the course of ANLL). In only one study [48] were transfused patients more likely to achieve remission. In a brief update [49] of the study of Ford *et al.* [9], the duration of complete first remission was prolonged in patients who managed to achieve remission while receiving prophylactic granulocyte transfusions. A similar finding was reported, anecdotally, by McCredie [56]. These observations require confirmation.

Third, the risks of prophylactic granulocyte transfusions, although incompletely defined, seem substantial. Reactions to granulocyte transfusions occurred in the majority of our patients [53] and in those of Schiffer *et al.* [11]. They were severe enough to prompt premature closure of the latter trial [11], and to disqualify 11% of our patients from further transfusions [53]. Recipient reactions to centrifuge-collected cells were ≅18% in a previous review [57]. The incidence of pulmonary infiltrates was significantly increased in our transfused patients. Infiltrates could not be related to the number of granulocytes infused, and the mechanisms remained undefined. Clearly, some of these patients were simply overloaded with fluid. Many had infections and were receiving nephrotoxic antibiotics intravenously. Blood products were being administered in large volumes. Finally, some patients were elderly or had underlying medical illnesses that might predispose them to fluid accumulation. These circumstances apply to many patients encountered in practice, and physicians must be aware of this potential danger. Diuretics should be used vigorously in these patients. Other diagnostic possibilities that have been raised in the literature include pulmonary infections, antibody-mediated intrapulmonary sequestration of granulocytes [62], pulmonary reaction related to the combined administration of GTX and amphotericin B [63], and the infusion of leukocyte aggregates that formed *in vitro* during preparation of the granulocyte units.

A major problem among adverse effects is the inescapable fact that most transfused patients become alloimmunized [9, 11, 58]. Although immunization to HLA is reduced by selecting HLA matched donors [48], this precaution will not eliminate the potential for immunization to granulocyte specific antigens. The success of the initial course of GTX in treating infections in man seems unrelated to leukocyte crossmatching in studies published to date. It is likely that the infections resolved and GTX were discontinued prior to the emergence of antibodies. However, the importance of matching has been documented by experimental studies in which results of GTX were inferior in immunized animals [59]. Similar studies have been reported in man in which *in vitro* granulocyte functions and the circulating kinetics of transfused granulocytes were affected adversely by either incomplete matching or by the presence of antileukocyte antibodies [15, 60]. On the other hand, antibody screening tests currently available demonstrate little value in predicting recipient response to GTX [61], and strong recommendations cannot be made to select donors by these tests.

Although not specifically addressed in the prophylactic GTX trials reviewed, knowledge of two additional risks have emerged that would apply both to prophylactic and therapeutic GTX. Firstly, five patients have been reported with graft-versus-host disease acquired coincident with transfusions of leukocytes obtained from normal donors [64–68]. The true incidence of this disorder may be even higher because it would be recognized with difficulty in patients with leukemia who may exhibit fever, pancytopenia, enlargement of the reticuloendothelial organs, liver dysfunction, gastrointestinal bleeding and diarrhea while undergoing intense therapy, particularly when infected. It is difficult to ascribe graft-versus-host disease in these patients to GTX because most received other blood products that contain large number of viable lymphocytes (e.g., platelet concentrates). This raises the issue as to whether all blood products should be irradiated for immunosuppressed patients, a task not easily accomplished at all blood banks. Secondly, an increased incidence of cytomegalovirus infections was found in a study of leukemic patients and bone marrow transplant recipients who received GTX [69]. Infection was acquired predominately in patients with negative cytomegalovirus titers prior to transfusion, suggesting that the virus was transmitted by the transfused cells rather than by reactivation of a latent infection. In probable confirmation, a mononucleosis syndrome has been reported in children with leukemia that was suspected to be caused by cytomegalovirus acquired via GTX [70].

6. CONCLUSIONS, CURRENT RECOMMENDATIONS, AND FUTURE DIRECTIONS

General agreement exists for the use of GTX in only one condition: the severely neutropenic patient with gram-negative sepsis that has failed to respond to antibiotics in whom prompt bone marrow recovery seems unlikely. Many factors belittle the benefit of GTX, *as they are prepared today,* in treating other types of infections or in the prevention of infections. Prophylactic GTX seem able to reduce the incidence of bacterial septicemia even when given in modest doses. Although desirable, it is unlikely that this benefit is of great worth to most patients with acute leukemia undergoing initial remission induction chemotherapy because even if these infections arise, they can be successfully treated by antibiotics and, when indicated, by therapeutic GTX [2, 31, 50]. Moreover, the occurrence of other types of infections seems to be little affected by prophylactic GTX. The majority of transfused patients experience one or more adverse effects of varying severity. Furthermore, GTX are expensive [13]. Finally, a definite influence of either prophylactic or therapeutic GTX on the ultimate course of adult acute leukemia has not been demonstrated.

We believe that the information presented in this review renders as totally unacceptable the tenets recently voiced, perhaps facetiously, by Higby [71] that '... the wide availability and increasing use of granulocyte transfusions is evidence that most physicians are convinced from the published literature and personal experience (as we are) that granulocyte transfusions are of benefit...' and 'if... granulocyte transfusions are effective in some patients with neutropenia but not others, we will hear arguments that at least they cannot hurt those in the nonbenefited groups.... ' Broad medical endorsement does not guarantee efficacy. The medical literature contains many examples of treatments accepted widely in the past that are currently believed either to offer marginal benefit or to expose patients to excessive risks. A few examples related to hematology-oncology include the futility of using androgens to treat severe aplastic anemia [72], the appearance of aplastic anemia in patients given chloramphenicol for minor infections that require no antibiotics [73], the occurrence of thyroid neoplasia following use of irradiation to treat diverse disorders of the head and neck [74], and the emergence of genital cancer following estrogen therapy [75, 76].

In our opinion, GTX should be considered as investigational therapy for most conditions, and the practicing physician must weigh the potential benefits and risks of adding GTX to conventional therapy. Therapeutic GTX are administered to patients refractory to antibiotic therapy, and it seems acceptable to take additional risks that cannot be justified in a prophylactic setting. The benfit and risk factors that must be considered are discussed briefly in the five paragraphs that follow.

a) The expected duration of severe neutropenia must be estimated (often by bone marrow examination) because virtually all infections will respond to antibiotics if there is a return of endogenous granulocyte production. Thus, GTX are not needed by patients whose marrow recovery seems imminent.

b) The status of the infection must be clearly documented. Patients with persistent severe neutropenia who have documented bacterial infections, particularly gram-negative sepsis, that are progressing despite antibiotics are candidates for therapeutic GTX. However, patients without culture-proven or strong clinical evidence of infection have not been benefited by GTX, and the risks do not seem justified.

c) Physicians must know the characteristics of the granulocyte units provided at their institutions. Although precise dose relationships have not been established, it is generally accepted that a minimum daily dose of therapeutic granulocytes should be $1 \times 10^{10}$. Granulocyte yields of this magnitude can be predictably obtained by centrifugation and gravity leukapheresis only when performed in the presence of an erythrocyte sedimenting agent such as hydroxyethyl starch, and when donors are stimulated by adrenal corticosteroids. Although large numbers of granulocytes can be collected by continuous-flow filtration leukapheresis, its popularity has waned, and it is currently recommended that this technique be employed only in investigative centers [77].

d) Clearly, GTX are associated with recipient risks. Fever occurs regularly during or shortly after GTX. More serious reactions may appear such as shaking chills, extreme hyperpyrexia, alterations of vital signs or sensorium, and pulmonary dysfunction. Patients with underlying pulmonary, cardiovascular, and renal diseases should be considered at increased risk for these complications, as should those suspected to be alloimmunized. Finally, the risks of bloodborne infections and graft-versus-host disease must be weighed.

e) Donor risks, inconveniences, and expenses must be considered. To provide satisfactory numbers of granulocytes by current methods, donors receive anticoagulants, adrenal corticosteroids, and hydroxyethyl starch. All present theoretical risks, although their clinical significance, if any, has not been established [14]. It seems reasonable, however, to avoid exposing healthy donors to risks except under circumstances in which the efficacy of GTX has been firmly established. Informed consent to participate in research should be obtained if donors are providing GTX for therapy of debatable merit.

Several obstacles must be overcome before the roles of GTX in acute leukemia can be fully defined. Alloimmunization is the major difficulty since the emergence of antibodies would present problems even if leukapheresis advances permitted one to infuse unlimited numbers of granulocytes. Long-term preservation of autologous granulocytes is a promising technique of the future [78]. Considerable success has been achieved using platelets stored in this fashion [79]. This technique should avoid problems with alloimmunization. Autologous GTX should be useful. First, it is impossible to identify sufficient numbers of HLA identical blood relatives to provide prolonged transfusion support for most patients. Second, even if HLA-matched, unrelated donors were available, it is debatable whether they could provide support as well as that from genetically-related family members due to the presence of so-called 'minor' antigenic differences between unrelated individuals. Third, the importance of granulocyte and platelet specific antigens is undefined, but it is reasonable to conclude that immunization could occur to these antigens even if HLA identical donors were used, thereby decreasing the effectiveness of the HLA-matched transfusions.

Additional obstacles lie with the process of leukapheresis itself. Machines currently in use collect 40–70% of the granulocytes flowing through them. It is unlikely that improving the efficiency to 100% will greatly affect granulocyte yields. Certainly, progress is being made, but within limitations [80]. Monumental advances (increasing yields by logs) must await technology that will permit larger volumes of blood to be rapidly processed from donors who (hopefully) will not have been subjected to the risks of anticoagulants, steroid stimulation, and erythrocyte sedimenting agents.

REFERENCES

1. Slichter SJ: Controversies in platelet transfusion therapy. Ann Rev Med 31:509–540, 1980.
2. Strauss RG: Therapeutic neutrophil transfusions, are controlled studies no longer appropriate? Am J Med 65:1001–1006, 1978.
3. Tobias JS, Brown BL, Brivkalns A, Yankee RA: Prophylactic granulocyte support in experimental septicemia. Blood 47:473–479, 1976.
4. Dale DC, Reynolds HY, Pennington JE, Elin RJ, Herzig GP: Experimental pseudomonas pneumonia in leukopenic dogs: comparison of therapy with antibiotics and granulocyte transfusions. Blood 47:869–876, 1976.
5. Chow HS, Sarpel SC, Epstein RB: Pathophysiology of candida albicans meningitis in normal, neutropenic, and granulocyte transfused dogs. Blood 55:546–550, 1980.
6. Higby DJ: Controlled prospective studies of granulocyte transfusion therapy. Exp Hematol 5 (Suppl):57–64, 1977.
7. Higby DJ, Burnet D: Granulocyte transfusions: current status. Blood 55:2–8, 1980.
8. McCullough J: Leukapheresis and granulocyte transfusion. Arch Pathol Lab Med 102:53–56, 1978.
9. Ford JM, Cullen MH: Prophylactic granulocyte transfusions. Exp Hematol 5 (Suppl):65–72, 1977.
10. Boggs DR: Transfusion of neutrophils as prevention or treatment of infection in patients with neutropenia. N Engl J Med 290:1055–1062, 1974.
11. Schiffer CA, Aisner J, Daly PA, Schmimpff SC, Wiernik PH: Alloimmunization following prophylactic granulocyte transfusion. Blood 54:766–774, 1979.
12. Strauss RG: Function of granulocytes collected for transfusion. In: Proceedings of Progress in pheresis: a national symposium (in press), 1980.

13. Rosenshein MS, Farewell VT, Price TH, Larson EB, Dale DC: The cost effectiveness of therapeutic and prophylactic leukocyte transfusion. N Engl J Med 302:1058–1062, 1980.

14. Strauss RG, Koepke JA, Maguire LC, Thompson JS: Clinical and laboratory effects on donors of intermittent-flow centrifugation platelet-leukapheresis performed with hydroxyethyl starch and citrate. Clin Lab Haematol 2:1–11, 1980.

15. Graw RG, Jr, Herzig G, Perry S, Henderson ES: Normal granulocyte transfusion therapy. N Engl J Med 287:367–371, 1972.

16. Herzig RH, Herzig GP, Graw RG, Jr, Bull MI, Ray KK: Successful granulocyte transfusion therapy for gram-negative septicemia. N Engl J Med 296:702–705, 1977.

17. Higby DJ, Yates JW, Henderson ES, Holland JF: Filtration leukapheresis for granulocyte transfusion therapy. N Engl J Med 292:761–766, 1975.

18. Fortuny IE, Bloomfield CD, Hadlock DC, Goldman A, Kennedy BJ, McCullough JJ: Granulocyte transfusion: a controlled study in patients with acute nonlymphocytic leukemia. Transfusion 15:548–558, 1975.

19. Vogler WR, Winton EF: A controlled study of the efficacy of granulocyte transfusions in patients with neutropenia. Am J Med 63:548–555, 1977.

20. Alavi JB, Root RK, Djerassi I, Evans AE, Gluckman SJ, MacGregor RR, Guerry D, Schreiber AD, Shaw JM, Koch P, Cooper RA: A randomized clinical trial of granulocyte transfusions for infection in acute leukemia. N Engl J Med 296: 706–711, 1977.

21. Curtis JE, Hasselback R, Bergsagel DE: Leukocyte transfusions for the prophylaxis and treatment of infections associated with granulocytopenia. Con Med Assoc J 117:341–345, 1977.

22. Schiffer CA, Buchholz DH, Aisner J, Betts SW, Wiernik PH: Clinical experience with transfusion of granulocytes obtained by continuous flow filtration leukopheresis. Am J Med 58:373–381, 1975.

23. Maybee DA, Millan AP, Ruymann FB: Granulocyte transfusion therapy in children. S Med J 70:320–324, 1977.

24. Pole JG, Davie M, Kershaw I, Barter DAC, Willoughby MLN: Granulocyte transfusion in treatment of infected neutropenic children. Arch Dis Child 51:521–527, 1976.

25. Higby DJ, Freeman A, Henderson ES, Sinks L, Cohen E: Granulocyte transfusions in children using filter-collected cells. Cancer 38:1407–1413, 1976.

26. Hahn DM, Schimpff SC, Young VM, Fortner CL, Standiford HC, Wiernik PH: Amikacin and cephalothin: empiric regimen for granulocytopenic cancer patients. Antimicrob Agents Chemother 12:618–624, 1977.

27. McCredie KB, Freireich EJ, Hester JP, Vallejos C: Leukocyte transfusion therapy for patients with host-defense failure. Transplant Proc 5:1285–1289, 1973.

28. Strauss RG, Goedken MM, Maguire LC, Koepke JA, Thompson JS: Gram-negative sepsis treated with neutrophils collected exclusively by intermittent flow centrifugation leukapheresis. Transfusion 20:79–81, 1980.

29. Buchholz DH, Blumberg N, Bove JR: Long-term granulocyte transfusion in patients with malignant neoplasms. Arch Intern Med 139:317–320, 1979.

30. Hershko C, Naparstek E, Eldor A, Izak G: Granulocyte transfusion therapy. Vox Sang 34:129–135, 1978.

31. Love LJ, Schimpff SC, Schiffer CA, Wiernik PH: Improved prognosis for granulocytopenic patients with gram-negative bacteremia. Am J Med 68:643–648, 1980.

32. Boggs DR: Neutrophils in the blood bank. N Engl J Med 296:748–750, 1977.

33. Schimpff SC: Therapy of infection in patients with granulocytopenia. Med Clin N Am 61:1101–1118, 1977.

34. Valdivieso M, Bodey GP, Burgess MA, Rodriguez V: Therapy of infections in neutropenic patients. Med Pediatr Oncol 2:99–108, 1976.

378

35. Bodey GP, Feld R, Burgess MA: β-lactum antibiotics alone or in combination with gentamicin for therapy of gram-negative bacillary infections in neutropenic patients. Am J Med Sci 271:179–186, 1976.
36. Love LJ, Schimpff SC, Hahn DM, Young VM, Standiford HC, Bender JF, Fortner CL, Wiernik PH: Randomized trial of empiric antibiotic therapy with ticarcillin in combination with gentamicin, amikacin or netilmicin in febrile patients with granulocytopenia and cancer. Am J Med 66:603–610, 1979.
37. Siber GR, Echeverria P, Smith AL, Paisley JW, Smith DH: Pharmacokinetics of gentamicin in children and adults. J Infect Dis 132:637–651, 1975.
38. Anderson ET, Young LS, Hewitt WL: Antimicrobial synergism in the therapy of gram-negative rod bacteremia. Chemotherapy 24:45–54, 1978.
39. Klastersky J, Cappel R, Daneau D: Clinical significance of in vitro synergism between antibiotics in gram-negative infections. Antimicrob Agents Chemother 2:470–475, 1972.
40. Klastersky J, Cappel R, Swings G, Vandenborre L: Bacteriological and clinical activity of the ampicillin/gentamicin and cephalothin/gentamicin combinations. Am J Med Sci 262:283–290, 1971.
41. Klastersky J, Danaeli D, Henri A: Antibiotic combinations for gram-negative infections in patients with cancer. Eur J Cancer 9:407–412, 1973.
42. Scott RE, Robson HG: Synergistic activity of carbenicillin and gentamicin in experimental psuedomonas bacteremia in neutropenic rats. Antimicrob Agents Chemother 10:646–651, 1976.
43. Andriole VT: Antibiotic synergy in experimental infection with pseudomonas. J Infect Dis 129:124–133, 1974.
44. Klastersky J, Swings G, Vandenborre L, Weerts D, deMaertelaer V: Effectiveness of the carbenicillin/cephalothin combination against gram-negative bacilli. Am J Med Sci 265:45–53, 1973.
45. Klastersky J, Cappel R, Daneau D: Therapy with carbenicillin and gentamicin for patients with cancer and severe infections caused by gram-negative rods. Cancer 31:331–336, 1973.
46. Singer C, Kaplan MH, Armstrong D: Bacteremia and fungemia complicating neoplastic disease. Am J Med 62:731–742, 1977.
47. Anderson ET, Young LS, Hewitt WL: Simultaneous antibiotic levels in 'breakthrough' gram-negative rod bacteremia. Am J Med 61:493–498, 1976.
48. Cooper MR, Heise E, Richards F, Kaufmann F, Spurr CL: A prospective study of histo-compatible leukocyte and platelet transfusions during chemotherapeutic induction of acute myeloblastic leukaemia. In: Leukocytes: separation, collection and transfusion, Goldman JM, Lowenthal RM (eds). New York: Academic Press, 1975, pp 436–449.
49. Ford JM, Cullen MH, Oliver RTD, Lister TA: Possible prolongation of remission in acute myeloid leukemia by granulocyte transfusions. N Engl J Med 302:583, 1980.
50. Mannoni P, Rodet M, Vernant JP, Brun B, Coquin-Radeau EI, Bracq C, Rochant H, Dreyfus B: Efficiency of prophylactic granulocyte transfusions in preventing infections in acute leukaemia. Blood Trans Immunohaematol 22:503–518, 1979.
51. Mannoni P, Rodet M, Radeau E: Granulocyte transfusion: Efficiency of prophylactic transfusions in care of patients with acute leukemia. In: Blood leukocytes functions and use in therapy. Stockholm: Almqvist and Wiksell International, 1977, p 72.
52. Mannoni P, Radeau E, Rodet M, Brun B, Dreyfus B: Prophylactic granulocyte transfusions in the supportive care of postchemotherapeutic aplasia. N Engl J Med 299:489, 1978.
53. Strauss RG, Connett JE, Gale RP, Bloomfield CD, Herzig GP, McCullough J, Maguire LC, Winston DJ, Ho W, Stump DC, Miller W, Koepke JA: A controlled trial of prophylactic granulocyte transfusions during initial induction chemotherapy for acute myelogenous leukemia. N Engl J Med 305:597–603, 1981.

54. Hester JP, McCredie KB, Freireich EJ: Advances in supportive care: blood component transfusions. In: Care of the Child with Cancer. Amer Cancer Soc 1979, pp 93–100.
55. McCullough J, Carter SJ, Quie PG: Effects of anticoagulants and storage on granulocyte function in bank blood. Blood 43:207–217, 1974.
56. McCredie KB: Platelet and granulocyte transfusion therapy. Postgrad Med 62:151–153, 1977.
57. Buchholz DH, Houx JL: A survey of the current use of filtration leukapheresis. Exp Hematol 7 (Suppl):1–10, 1979.
58. Thompson JS, Herbick JM, Burns CP, Strauss RG, Blaschke JW, Koepke JA, Maguire LC, Goedken MM: Granulocyte antigens detected by cytotoxicity (GCY) and capillary agglutination (CAN). Transplant Proc 10:885–888, 1978.
59. Appelbaum FR, Trapani RJ, Graw RG, Jr: Consequences of prior alloimmunization during granulocyte transfusion. Transfusion 17:460–464, 1977.
60. Goldstein IM, Eyre HJ, Terassaki PI, Henderson ES, Graw RG, Jr: Leukocyte transfusions: role of leukocyte alloantibodies in determining transfusion response. Transfusion 11:19–24, 1971.
61. Ungerleider RS, Appelbaum FR, Trapani RJ, Deisseroth AB: Lack of predictive value of antileukocyte antibody screening in granulocyte transfusion therapy. Transfusion 19:90–94, 1979.
62. Thompson JS, Severson CD, Parmely MJ, Marmorstein BL, Simmons A: Pulmonary 'hypersensitivity' reactions induced by transfusion of non-HLA leukoagglutinins. N Engl J Med 284:1120–1125, 1971.
63. Wright DG, Robichaud KJ, Pizzo PA, Diesseroth AD: Lethal pulmonary reactions associated with the combined use of amphotericin B and leukocyte transfusions. Blood 54 (Suppl):130a, 1979.
64. Ford JM, Lucey JJ, Cullen MH, Tobias JS, Lister TA: Fatal graft-versus-host disease following transfusion of granulocytes from normal donors. Lancet:1167–1169, 1976.
65. Salfner B, Borberg H, Kruger G, Schumacher K, Siebel E: Graft-versus-Host-reaktion nach Granulozytentransfusion von einem Normalspender. Blut 36:27–34, 1978.
66. Betzhold J, Hong R: Fatal graft-versus-host disease after a small leukocyte transfusion in a patient with lymphoma and varicella. J Pediatr 62:63–66, 1978.
67. Rosen RC, Huestis DW, Corrigan JJ, Jr: Acute leukemia and granulocyte transfusion: fatal graft-versus-host reaction following transfusion of cells obtained from normal donors. J Pediatr 93:268–270, 1978.
68. Cohen D, Weinstein H, Mihm M, Yankee R: Nonfatal graft-versus-host disease occurring after transfusion with leukocytes and platelets obtained from normal donors. Blood 53:1053–1057, 1979.
69. Winston DJ, Ho WG, Howell CL, Miller MJ, Mickey R, Martin WJ, Young LS, Lin CH, Gale RP: Cytomegalovirus infections associated with leukocyte transfusions. Ann Int Med 93:671–675, 1980.
70. Ritchey AK, Andiman W, McIntosh S, Berman B, Luce D: Mononucleosis syndrome following granulocyte transfusion in patients with leukemia. J Pediatr 97:267–269, 1980.
71. Higby DJ: Correspondence. Blood 56:325, 1980.
72. Camitta BM, Thomas ED, Nathan DG, Gale RP, Kopecky KJ, Rappaport JM, Santos G, Gordon-Smith EC, Storb R: A prospective study of androgens and bone marrow transplantation for treatment of severe aplastic anemia. Blood 53:504–514, 1979.
73. Yunis AA: Chloramphenicol-induced bone marrow suppression. Sem Hematol 10:225–234, 1973.
74. McConahey WM, Hayles AB: Thyroid neoplasia and radiation to the head, neck and upper thorax of the young. J Pediatr 89:169–170, 1976.

75. Herbst AL, Kurman RJ, Scully RE, Poskanzer DC: Clear-cell adenocarcinoma of the genital tract in young females. N Engl J Med 287:1259–1264, 1972.
76. Antunes CMF, Stolley PD, Rosenbshein NB, Davies JL, Tonascia JA, Brown C, Burnett L, Rutledge A, Pokempner M, Garcia R: Endometrial cancer and estrogen use. N Engl J Med 300:9–13, 1979.
77. Schiffer CA: Filtration leukapheresis: Summary and perspectives. Exp Hematol 7 (Suppl):42–47, 1979.
78. Boonlayangoor P, Telischi M, Boonlayangoor S, Sinclair TF, Millhouse EW: Cryopreservation of human granulocytes: study of granulocyte function and ultrastructure. Blood 56:237–245, 1980.
79. Daly PA, Schiffer CA, Aisner J, Wiernik PH: Successful transfusion of platelets cryopreserved for more than 3 years. Blood 54:1023–1027, 1979.
80. Hester, JP, Kellogg RM, Mulzet AP, Kruger VR, McCredie KB, Freireich EJ: Principles of blood separation and component extraction in a disposable continuous-flow single-stage channel. Blood 54:254–268, 1979.

# 12. Bone Marrow Transplantation in Adult Acute Leukaemia: Who Should Be Transplanted, and When?

H. E. M. KAY

## CONTENTS

*C. D. Bloomfield (ed.), Adult leukemias 1, 381–406. All rights reserved.*
*Copyright © 1982 Martinus Nijhoff Publishers, The Hague/Boston/London.*

## 1. ROLE OF BONE MARROW TRANSPLANTATION IN THE TREATMENT OF LEUKAEMIA

There are three ways in which the transplantation of allogeneic marrow may assist the treatment of leukaemia. The main purpose, and one which applies to syngeneic as well as to allogeneic transplants, is to enable an eradicative dose of cytotoxic treatment to be delivered to the patient without causing death through haemopoietic insufficiency.

### 1.1. Increased Cytotoxic Treatment

For many cytotoxic agents, the bone marrow is the tissue most susceptible to a lethal dose, and although such damage may not be totally irreversible insofar as small numbers of stem cells could survive such a dose, the time taken to restore haemopoiesis is too long, even with maximum supportive therapy, to allow somatic survival. Where bone marrow can be given so as to shorten the duration of haemopoietic insufficiency, the dose of cytotoxic agent(s) can be raised until the lethal threshold of the next tissue—gut, lung, skin, etc.—is reached. It should be emphasised that these thresholds are not absolutely fixed and independent measures since recovery of say, the intestinal mucosa will be enhanced by the early restoration of leucopoiesis and thrombocytopoiesis. Table 1 sets out the thresholds of lethal toxicity for most of the current and potential anti-leukaemic agents. From that it will be seen that for some, such as irradiation, the therapeutic margin is appreciably increased, but that for many agents toxicity to other tissues remains the limitation, so that bone marrow transplantation cannot assist in raising their dose to more effective leukaemicidal levels. On the other hand, it is possible that other agents, more specifically myelotoxic, but with a negligible therapeutic margin between the killing of normal and leukaemic cells, could be brought into the therapeutic armamentarium, e.g. chloramphenicol or dibromomannitol. All agents, however, must have a reasonably short duration of activity so that the marrow transplant can be undertaken soon after they are given and thus without undue prolongation of the period of pancytopenia.

*Table 1.* Limiting toxicity of anti-leukaemic agents.

| | Haemo-poietic | Mucosal | Cardiac | Lung | Neuro | Other |
|---|---|---|---|---|---|---|
| Steroids | 0 | | | | | Various |
| Vincristine | (+) | | | | + | |
| Anthracyclines | + | (+) | + | | | |
| Asparaginase | (+) | | | | + | + |
| Ara-C | + | + | | | | |
| MP and TG | + | (+) | | | | Hepatic |
| Methotrexate | (+) | + | | + | + | |
| Cyclophosphamide | + | | + | (+) | | Bladder |
| Radiation | + | + | (+) | + | (+) | + |
| BCNU | + | (+) | | | | Hepatic |

Conventional treatment of acute leukaemia depends upon the recovery of a population of normal stem cells which are co-existing with the leukaemic clone, although in a state of partial or complete suppression. However, it is possible that in some forms of leukaemia, especially those with a chronic or pre-leukaemic phase, no residual population of normal stem-cells survives, or that it does so in numbers so small that even mild cytotoxic treatment will cause its total elimination. Where that happens, bone marrow transplantation affords the only possible means of successful radical therapy and it must be an important objective of current research to identify instances where normal stemcells are absent. Are cases of AML without any normal karyotypes (AA) of this sort for example? In CGL it is possible to regain karyotypically normal cells in some cases, but in others this is not possible [1]. To what extent this reflects the lack of selectivity of anti-leukaemic agents, and to what extent it denotes actual lack of normal cells at the time of diagnosis remains to be discovered. Whichever is the main cause, such cases have a high priority as candidates for bone marrow transplants.

## 1.2. Immune Factors

A second benefit which may be gained from a bone marrow transplant is that the grafted cells may be able to react against those residual leukaemic cells which have survived the attack by cytotoxic agents. The therapeutic benefit, therefore, depends upon the presence of antigen(s) on the leukaemic cells which can be recognised and attacked by donor cells, and on the presence of sufficient immuno-reactive donor cells in relation to the number of residual leukaemic cells for such an attack to be effective. These conditions may or may not be fulfilled.

*1.2.1. Experimental Data.* In experiments using transplanted leukaemia, the probability of antigenic differences between leukaemic cells and donor immunocytes is so great that such experiments have very little value in predicting or interpreting the outcome of clinical observations. However, in many species it has been shown that spontaneous leukaemia has a virus infection as one of its causes and that viral antigens may be detectable on the leukaemic cells. The spontaneous AKR leukaemia of the mouse could be expected for that reason to be capable of provoking an immune response in donor cells which were not already tolerant of the AKR virus-induced antigens [2]. Transplantation within the AKR strain of syngeneic cells would not, of course, be expected to give rise to an immune response since the donor cells would already be tolerant of the antigens and some, indeed, would already be carrying virus themselves. Transplants from another strain, however, could be expected to respond, and in experiments using SJL/J mice as donors, prolonged leukaemia-free survivals have been obtained [3, 4]. The two strains are H-2 different so that Graft versus Host (GvH) reactions can occur; indeed if the animals are conventionally housed, there is severe and mostly fatal GvH, but if the animals have been isolated and decontaminated, GvH is avoided and in this way 50% survive and remain free of leukaemia. This procedure has been termed adoptive immunotherapy and illustrates the benefit of an allogeneic rather than syngeneic graft in the therapy of spontaneous leukaemia [5], but it should be noted that this is not conclusive evidence for an immune reaction as distinct from a failure for the leukaemia to be reactivated in the donor cells (see below).

*1.2.2. Clinical Data.* In the treatment of human leukaemia by transplantation, a similar comparison can be made between the results of allogeneic and syngeneic (identical twin) transplants. With an allogeneic transplant, there is the chance of a specific graft-versus-leukaemia reaction, and also the chance that a GvH reaction would indirectly affect the viability of residual leukaemic cells. The results of the Seattle transplants go some way towards answering the question. Their data from identical twin transplants and allogeneic transplants in AML and ALL show a higher rate of relapse in the identical twins and in the absence of GvH than when GvH of Grade II or more has occurred; this is so even when allowance has been made for the improved survival without GvH, and thus the longer opportunity for recurrent leukaemia to be diagnosed. The effect is seen in ALL whether transplanted in remission or relapse, and in AML transplanted in relapse but not in remission [7]. Similarly, in the series at Los Angeles, leukaemic relapse has not occurred in a large number of allogeneic transplants for AML but has been noted in two out of three syngeneic transplants [8]. It is conceivable, but unlikely that in this instance and in the Seattle syngeneic transplants, the increased relapse incidence was in part due to the lack of methotrexate (which is given to prevent GvH in allogeneic grafts but may have some additional anti-leukaemic effect). Cases have also been reported where the course of the disease was strongly suggestive of a graft-versus-leukaemia reaction which partially but temporarily controlled the recurrence of the leukaemia [9]. These observations can certainly be interpreted in favour of immune responses, leukaemia-specific or not, which defer or prevent leukaemic recurrence and it is possible that immunotherapy as practised in AML has a similar basis [10].

### 1.3. Susceptibility to Leukaemogenic Agents

A third source of benefit from allogeneic grafts, which is not easy to dissociate from the possible immune factors, arises from a putatively lower susceptibility of the grafted marrow to a persistent leukaemogenic agent. In different strains of mouse, the suspectibility to leukaemogenesis by viruses varies widely [11], and it is reasonable to suppose that the same might be true in man. The fact that in five (probably six) cases [12] leukaemia has recurred in the cells of the donor marrow emphasises the liability of donor cells to leukaemogenesis, and it is safe to assume that more such 'recurrences', where the origin of the leukaemia cells could not be, or were not, identified, were actually instances of leukaemia *de novo* in the donor cells. Syngeneic (twin) cells should be maximally liable to the same agent which caused the original leukaemia, whereas allogeneic cells, even when MHC-identical, might well have a reduced susceptibility to the agent. This then is an alternative or supplementary explanation of the difference in leukaemia recurrence rates between recipients of syngeneic and allogeneic marrow.

### 2. PRACTICE OF BONE MARROW TRANSPLANTATION

### 2.1. Histocompatibility

In most centres, transplant-donations are restricted to identical twins and to sibs where there is MHC-identity. This degree of compatibility can be determined usually with ease by HLA-typing of recipient, sibs and parents, followed by tests for mixed lymphocyte reactivity. Homozygosity, silent alleles, non-available parents, lymphopenia or non-specific lack of reactivity can raise difficulties in a few cases. Graft rejection is never a serious problem with leukaemic patients, since the treatment designed to eradicate the leukaemia—in particular whole body irradiation—is sufficiently immunosuppressive to allow a take of the graft even when there may have been sensitisation through previous blood transfusion. On the other hand, GvH reactions are frequent and often severe, partly no doubt because of the damage inflicted by the anti-leukaemic treatment, so that tests designed to predict the probability of GvH are desirable. Unfortunately, although such tests are valid in mice, where positive results in cell-mediated lympholysis (CML) tests are correlated with GvH [13], no close correlation has been found in man. The standard practice, therefore, is limited to MHC serological testing for the A, B, C and DR loci, the mixed lymphocytic reaction performed as two one-way tests, with or without a two-way test. The results is expressed as either a stimulation index or as a relative response index.

## 2.2. Graft Acceptance

Multiple aspirations of marrow from healthy donors yield $>2 \times 10^8$ cells/kg without difficulty and the cells are infused after some sort of filtration to separate potential emboli as soon as possible. Acceptance is only imperilled after anti-leukaemic regimens if very low cell numbers are infused, but the cellular components of the graft may be important. Thus, it has been shown [14] that viable lymphocytes can enhance the acceptability of a graft, but conversely these will engender GvH reactions. It remains to be seen whether treatment of donor marrow suspensions with an anti-T-cell serum can, as in experimental animals, produce viable grafts without the risk of GvH reactions, but preliminary experience suggests that this is possible [15].

## 2.3. Graft versus Host Disease (GvHD) [16, 17]

One of the main obstacles to successful marrow grafting is the frequency of graft versus host reactions, many of which are fatal or lead to permanent disability. Experimental evidence shows conclusively that an essential factor in their genesis is the transfusion of foreign non-rejected T-lymphocytes, but many other aspects of the pathogenesis remain obscure. Other causative factors include infections [18] and the degree of tissue damage due to cytotoxic treatments [19]. In experiments, the latter have usually been acute effects and the possible role of cumulative drug-induced damage, which would, of course, be important in human leukaemia, has not yet been sought. The role of infection is evident from experiments where pathogenfree mice remain exempt from GvH reactions which allogeneic grafts otherwise induce [3, 20, 21], and recent experiments with monkeys show much the same [22]. The role of particular organisms, including viruses, has only been partially explored and it is not clear how these infections influence GvHD. One hypothesis proposes that an incompatible graft induces a state of immuno-deficiency which is responsible for fatal infections, but it may well be that the infection itself actually provokes a reaction by the immunoreactive cells of the grafted recipient: probably both types of event occur.

The frequency and severity of GvH reactions is, in general, proportional to the degree of histo-incompatibility, but conspicuous exceptions can occur. MHC-incompatibility can be associated rarely with GvH-free grafts [23, 24] and conversely, acute fatal reactions can occur with complete MHC-identity. In such cases, the existence of minor histo-compatibility genes can be invoked, although little is known about these except their existence. GvH is more likely where the donor is female [25], a fact which is not satisfactorily explained. It is not due to Y-borne antigens in the male, since the incidence is equally high where the recipient is female. Data from the Seattle transplants suggest that age is also a critical factor in liability to GvHD, especially chronic GvH. This is relatively uncommon in children but over the age of 30, seven out of eight long survivors had some degree of GvHD [26].

The actual pathogenesis of the GvH reaction remains tantalisingly elusive, perhaps because more than one mechanism of classical immunity or of genetic resistance (i.e. via NK cells) may be involved.

There is a little evidence that antibody is directly involved in that Coombs-positive haemolysis has been recorded in chronic GvH and rarely anti-nuclear and other auto-antibodies are found [27]. The accumulation of IgM, together with complement components at the dermoepidermal junction is noted in only a proportion of cases [28], and the main manifestations of the disease are unlikely to be the result of antibody attack. T-lymphocytes still remain the prime suspect, especially as GvH can often be prevented if they are removed from the graft inoculum by means of anti-T-cell sera [29, 30]. However, where T-cells are given, they usually disappear from the bloodstream fairly quickly and are not easy to demonstrate at the site of GvH lesions. Necrotic cells in the epidermis may sometimes have lymphocytic satellites and that could perhaps represent direct cytotoxicity. Another approach has been to examine the numbers and proportions of suppressor and helper T-cells; in one study it was shown that in acute GvH there was an imbalance with a deficit of suppressor cells, whereas in chronic GvH suppressor cells might be either decreased or increased [31].

In another study, chronic GvH was shown to be associated with an excess of non-specific suppressor cells and in most cases, with a deficiency of specific (anti-host) suppressor cells [32]. Alternatively, it has been suggested that the cell which actually promotes the destruction of the GvH reaction is a natural killer cell (NK) of recipient origin [33]. Thus, in all seven patients where there was a normal quantity of NK cells before transplant GvH reactions occurred, whereas in six patients where there was a lower than normal number, GvH reactions were entirely avoided, even though in two cases there was MHC-incompatibility [34].

## 2.4. Management and Prevention of GvH

The treatment of established GvH is by no means satisfactory. In acute GvH, high dose steroids sometimes appear to be effective; antithymocyte globulin has been tried, and Cyclosporin-A has suppressed the skin rash; but although beneficial in some patients, the effects are usually weak or temporary. In chronic GvH, azathioprine and steroids are probably valuable, especially if given early [35]. The future of marrow grafting undoubtedly depends upon the prevention of GvH. In leukaemia, three approaches are in use. Methotrexate, given at weekly intervals for 14 weeks after the transplant, has been the standard regimen formulated by Thomas at Seattle [36], and is derived from extensive experimental data with a variety of immunosuppressive agents. Its efficacy in man has never been put to formal test and as it is not fully effective and has disadvantageous toxic side-effects, it is likely to be superseded by other methods.

Secondly, anti-thymocyte globulin can be used to eliminate from bone marrow suspension those thymic cells on which the GvH reaction depends. This approach succeeds in dogs [37] and monkeys [22] and has now been applied in man with some encouraging initial resulsts [30]; the advent of ample supplies of carefully selected anti-T sera of monoclonal origin should enable this technique to be tested decisively. Alternative methods of T-cell elimination employ density separation techniques or incubation with methyl prednisolone [38]. The former has not found clinical acceptance; the latter has yet to be tried.

The third method depends upon Cyclosporin-A (CsA) a relatively new type of immunosuppressive agent of great potential. It has several toxic side-effects, but they are mostly mild and reversible. Initial clinical experience shows that it is usually fully preventive of GvHD for MHC-compatible grafts and may permit grafts of less than full compatibility [39]. One of the practical problems not yet solved is that the drug is very poorly water-soluble but readily fat-soluble. It is best given by mouth in olive oil and appears to be usually well-absorbed, presumably in chylomicrons. However, there appears to be wide variation in its concentration in the blood and tissues, and the variation in the incidence of toxic effects—especially renal nitrogen retention—may indicate widely different rates of metabolism, excretion and hence pharmacological effect. Standardisation of tissue-delivered dose is thus essential before it can be fully evaluated; meanwhile the occurrence of three cases of lymphoma when CsA was used in connection with renal transplants points to a new hazard [40]. In marrow transplant patients it appears that the drug can probably be discontinued at about six months from transplant.

## 2.5. Supportive Treatment

In marrow transplantation, the ability to provide full supportive treatment is a sine qua non. The period of pancytopenia usually lasts about three weeks after whole body irradiation, but the period will start earlier and hence will be longer if irradiation has been preceded by an intensive combination of cytotoxic drugs. Where patients are uninfected and in first remission, little support may be required: thus in 22 consecutive first remission AMLs, no granulocyte transfusions were needed [41] but some platelets and red cells, and some antibiotic cover are always necessary. Protective isolation and gut antibiotics are advantageous, not only to prevent dangerous infections [42], but to reduce the hazard of GvH (see above). After discharge from hospital, there is still a period of risk from exogenous and endogenous infections since the immune system takes many months to complete its recovery [43]. Indeed, susceptibility to pneumococcal infections persists for many months, so that prophylactic co-trimoxazole for six months (to prevent also pneumocystitis infection) and oral penicillin thereafter are advisable.

## 2.6. Pneumonitis

Pneumonitis has been a major hazard in most centres [44]. At Seattle, 10% have had pneumocystis infection and 40% have had evidence of CMV infection, but for the latter and for the 50% where no organism is found, the aetiology of the pneumonitis is obscure. At Baltimore, an association between pneumonitis and GvH elsewhere has led to the suggestion that the pneumonitis is a pulmonary manifestation of GvH [45]. Other circumstances, such as age and damage to the lung by radiation (see below) and cytotoxic agents, play a part in the genesis of pneumonitis, and where cumulative damage can be inferred from previous treatment by busulphan and alkylating agents, the case for advocating a marrow transplant is weakened. Conversely, the ability to protect the lungs by shielding or dose-fractionation may enlarge the scope of transplantation.

## 2.7. Late Complications

Late complications include chronic graft-versus-host disease, growth retardation, severe dental caries, cataract formation and infertility [46]. It must also be anticipated that some of the patients may develop second neoplasms in years to come. By far the most distressing complication is chronic graft-versus-host disease [47-49], which is most often manifest as a scleroderma-like condition of the skin, especially affecting the limbs and leading to contractures and a painful atrophy of the skin, with fissure formation. The mucous membrane of the mouth is similarly affected. Keratitis sicca and parotitis, as in Sjögren's syndrome, and lupus-like lesions may occur. Treatment with azathioprine and steroids may sometimes be of benefit.

## 2.8. *Present Practice in Bone Marrow Transplantation*

The foregoing paragraphs have given a brief summary of practice, as it exists in 1980, in a number of centres in North America and Europe, but it should be emphasised that rapid and major changes may be on the way. Hitherto, procedures have been very much dominated by the pioneering work of Thomas of Seattle, but greater diversity must now be expected. New immunosuppressive regimes, tissue-shielding, fractionation and greater precision in whole body irradiation; greater understanding of the role of lymphocytes and other cells in GvH; new antibiotics including antiviral agents; and the preference for earlier, trouble-free grafts will reduce the risks for the matched graft. On the other hand, the wish to graft older adults and to step outside the restrictions of complete MHC-compatibility will continue to bring complications.

## 3. ERADICATION REGIMENS

### 3.1. *Radiation*

Most attempts to eradicate leukaemia before transplantation have, hitherto, included radiation as one of the agents. This practice has historical precedents extending back to the first successful experiments in mice [59] and has some practical advantages. These are that most leukaemias, experimental and human, are sensitive or very sensitive to radiation, that radiation is not critically dependent on the state of cell-cycle for its lethal effect and that radiation will kill leukaemic cells in the CNS and other putative sanctuary sites.

In experimental leukaemias, a lethality dose-response curve with a small shoulder, a Do value of about 140 rads, and the absence of resistant hypoxic cells enables eradication of $10^3$ cells to be effected with single doses of about 900 rads [51]. In man, these parameters are not known, but the response to radiation of local leukaemic deposits, the successful treatment and prophylaxis of ALL in the CNS and testes, suggest that human leukaemia should be at least equally sensitive. Three important variables must be considered: uniformity of dose, dose-rate and fractionation.

*3.1.1. Uniformity* [52, 53]. Theoretically, uniformity is desirable so as to give an equal dose to each leukaemic cell, wherever it may be, and so as to avoid local radiation damage to normal tissues. Owing to the conformation and variable opacity of the body, uniformity cannot be ensured but so far as cell-killing is concerned, a variation of 10 % or so from the mean dose may not be important. Such variations can occur with many forms of apparatus where the beam gives a slightly lower dose to the feet and the top of the head. However, one should ensure that the most susceptible normal tissues, the lung and the gut, do not receive an excessive dose and that the hands are properly positioned in relation to the rest of the body so that they too are not over-exposed.

Ideally, two opposed sources should be used to give as great a uniformity as possible without having to move the patient too often, but with proper re-positioning and with placing of dosimeters in various parts of the body, reasonable uniformity can be attained with a single beam source [54]. The only tissue that may require shielding is the lungs; there is no doubt that the incidence and severity of pneumonitis could be lessened by shielding but the presence of haemopoietic tissue in the ribs and thoracic vertebrae dictates that these tissues must receive a full dose.

*3.1.2. Dose-Rate* [55]. The importance of dose-rate in the killing of human leukaemia cells is unknown. In experimental work with animal leukaemias it has been customary and convenient to give the irradiation fairly rapidly at rates of about 100 rads/min. This is impractical for man and might be unacceptable on account of gastro-intestinal toxicity. At present, there is great variation in radiation dose-rate as between different centres. The standard dose-rate at Seattle has been approximately 8 rads/min, while faster rates of 27 rads/min are given in Minneapolis, and slower rates of 2.5 rads/min at the Royal Marsden Hospital. If a single fraction is used, this dictates a maximum total dose of 900–1000 rads at 8 rads/min and of 750 rads at 27 rads/min. It is obviously more laborious to use a slow rate, but with experience, the eight hours or so needed for the slower irradiation is well-tolerated by the patient and is manageable for the staff. What is not known as yet, is the difference in effects—both the eradication or relapse rate, and the relative toxicity to normal tissues, especially the lungs. Preliminary data suggest that the lung damage is appreciably less with slow irradiation since the incidence of pneumonitis at 2.5 rads/min has been small (two out of 60 cases) but the relapse rate is rather higher, possibly 20 % [56].

*3.1.3. Dose Fractionation.* The chief advantage of giving whole body irradiation in one unfractionated dose is that the donor marrow can then be given immediately, and the period of pancytopenia is kept to a minimum. If the dose is given in a few fractions spread over a period of up to one week, then the pancytopenia is prolonged, but the toxicity to normal tissues is reduced and so a larger aggregate dose, which may be at least equally effective in eradicating the leukaemia, can be given. The risks with fractionated dosage are that there will be some recovery of reversible damage in the leukaemic cells between doses, and also that some regeneration of cell numbers will also occur. The latter might be a very important factor in some T-cell and B-cell leukaemias where proliferation rates are very high. It will be recalled that Burkitt's lymphoma was originally thought to be a radio-resistant tumour, but that was because the number of cells killed by each daily fraction was made good by proliferation between each fraction [57].

### 3.2. Pre-Transplant Leukaemia-Eradication Regimes

A variety of regimens have been tried as a precedent to marrow transplantation in leukaemia. In evaluating them, it is of course important to consider the condition of the patient before the transplant regime is initiated. From all the reports, especially from Thomas's group [58], it can be concluded that a state of complete remission is almost essential before the final pre-transplant regimen. Rapid recurrence, and even failure to eradicate the leukaemia, is so common if there is overt residual leukaemia before the pre-transplant regimen that it is generally considered not worthwhile to proceed further. However, this begs two questions; how far back does one extend the pre-transplant regimen—what one might term the 'run-up'?—and how much previous treatment has been given, not only to achieve, but to consolidate the complete remission? It is, of course, well-recognised that the state of 'complete' remission encompasses the presence of leukaemic cells up to a number of $10^9$, or even $10^{10}$, and in any series, the patients will be scattered throughout this whole range. The ability of the pre-transplant regime to effect a cure must depend to a large extent on the take-off point, i.e. the number of cells which must be eliminated and this depends in turn on the prior chemotherapy. Wherever possible, therefore, the whole of the anti-leukaemic treatment should be considered and that is possible where, for example, transplants are undertaken early in remission after a standard form of remission induction and consolidation treatment. Where transplants are undertaken after relapse, the best that can be done is to state the total treatment given to achieve the second remission. In the absence of this information, comparison of the pre-transplant regimens can be misleading.

### 3.2.1. Irradiation Alone [36, 58]. 

Radiation without high-dose cyclophosphamide was relied on in 10 early cases at Seattle, of whom one is a long-term survivor, but failures, which included two cases where relapse had occurred in donor cells, showed that additional agents were needed.

*3.2.2. Cyclophosphamide and Irradiation* [58]. This regime, where two doses of cyclophosphamide at 60 mg/kg i.v. are given five and four days before TBI, has become the standard practice at many centres, both for ALL and AML. It has the merits of simplicity, low toxicity and it is, by and large, effective. In three series of AML in first remission, the survivors in remission at 162 days or more number 34/57, or about 60% [59–62]. The failures have been mainly due to GvH, pneumonitis, and relapse with a slightly different incidence in each series, but with a conspicuous lack of success in the older patients, where not one of five aged over 40 survived. Fewer patients in second remission can be salvaged by this regime, and fewer still if the marrow still shows relapse. In ALL, the situation is less precise because transplants are undertaken at a later stage and the disease is more heterogeneous, but at Seattle [63] 11 out of 22 transplanted in remission were still in remission at 15 to 33 months, as were four out of 26 transplanted in relapse.

*3.2.3. Regimes with Additional Agents.* Cytotoxic drugs have been added to the foundation of cyclophosphamide + TBI in the form of Ara-C, daunorubicin, BCNU, etc. but insufficient numbers have been treated alike to assess the value of the modifications. The regime at UCLA, known as SCARI [64], adds daunorubicin, Ara-C, and thioguanine and it would appear that the subsequent relapse rate is reduced to zero though at an unacceptable cost of early complications. However, if such a regime were used for first remission patients and if modern means were employed to avoid GvHD, the results might be very much better than in the original series.

*3.2.4. Other Regimes.* An alternative approach has been to reduce the dose of whole body irradiation and to substitute additional drugs, especially busulphan [65]. A few long survivors are reported, but the incidence of GvH and pneumonitis is not, apparently, reduced and there is as yet no series of early cases (e.g. first remission AML), for comparison so that the necessity of maximum doses of TBI could be assessed. Other regimes relying on combinations of cytotoxic drugs, e.g., BACT [66] or TACC [67] have not yet been given to enough patients for comparative evaluation.

## 4. COMPARISON OF TREATMENT STRATEGY IN ADULT LEUKAEMIA

The prospect that many cases of leukaemia can be radically and effectively treated with the aid of bone marrow transplants is at present fringed by a wide margin of uncertainty where the balance of factors on which a therapeutic decision rests is evenly disposed. Moreover, the practice and facility of transplantation is changing so rapidly while the results of treatment, both by transplants or conventionally, take so many months or years to assess that many uncertainties are bound to persist for the foreseeable future. Thus, although the future development of marrow transplantation seems hopeful because immunological research is revealing fresh opportunities to combat the complications and to extend the scope of transplants, it is always possible that new and more selective drugs or the better deployment of existing agents might remove the necessity for transplants in an increasing fraction of cases of leukaemia.

## 4.1. Practical Considerations

If, as seems highly possible, transplant-dependent regimes can be determined which give, say, 90% eradication for AML and perhaps 70% for ALL in young adults, and if, as seems only slightly less probable, transplants from non-MHC-identical or unrelated donors can be performed with only minor morbidity, then the major limitations might for a short while become the availability of facilities and the lack of expertise.

The financial considerations, however, should not be a limitation. Given that facilities exist, or can be provided, the cost of a bone-marrow transplant and its attendant treatment, compares favourably with those of conventional treatment, at least for first remission AML, and probably for other circumstances also. Figures of £ 6 000 [41] or $ 60 000 [68] need to be enlarged to take account of inflation, but when compared for cost-effectiveness with other current objectives in medicine, the financial burden is trivial. Nor should ethical considerations and the availability of donors be a serious hindrance to the practice of bone marrow transplants, especially if the MHC-barrier can be crossed.

## 4.2. Age

One of the outstanding facts of human marrow transplantation is the declining success with advancing age. This is not so much because of failure to engraft, but because the older patient is more liable to GvH and pneumonitis; there are very few long-term successes over the age of forty and it seems probable that there is a progressive likelihood of failure from adolescence onward. The cause is obscure, partly because there is no appropriate animal model; nor is it yet clear whether it is the age of the donor or recipient which is decisive—a matter which may be resolved when more haplotype-matched parent-to-child and child-to-parent grafts have been performed. Speculation that thymic involution is the key factor is plausible and could lead to a solution through the implantation of thymic tissue or by the use of thymic extracts.

Meanwhile, where a leukaemic patient is being considered for a transplant there need be no hesitation up to the age of thirty, there should be a cautious optimism for the next decade, but over the age of forty, the transplant should only be advised if other factors are favourable and no plausible alternative exists.

## 4.3. Acute Myeloid Leukaemia (AML)

In newly-diagnosed AML, an overall remission-rate of 70–80% can now be expected and with optimum non-transplant regimes the first remission may extend to four years in about 30–40% of cases [69, 70]. A somewhat larger series of cases from CALGB is expected to show a similar trend [71]. After relapse on treatment a second remission can often be obtained but the long-term outlook then is dismal. Where relapse occurs after stopping treatment, however, a long second remission may be possible.

These conditions suggest some alternative strategies. The first and simplest is to undertake a transplant as soon as possible after remission has been obtained. The majority below the age of 30 should do well but some patients may die of GvH or infection who would otherwise have done better on cytotoxic drugs only and a few may relapse after the transplant. Obviously their outlook is very poor although the possibility that the relapse can be treated by conventional means should not be overlooked.

A second option is to treat all with cytotoxic drugs alone and to keep marrow transplantation in reserve for those who relapse. It is much more difficult to estimate the overall success of this strategy because although the rate of success in the original post-relapse Seattle transplants was established to be about 15%, subsequent improvements in technique, especially the avoidance of GvHD, could lead to a higher proportion of second option transplant successes. However, even if we put the rate of long-term non-transplant 'cures' as high as 30% and the rate of second remission transplant successes at 30% of the remainder the aggregate salvage rate of $30 + (30 \times 70)/100 = 51\%$, is still somewhat lower than the current rate of 60% for first remission transplants.

Such calculations, which are in any case based on changing rates, are obviously speculative and furthermore take no account of the possible identification of groups for whom a transplant is, or is not, a desirable first option.

## 4.4. Sub-types of AML

Certain sub-types of AML may be curable by conventional treatment without the need for a graft (see chapter by Keating). Favourable factors (in addition to youth) are promyelocytic (M3) type where remission, if obtained, is often relatively long [72], absence of karyotype anomalies [73, 74] or the presence of t(8;21) [75] in the leukaemic cells. Conversely, in monocytic (M5) disease remissions are short [76] and in cases where cells with a normal karyotype are absent from the initial marrow long remissions are rare [73]. Two definable subcategories could be mentioned. In those cases where leukaemia has followed treatment or accidental poisoning with cytotoxic agents [77] the chance that residual normal cells are still present and able to re-establish a long remission with normal haemopoiesis is probably small. A history of poisoning or the presence of multiple and perhaps specific chromosome abnormalities may be able to denote such cases (see Chapter by Golomb). A secondary category are those patients where a history of pre-leukaemia or specific chromosomal evidence [78] indicates that completely normal haemopoiesis probably is unattainable. Such patients, who are admittedly in a small minority in the transplantable age-range, are thus theoretically prime candidates for a transplant. In practice the difficulty of obtaining a complete remission in these cases and the possibility that other systems may also be sub-clinically damaged, e.g., lung, skin, thymic epithelium etc., may make grafting difficult and hazardous.

Another approach to the problem of case-selection might lie in the accurate prediction of a good response to treatment through the use of *in vitro* techniques. Some correlation between prognosis and *in vitro* growth characteristics is well-established [79] and it may be possible to assess directly the susceptibility of leukaemic cells to particular drugs or drug combinations (see chapter by Preisler). A number of attempts have been made [e.g., 80–83] but none are yet in any sort of routine use for leukaemia (cf. myeloma where such a system is in practice) [84]. For example, the demonstration of a high degree of sensitivity to the combination of cytosine arabinoside and thioguanine might well become a pointer to a strategy of conventional treatment with transplantation held in reserve as a second option.

## 4.5. Acute Lymphoblastic Leukaemia (ALL)

An apparent cure rate in childhood ALL of between 50% and 80% [85] is not matched in adult ALL. This is partly because all the adverse factors are commoner in adult ALL, i.e. high leucocyte count, T, B and 'null' (as distinct from common) cell phenotype, L2 cytological type, male sex and the $Ph^1$ anomaly [86]. As a consequence, long-term remission rates in adult ALL are usually less than 30% (see Chapter by Esterhay and Wiernik) and such differences as exist from one series to another are as likely to be due to differences in the composition of the series as in the merits of particular treatments. It has generally been held that the chance of a cure in any case of ALL contradicts the desirability of early transplantation, and it is only recently that transplantation policies have encompassed poor risk ALLs for an elective transplant in first remission. Indeed the total information to date from which bone marrow transplantation in ALL could be evaluated is very meagre. Only in the series from Seattle and City of Hope can any sort of quantitative conclusion be derived [63, 61]; other reports have been anecdotal, often without data such as age and mostly recording failures [65, 87–89], but it is safe to assume that any successful series, however small, would have found an eager publisher. Even at Seattle [63] the number of adults ($\geqslant 15$ years) is small and by comparison with children the results are poor. Thus, although at 464 days from transplant (in remission) there were 11 survivors (9 disease-free) out of 22 patients at all ages, all seven of those over 15 had either relapsed (five cases) or died of infection (two cases). However, out of 14 adult transplants in relapse, three are long-term disease-free survivors, six having succumbed to relapse and to GvHD or pneumonia. The relapse-preventing effect of GvH in these cases is worthy of note as is also the result of more recent mis-matched transplants in ALL—three survivors out of five transplanted in remission, and one out of eight in relapse [90]. At City of Hope [61] six out of 11 adults with ALL were still in remission at 262 days or more; these include three patients transplanted in first remission, and four cases of T-cell ALL of which two are 'long' remitters.

A report [91] of two cases of adult T-cell ALL refractory to treatment in which bone-marrow grafts were successful, at least insofar as there was no relapse at 8 and 20 months, offers some encouragement and one or two similar patients transplanted without prior remission [61, 92] may be heralds of a new therapeutic opportunity. Success in transplantation for 'American Burkitt's Lymphoma' may also indicate that B-cell ALL is amenable to a similar approach [93]. Indeed, in cases where remission cannot be obtained or where high counts and bulk disease indicate the probability of very early relapse with rapidly proliferative disease, immediate grafting may offer the best chance of eradication.

Otherwise there are at present insufficient data to dogmatise on the criteria which should influence a decision, but as it is rare for long remissions to occur in Ph$^1$+ve ALL [94] and as the prognosis is universally poor in B-ALL and in high count T-ALL in males (but not always in females) these are categories for whom an early transplant is appropriate. In other cases it is at present usually preferable to hope for a long remission and, if relapse occurs, to transplant in second remission. With increasing experience, however, we must expect that more and more poor risk patients are, if they have compatible donors, placed in the early transplant group.

One dilemma which must be resolved is the timing and form of treatment to the CNS. While there is no impediment to giving intrathecal methotrexate before cranial irradiation, and with some caution afterwards, the juxtaposition which must be avoided is that of standard cranial irradiation (1800 or 2400 rads) followed within a few weeks by TBI, 1000 rads in a single dose [95] with perhaps the obligation to supplement with intrathecal methotrexate afterwards. Although encephalopathy is a greater hazard to children, it can certainly occur in adults.

## 5. PROSPECTS FOR THE MIS-MATCHED GRAFT IN ACUTE LEUKAEMIA

Hitherto, the vast majority of bone marrow transplants have been made between MHC-identical subjects, usually matched siblings, and the majority of early attempts at mismatched grafts, especially for marrow aplasia, have been attended by graft rejection or fatal GvH. However, in leukaemia, where a high dose of TBI is given, incompatible grafts are not rejected and GvH may soon be avoidable through the use of some newly evolved procedures and agents. Since the majority of patients do not have a MHC-matched donor, the prospect of a mismatched graft is now receiving attention. Two types of donors can be considered. On the one hand it may be possible to find unrelated donors who share the same HLA antigens as the recipient and although many of these will give positive reactions in MLR tests, some will give weak or negative responses. In these circumstances a marrow graft in leukaemia can succeed [96] or at least be accepted [97] and whereas in other diseases graft-rejection has been a major obstacle, in leukaemia acceptance should be the rule. Thus with the establishment of panels of volunteer marrow donors it should be posssible to find suitable donors for many patients with the commoner MHC phenotypes.

A second alternative is the related haplotype-similar graft. It is assumed that haplotype matching would nearly always be possible if siblings, parents, children or other family members were to act as donors, and very often by chance a partial identity of the opposite haplotype would occur.

There have been random reports of successful mismatched grafts in leukaemia [98] or in other diseases [99] and Clift [100] has reviewed the results of 29 mismatched transplants in a rather heterogeneous group of leukaemias at Seattle; in all cases there was haplo-identity and in nearly all, some of the allelic antigens were matched. Many of the patients were late relapsed cases and the outcome for these was poor, with a high incidence of severe GvHD. However, among those transplanted in remission, 8/13 were alive 148–790 days from transplant—a result which is scarcely different from the fully matched leukaemias; while at the Royal Marsden Hospital [101] of eight patients receiving mismatched grafts with the aid of Cyclosporin-A, four are survivors at 145–300 days, despite some unusual complications. It is not yet clear whether incompatibility at particular loci, e.g. HLA-A, B or D, are equally important or whether one part, e.g. the D locus, is predominant in precipitating GvH reactions.

The situation presents a similar dilemma to that for the matched transplant. If a mismatched transplant is to have the best chance of success, it should be made early before relapse and the cumulative effects of multiple treatments have prejudiced the chances.

## 6. TRANSPLANTATION OF AUTOLOGOUS BONE MARROW IN LEUKAEMIA [102]

An alternative strategy in the management of ALL and AML, as well as CML, is the use of autologous marrow which has been withdrawn and held in a viable state while intensive treatment is given. In acute leukaemias the marrow must obviously be taken in remission, i.e. at a time when the number of leukaemic cells is at a minimum. Then two options are open: the marrow may be stored in liquid nitrogen so that should relapse occur, intensive treatment can be followed by re-infusion of remission marrow; or the intensive treatment can be given immediately and the marrow, cryopreserved or not depending on the period of intensive treatment, is re-infused. The marrow withdrawn may be returned without any selective treatment in the hope that the aspirate contains no viable leukaemic cells [103–105] or it may be treated by density gradient centrifugation [106], or by antisera to remove selectively the leukaemic cells [107–109]. The antisera can be used to induce cell lysis (with or without complement) or could be placed on a surface (e.g. glass beads) so as to absorb the leukaemic cells, or possibly opsonisation alone, with the hope of phagocytic removal after re-infusion, would be effective. If there were leukaemic-specific antisera, these would be logical procedures and could well succeed. However, no convincingly leukaemia-specific antibodies have yet been described and in AML relapse has almost invariably followed re-infusion of the serum-treated remission marrow. Two remissions of over six months [109] and a single survivor in remission at 630 days (after untreated remission marrow) is the best that can be reported [110] but it must be realised that sporadic cases must be expected to do well because they were already 'cured' at the time the remission marrow was withdrawn. Control studies for this procedure will be very important. In the absence of specific anti-leukaemic sera, the manoeuvre depends for success upon the leukaemic population being either foreign to the marrow, as in T-ALL, or else as in the case of common-ALL (C-ALL), that the final recovery of normal haemopoiesis can occur from stem cells which lack the C-ALL antigen—presumptively those at an even earlier stage of ontogeny.

Neither of these schemes has yet been fully realised, although remissions of 120 and 150 days [107, 108] have been reported in C-ALL relapse treated in the latter way. Development of more specific monoclonal antisera and experience with the techniques of cell removal may bring these methods into more general application, but paradoxically they are more likely to succeed with almost any other disease than leukaemia, since sera directed against other types of neoplastic cell are least likely to impair the normal haemopoietic cells which promote recovery [102].

## 7. CONCLUSION

The role of bone marrow transplantation in adult acute leukaemia can now be perceived in a very rough outline only. Furthermore, developments in technique, especially means to avoid graft-versus-host reactions, should shortly extend the opportunities for successful transplantation. At the same time, the diagnostic dissection of acute leukaemia into definable groups with known prognostic limitations should enable greater precision in the selection of transplant or non-transplant regimens. Two major obstacles lie in the way of extending transplant-based therapies—age and histocompatibility barriers. For non-transplant treatment, the limitation may remain the restricted ability to devise selective anti-leukaemic agents and regimens. We stand, at present, like a racing commentator seeing two horses of half-proven worth near the outset of a race, where the size and nature of the fences and ditches to come can only be guessed. It is an exciting prospect.

## REFERENCES

1. Cunningham I, Gee T, Dowling M, Chaganti R, Bailey R, Hopfan S, Bowden L, Turnbull A, Knapper W, Clarkson B: Results of treatment of $Ph^1+$ chronic myelogenous leukemia with an intensive treatment regimen (L-5protocol). Blood 53:375-395, 1979.
2. Chester SJ, Esparza AR, Flinton LJ, Simon JD, Kelley RJ, Albala MM: Further development of a successful protocol of graft *versus* leukemia without fatal graft-*versus*-host disease in AKR mice. Cancer Res 37:3494-3496, 1977.
3. Truitt RL: Use of decontamination and a protected environment to prevent secondary disease following adoptive immunotherapy of acute leukemia in mice. In: Experimental Hematology Today, Baum SJ, Ledney GD (eds). New York: Springer-Verlag, 1978, pp 195-201.
4. Bortin MM, Truitt RL, Rimm AA, Bach FH: Graft-versus-leukaemia reactivity induced by alloimmunization without augmentation of graft-versus-host reactivity. Nature 281:490-491, 1979.
5. Emeson EE, Weintraub FM: Prevention of AKR leukemia by transplanting H-2 incompatible allogeneic bone marrow requires the maintenance of chimerism. VIII International Congress of the Transplantation Society, 1980.
6. Weiden PL, Flournoy N, Thomas ED, Prentice R, Fefer A, Buckner CD, Storb R, Antileukemia effect of graft versus host disease in human recipients of allogeneic marrow grafts. N Engl J Med 300:1068-1075, 1979.

7. Weiden PL, Flournoy N, Sanders J, Sullivan K, Thomas ED. Improved survival in patients with graft-vs-host disease (GVHD) after allogeneic marrow transplantation for acute leukemia. VIII International Congress of the Transplantation Society, 1980.

8. Gale RP. Personal communication, 1980.

9. Odom LF, Githens JH, Morse H, Sharma B, August CS, Humbert JR, Peakman D, Rusnak ST, Johnson FB: Remission of relapsed leukaemia during a graft versus host reaction. Lancet ii:537–540, 1978.

10. Taylor GM, Bradley BA: Graft-versus-leukaemia without graft-versus-host? Lancet ii:959–960, 1979.

11. Moloney JB: The rodent leukaemias: virus-induced murine leukaemias. Ann Rev Med 15:383, 1964.

12. Elfenbeim GJ, Brogaonkar DS, Bias WB, Burns WH, Saral R, Sensenbrenner LL, Tutscha PJ, Zaczek BS, Zander AR, Epstein RB, Rowley JD, Santos GW: Cytogenetic evidence for recurrence of acute myelogenous leukemia after allogeneic bone marrow transplantation in donor hematopoietic cells. Blood 52:627–636, 1978.

13. Elina WL: Correlation of graft versus host mortality and positive CML assays in the mouse. Transplant Proc 8:343, 1976.

14. Deeg HJ, Storb R, Weiden PL, Shulman HM, Grahman TC, Torok-Storb BJ, Thomas ED: Abrogation of resistance and enhancement of DLA-nonidentical unrelated marrow grafts in lethally irradiated dogs by thoracic duct lymphocytes. Blood 53:552–557, 1979.

15. Rodt H, Kolb HJ, Netzel B, Haas RJ, Bender-Gotze CH, Emmerich B, Wilms K, Thierfelder S: Prevention of GvHD by incubation of bone marrow grafts with anti-T-lymphocyte globulin. VIII International Congress of the Transplantation Society, 1980.

16. Lerner KG, Kao GF, Storb R, Buckner CD, Clift RA, Thomas ED: Histopathology of graft vs. host reaction (GvHR) in human recipients of marrow from HL-A-matched sibling donors. Transplan Proc 6:367–371, 1974.

17. Grebe SC, Streilein JW: Graft versus host reactions: a review. In: Advances in Immunology, Dixon FJ, Funkel HG (eds). New York: Academic Press, 1976, pp 119–221.

18. Bealmear PM, Loughman BE, Nordin AA, Wilson R: Evidence for graft vs. host reaction in the germfree allogeneic radiation chimaera. In: Germfree research: biological effects of gnotobiotic environment, Heneghan JB (ed). New York: Academic Press, 1973, p 471.

19. Barnes DW, Loutit JF, Micklem HS: 'Secondary disease' of radiation chimaeras: a syndrome due to lymphoid aplasia. Ann NY Acad Sci 99:374, 1962.

20. van Bekkum DW, Roodenburg J, Heidt PJ, van der Waaij D: Mitigation of secondary disease of allogeneic mouse radiation chimeras by modification of the intestinal microflora. J Natl Cancer Inst 52:401–404, 1974.

21. Pollard M, Chang CF, Srivastava KK: The role of microflora in the development of graft versus host disease. Transplant Proc 7:533, 1975.

22. Wagemaker G, Vriesenendorp HM, van Bekkum DW, Walma EP, Zurcher C, Heidt PJ, Balner H: Successful allogeneic bone marrow transplantation in rhesus monkeys across major histocompatibility barriers. VIII International Congress of the Transplantation Society, 1980.

23. O'Reilly RJ, Dupont B, Phwa S, Crimes E, Smithwick Em, Pahwa R, Schwartz S, Hansen JA, Siegal FP, Sorell M, Svejgaard A, Jersild C, Thomsen M, Platz P, L'Esperance P, Good RA: Reconstitution in severe combined immunodeficiency by transplantation of marrow from an unrelated donor. N Engl J Med 297:1311–1318, 1977.

24. Dupont B, O'Reilly RJ, Pollack MS, Good RA: Histocompatibility testing for clinical bone marrow transplantation and prospects for identification of donors other than HLA genotypically identical siblings. In: Recent trends in the immunology of bone marrow transplantation, Thierfelder S (ed). Berlin: Springer, 1979.

25. Bortin MM, Rimm AA: Allogeneic bone marrow transplantation for 144 patients with severe aplastic anemia. JAMA (in press).

26. Storb R: Recent results in marrow transplantation for the treatment of aplastic anaemia and acute leukemia in Seattle. In: Immunobiology of bone marrow transplantation, Thierfelder S, Rodt H, Kolb HJ (eds). New York: Springer-Verlag, 1980, pp 367–374.

27. Slavin RE, Santos GW: The graft versus host reaction in man after bone marrow transplantation: pathology, pathogenesis, clinical features, and implication. Clin Immunol Immunopathol 1:472–498, 1973.

28. Tsoi M-S, Storb R, Jones E, Weiden PL, Shulman W, Witherspoon R, Atkinson K, Thomas ED: Deposition of IgM and complement at the dermo-epidermal junction in acute and chronic cutaneous graft-vs-host disease in man. J Immunol 120:1485–1492, 1978.

29. Thierfelder S, Thiel E, Hoffmann-Fezer G, Rodt H: Bone marrow transplantation into recipients sensitized against donor-type T cells. In: Immunobiology of bone marrow transplantation, Thierfelder S, Rodt H, Kolb HJ (eds). New York: Springer-Verlag, 1980, pp 205–217.

30. Rodt H, Kolb HJ, Netzel B, Haas RJ, Bender-Gotze CH, Emmerich B, Wilms K, Thierfelder S: Prevention of GvHD by incubation of bone marrow grafts with anti-T-lymphocyte globulin. VIII International Congress of the Transplantation Society, 1980.

31. Reinherz EL, Parkman R, Rappaport J, Rosen FS, Schlossman SF: Aberrations of suppressor T cells in human graft versus host disease. N Engl J Med 19:1061–1067, 1979.

32. Tsoi M-S, Storb R, Dobbs S, Thomas ED: Specific suppressor cells and immune response to host antigens in long-term allogeneic marrow recipients: implications for the mechanisms of graft-vs-host tolerance and chronic GVHD. VIII International Congress of the Transplantation Society, 1980.

33. Lafferty KJ, Talmage DW: Theory of allogeneic reactivity and its relevance to transplantation biology. Transplant Proc 8:349–353, 1976.

34. Lopez C, Kirkpatrick D, Sorell M, O'Reilly RJ, Ching C: Association between pre-transplant natural kill and graft-versus-host disease after stem-cell transplantation. Lancet ii:1103–1106, 1979.

35. Thomas ED, Storb R, Sullivan KM: Bone marrow transplantation. Hematology Transfusion 1980. The Education Program of the American Society of Hematology, Montreal, 1980.

36. Thomas ED, Storb R, Clift RA, Fefer A, Johnson FL, Neiman PE, Lerner KG, Glucksberg H, Buckner CD: Bone marrow transplantation. N Engl J Med 292:832–895, 1975.

37. Kolb HJ, Bodenberger U, Rodt HV, Rieder I, Netzel B, Grosse-Wilde H, Scholz S, Thierfelder S: Bone marrow transplantation in DLA-Haploidentical canine littermates. Fractionated total boby irradiation (FTBI) and in vitro treatment of the marrow graft with anti-T-cell globulin (ATCG). In: Immunobiology of bone marrow transplantation. Thierfelder S, Rodt H, Kolb HJ (eds). New York: Springer Verlag, 1980, pp 61–71.

38. Tutschka PJ, Korbling M, Hess AD, Beschorner WE: Prevention of graft versus host disease (GVHD) by chemoseparation of marrow cells. VIII International Congress of the Transplantation Society, 1980.

39. Powles RL, Clink HM, Spence D, Morgenstern G, Watson JG, Selby PJ, Woods M, Barrett A, Jameson B, Sloane J, Lawler SD, Kay HEM, Lawson D, McElwain TJ, Alexander P: Prevention of graft versus host disease following allogeneic bone marrow transplantation in man using cyclosporin A. Lancet ii:327–329, 1980.

40. Calne RY, Rolles K, White DJG, Thiru S, Evans DB, McMaster P, Dunn DC, Craddock GN, Henderson RG, Aziz S, Lewis P. Cyclosporin A initially as the only immunosuppressant in 34 recipients of cadaveric organs: 32 kidneys, 2 pancreases, and 2 livers. Lancet ii:1033–1036, 1979.

41. Kay HEM, Powles RL, Lawler SD, Clink HM. Cost of bone-marrow transplants in acute myeloid leukaemia. Lancet i:1067–1069, 1980.

42. Storring RA, Jameson B, McElwain TJ, Wiltshaw E, Spiers ASD, Gaya H. Oral non-absorbed antibiotics prevent infection in acute non-lymphoblastic leukaemia. Lancet ii:837–840, 1977.

43. Atkinson K, Storb R, Prentice RL, Weiden PL, Witherspoon RP, Sullivan K, Noel D, Thomas ED: Analysis of late infection in 89 long-term survivors of bone marrow transplantation. Blood 53:720–731, 1979.

44. Neiman PE, Reeves W, Ray G et al. A prospective study of interstitial pneumonia and opportunistic viral infection among recipients of allogeneic bone marrow grafts. J Infect Dis 136:754–767, 1977.

45. Beschorner WE, Sari R, Hutchins GM, Tutschka PJ, Santos GW. Lymphocytic bronchitis associated with graft-versus-host disease in recipients of bone-marrow transplants. N Engl J Med 299:1030–1036, 1978.

46. Stewart PS, Buckner CD, Clift RA, Sanders JE, Storb R, Leonard JM, Thomas ED: Allogeneic marrow grafting for acute leukemia: a follow-up of long term survivors. Exp Hematol 7:509–517, 1979.

47. Graze PR, Gale RP. Chronic graft versus host disease: a syndrome of disordered immunity. Am J Med 66:611–620, 1979.

48. Gratwohl AA, Moutsopoulos HM, Chused TM, Akizuki M, Wolf RO, Sweet JB, Deisseroth AB: Sjogren-type syndrome after allogeneic bone marrow transplantation. Ann Intern Med 87:703–706, 1977.

49. Lawley TJ, Peck GL, Moutsopoulos HM, Gratwohl AA, Deisseroth AB: Scleroderma, Sjogren-like syndrome, and chronic graft versus host disease. Ann Intern Med 87:707–709, 1977.

50. Barnes DWH, Loutit JF. Treatment of murine leukaemia with x-rays and homologous bone marrow. II. Br J Haematol 3:241, 1957.

51. Berry RJ, Hypoxic protection and recovery in tumour cells irradiated at low dose rates and assessed in vivo. Br J Radiol 41:921–926, 1968.

52. Lam WC, Lindeug BA, Order SE, Grant DG: The dosimetry of Cobalt-60 total body irradiation. Int J Radiol Oncol Biol Phys 5:905–911, 1979.

53. Lam WC, Order SE, Thomas DE: Uniformity and standardization of single and opposing Cobalt-60 sources for total body irradiation. Int J Radiol Oncol Biol Phys 6:245–250, 1980.

54. Lawrence G, Rosenbloom ME, Hickling P. A technique for total body irradiation in the treatment of patients with acute leukaemia. Br J Radiol 53:894–897, 1980.

55. Berry RJ: Effects of radiation dose-rate. From protracted, continuous irradiation to ultra-high dose-rates from pulsed accelerators. Br Med Bull 44–47, 1973.

56. Powles RL et al.: Unpublished.

57. Norin T, Onyango J: Radiotherapy in Burkitt's lymphoma: conventional or superfractionated regime – early results. Int J Radiol Oncol Biol Phys 2:399–406, 1977.

58. Thomas ED, Buckner CD, Banaji M, Clift RA, Fefer A, Flournoy N, Goodell BW, Hickman RO, Lerner KG, Neiman PE, Sale GE, Sanders JE, Singer J, Stevens M, Storb R, Weiden PL: One hundred patients with acute leukemia treated by chemotherapy, total body irradiation and allogeneic marrow transplantion. Blood 49:511–533, 1977.

59. Thomas ED, Buckner CD, Clift RA, Fefer A, Johnson FL, Neiman PE, Sale GE, Sanders JE, Singer JW, Shulman H, Storb R, Weiden PL: Marrow transplantation for acute non-lymphoblastic leukemia in first remission N Engl J Med 301:597–599, 1979.

60. Powles RL, Morgenstern G, Clink HM, Hedley D, Bandini G, Lumley H, Watson JG, Lawson D, Spence D, Barrett A, Jameson B, Lawler S, Kay HEM, McElwain TJ: The place

of bone marrow transplantion in acute myelogenous leukaemia. Lancet i:1047–1050, 1980.

61. Blume KG, Beutler E, Bross KJ, Chillar RK, Ellington OB, Fahey JL, Farbstein MJ, Forman SJ, Schmidt GM, Scott EP, Spruce WE, Turner MA, Wolf JL: Bone-marrow ablation and allogeneic marrow transplantation in acute leukemia. N Engl J Med 302:1041–1046, 1980.

62. Mannoni P, Vernant JP, Rodet M, Rochant H, Bracq CH, Tournesac A, Feuilhade F, Bierling P, Dreyfus B: Marrow transplantation for acute nonlymphoblastic leukemia in first remission. Blut 41:220–225, 1980.

63. Thomas ED, Sanders JE, Flournoy N, Johnson FL, Buckner CD, Clift RA, Fefer A, Goodell BW, Storb R, Weiden PL: Marrow transplantation for patients with acute lymphoblastic leukemia in remission. Blood 54:468–476, 1979.

64. U.C.L.A. Bone Marrow Transplantation Team. Bone marrow transplantation in acute leukaemia. Lancet ii:1197–1200, 1977.

65. Tutschka PJ, Santos GW, Elfenbein GJ: Marrow transplantation in acute leukemia following busulfan and cyclophosphamide. In: Immunobiolgy of bone marrow transplantation. Thierfelder S, Rodt H, Kolb HJ (eds). New York: Springer Verlag, 1980, pp 375–380.

66. Graw RG, Jr, Lohrmann HP, Bull MI, Decter J, Herzig GP, Bull JM, Leventhal BG, Yankee RA, Herzig RH, Krueger GRF, Bleyer WA, Buja LM, McGinnis MH, Alter HJ, Whang-Peng J, Gralnick HR, Kirkpatrick CH, Henderson ES: Bone marrow transplantation following combination chemotherapy immunosuppression (B.A.C.T.) in patients with acute leukemia. Transplant Proc 6:349–354, 1974.

67. Gorin NC, David R, Stachowiak J, Hirsch Marie F, Petit JC, Muller JY, Leblanc G, Parlier Y, Salmon CH, Duhamel G: High dose combination chemotherapy (TACC) with and without autologous bone marrow transplantation for the treatment of acute leukemia, and other malignant diseases. In: Proceedings of the Second European Symposium on Bone Marrow Transplantation. Bone Marrow Transplantation in Europe, Touraine J-L (ed). Amsterdam, Excerpta Medica, 1979, pp 88–97.

68. Gale RP: Transplantation in acute leukaemia. Transplant Proc 11:1920, 1979.

69. Peterson, BA, Bloomfield CD: Long-term disease-free survival in acute non-lymphocystic leukemia. Blood 57:1144–1147, 1981.

70. Weinstein HJ, Mayer RJ, Rosenthal DS, Camitta BM, Coral FS, Nathan DG, Frei E.: Treatment of acute myelogenous leukaemia in children and adults. N Engl J Med 303:473–478, 1980.

71. Bloomfield CD: Treatment of adult acute nonlymphocytic leukemia – 1980. Ann Intern Med 93:133–135, 1980.

72. Weil M, Jacquillat CI, Gemon-Auclerc MF, Chastang CL, Izrael V, Boiron M, Bernard J.: Acute granulocytic leukemia. Arch Intern Med 136:1389–1395, 1976.

73. Sakurai M, Sandberg AA: Chromosomes and causation of human cancer and leukemia. XI. Correlation of karyotypes with clinical features of acute myeloblastic leukemia. Cancer 37:285, 1976.

74. Nilsson PG, Brandt L, Mitelman F: Prognostic implications of chromosome analysis in acute non-lymphocytic leukemia. Leukemia Res 1:31–34, 1977.

75. Trujillo JM, Cork A, Ahearn MJ, Youness EL, McCredie KB: Hematologic and cytologic characterization of 8/21 translocation acute granulocytic leukemia. Blood 53:695, 1979.

76. Tobelem G, Jacquillat C, Chastang C, Auclerc M-F, Lechevallier T, Weil M, Daniel M-T, Flandrin G, Harrousseau J-L, Schaison G, Boiron M, Bernard J: Acute monoblastic leukemia: a clinical and biologic study of 74 cases. Blood 55:71, 1980.

77. Auclerc G, Jacquillat C, Auclerc MF, Weil M, Bernard J: Post-therapeutic acute leukemia. Cancer 44:2017–2025, 1979.

78. Nowell P, Finan J: Chromosome studies in preleukemic states. Cancer 42:2254–2261, 1978.

79. Curtis JE, Till JE, Messner HA, Souson P, McCulloch EA: Comparison of outcomes and prognostic factors for two groups of patients with acute myeloblastic leukemia. Leukaemia Res 3:409–416, 1979.

80. Gordon MY, Blackett NM: The sensitivities of human and murine hemopoietic cells exposed to cytotoxic drugs in an *in vivo* culture system. Cancer Res 36:2822–2826, 1976.

81. Sonis ST, Falcai R, MacLennan ICM: Assessment of drug sensitivity of human leukaemic myeloblasts. Br J Cancer 36:307, 1977.

82. Raich PC: Prediction of therapeutic response in acute leukaemia. Lancet 1:74–76, 1978.

83. Preisler HD: Prediction of response to chemotherapy in acute myelocytic leukemia. Blood (in press).

84. Salmon SE, Hamburger AW, Soehnlen B *et al.*: Quantitation of differential sensitivity of human-tumor stem cells to anticancer drugs. N Engl J Med 298:1321–1327, 1978.

85. Mauer AM: Therapy of acute lymphoblastic leukemia in childhood. Blood 56: 1–10, 1980.

86. Priest JR, Robinson LL, McKenna RW, Lindquist LL, Warkentin PI, LeBien TW, Woods WG, Kersey JH, Coccia PF, Nesbit ME, Jr, Philadelphia chromosome positive childhood acute lymphoblastic leukemia. Blood 56:15–22, 1980.

87. Speck B, Weber W, Cornu P, Nissen C, Groff P, Sartorius J: Current status and perspectives in the treatment of acute leukemia by bone marrow transplantation. In: Bone Marrow Transplantation in Europe. Touraine J-L (ed). Amsterdam, Excerpta Medica, 1979, pp 65–70.

88. Granena A, Rozman C, Casals F, Feliu E, Aranalde J, Montserrat E, Hernandez L: Bone marrow transplantation (BMT) in acute leukaemia with BACT conditioning: results in 7 cases. In: Bone marrow transplantation in Europe. Touraine J-L (ed). Amsterdam, Excerpta Medica, 1979, pp 98–103.

89. Unpublished data from London Bone Marrow Transplant centres.

90. Buckner CD, Clift RA, Fefer A, Meyers JD, Sullivan KM, Storb R, Weiden PI, Witherspoon RP, Thomas EDb: Bone Marrow Transplantation. In: Recent advances in haematology. Hoffbrand AV (ed). Edinburgh: Churchill Livingstone (in press).

91. Garrett TJ, Grossbard E, Hopfan S, Koziner B, Clarkson BD, Good RA, O'Reilly R: Bone marrow transplantation for the therapy of refractory adult T cell acute lymphoblastic leukemia. Cancer 45:2006–2008, 1980.

92. Prentice HG: Personal communication.

93. Kim TH, Kersey J, Sewchand W, Nesbit ME, Krivit W, Levitt SH: Total-body irradiation with a high-dose-rate linear accelerator for bone-marrow transplantation in aplastic anemia and neoplastic disease. Work in Prog 122:523–525, 1977.

94. Bloomfield CD, Brunning RD, Smith KA, Nesbit ME: The prognostic significance of the Philadelphia chromosome in acute lymphocytic leukemia. Cancer Genet Cytogenet 1:229, 1980.

95. Atkinson K, Clink H., Lawler S, Lawson DN, McElwain TJ, Thomas P, Peckham MJ, Powles R, Mann JR, Cameron AH, Arthur R: Encephalopathy following bone marrow transplantation. Eur J Cancer 13:623–625, 1977.

96. Hansen JA, Clift RA, Thomas ED, Buckner CD, Storb R, Giblett ER: Transplantation of marrow from an unrelated donor to a patient with acute leukemia. N Engl J Med 303:565–567, 1980.

97. Barrett AJ: Personal communication.

98. Feig SA, Opelz G, Winter HS, Falk PM, Neerhout RC, Sparkes R, Gale RP and UCLA

Bone Marrow Transplantation Group: Successful bone marrow transplantation against mixed lymphocyte culture barrier. Blood 48:385, 1976.

99. Dupont B, O'Reilly RJ, Pollack MS, Good RA: Histocompatibility testing for clinical bone marrow transplantation and prospects for identification of donors other than HLA genotypically identical siblings. In:Immunobiology of bone marrow transplantation. Thierfelder S (ed). New York: Springer-Verlag, 1980.

100. Clift RA, Hansen JA, Thomas ED: The role of HLA in marrow transplantation. VIII International Congress of the Transplantation Society, 1980.

101. Royal Marsden Transplant Team. Unpublished data.

102. Proceedings of Conference on Autologous Bone Marrow Transplantation. Exp Hematol 7 (Suppl 5), 1979.

103. Gorin NC, Najman A, Salmon CH, Muller JY, Petit JC, David R, Stachowiak J, Hirsch Marie F, Parlier Y, Duhamel G: High dose combination chemotherapy (TACC) with and without autologous bone marrow transplantation for the treatment of acute leukaemia and other malignant diseases. Eur J Cancer 15:1113, 1979.

104. Fay JW, Silberman HR, Moore JO, Noel KT, Huang AT: Autologous marrow transplantation for patients with acute myelogenous leukemia – a preliminary report. In: Exp Hematol 7 (Suppl 5), Heim LR (ed), pp 302–308, 1979.

105. Mahmood T, Robinson WA, Entringer M: Autologous bone-marrow and peripheral blood buffy coat cell infusion in the treatment of chronic myeloid and acute leukemia. In: Exp Hematol 7 (Suppl 5), Heim LR (ed), pp 321–326, 1979.

106. Dicke KA, Zander AR, Spitzer G, Verma DS, Peters LJ, Vellekoop L, Thomson S, Stewart D, Hester JP, McCredie KB: Autologous bone marrow transplantation in relapsed adult acute leukemia. In: Exp Hematol 7 (Suppl 5), Heim LR (ed), 1979, pp 170–187.

107. Wells JR, Billing R, Herzog P, Feig SA, Gale RP, Terasaki P, Cline MJ. Autotransplantation after in vitro immunotherapy of lymphoblastic leukemia. In: Exp Hematol 7 (Suppl 5), Heim LR (ed), 1979, pp 164–169.

108. Netzel B, Haas RJ, Rodt H, Kolb HJ, Thierfelder S: Antileukemic, autologous bone marrow transplantation in childhood acute lymphoblastic leukemia. VIII International Congress of the Transplantation Society, 1980.

109. Herzig GP: Personal communication, 1980.

110. Gorin NC, David R, Stachowiak J, Parlier Y, Najman A, Duhamel G: High dose chemotherapy and autologous bone marrow transplantation. A study on 24 patients. 18th Congress of the International Society of Hematology, Montreal, 1980.

# Index